Charting the Journey

Charting the Journey

AN ALMANAC OF PRACTICAL RESOURCES FOR CANCER SURVIVORS

The National Coalition for Cancer Survivorship

Edited by Fitzhugh Mullan, M.D., Barbara Hoffman, J.D., and the Editors of Consumer Reports Books

CONSUMERS UNION   MOUNT VERNON, NEW YORK

Copyright © 1990 by The National Coalition for Cancer Survivorship
Published by Consumers Union of United States, Inc., Mount Vernon, New York
10553
All rights reserved, including the right of reproduction
in whole or in part in any form.

Library of Congress Cataloging-in-Publication Data
Charting the journey : an almanac of practical resources for
  cancer survivors / the National Coalition for Cancer Survivorship ;
  edited by Fitzhugh Mullan and Barbara Hoffman and the editors of
  Consumer Reports Books.
      p. cm.
    Includes bibliographical references.
    Includes index.
    ISBN 0-89043-304-6
      1. Cancer—Patients—Handbooks, manuals, etc. I. Mullan,
  Fitzhugh. II. Hoffman, Barbara. III. National Coalition for Cancer
  Survivorship (U.S.)
      [DNLM: 1. Adaptation, psychological. 2. Neoplasms—psychology.
  QZ 200 C486]
  RC262.C44 1990
  362.1'96994—dc20
  DNLM/DLC
  for Library of Congress   90-2013
                                                                  CIP
                                                                  Rev.

Design by Glen M. Edelstein

First printing, October 1990
Manufactured in the United States of America

CONSUMER REPORTS BOOKS

Ruth Dvorkin	Director
Sarah Uman	Executive Director
Roslyn Siegel	Acquisitions Editor
Julie Henderson	Assoc. Acquisitions Editor
Neil R. Wells	Editorial Assistant
Meta Brophy	Editorial Production Manager
Benjamin Hamilton	Production Editor
Marlene Tungseth	Production Editor
Jane Searle	Production Coordinator
Michele Harris	Director of Marketing and Sales
Rea Christoffersson	Direct Mail Manager
Helene Kaplan	Sr. Marketing Analyst
Sandra Jackson	Sales Administrative Assistant
Lila Lee	Assistant to the Director
Ruth Cooper	Receptionist

A direct-mail edition of this book has been published simultaneously under the title *An Almanac of Practical Resources for Cancer Survivors.*

Charting the Journey is a Consumer Reports Book published by Consumers Union, the nonprofit organization that publishes *Consumer Reports,* the monthly magazine of test reports, product Ratings, and buying guidance. Established in 1936, Consumers Union is chartered under the Not-For-Profit Corporation Law of the State of New York.

The purposes of Consumers Union, as stated in its charter, are to provide consumers with information and counsel on consumer goods and services, to give information on all matters relating to the expenditure of the family income, and to initiate and to cooperate with individual and group efforts seeking to create and maintain decent living standards.

Consumers Union derives its income solely from the sale of *Consumer Reports* and other publications. In addition, expenses of occasional public service efforts may be met, in part, by nonrestrictive, noncommercial contributions, grants, and fees. Consumers Union accepts no advertising or product samples and is not beholden in any way to any commercial interest. Its Ratings and reports are solely for the use of the readers of its publications. Neither the Ratings nor the reports nor any Consumers Union publications, including this book, may be used in advertising or for any commercial purpose. Consumers Union will take all steps open to it to prevent such uses of its materials, its name, or the name of *Consumer Reports.*

The ideas, procedures, and suggestions contained in this book are not intended to replace the services of a physician. All matters regarding your health require medical supervision. You should consult with your physician before adopting any of the procedures in this book. Any applications of the treatments set forth in this book are at the reader's discretion, and neither the author nor the publisher assumes any responsibility or liability therefor.

INTRODUCTION

The quotation from "Seasons of Survival: Reflections of a Physician with Cancer" by Fitzhugh Mullan, *New England Journal of Medicine* 313 (1985): 270–73, is reprinted with the permission of the *New England Journal of Medicine*.

CHAPTER 1

The quotation from "The Median Isn't the Message" by Stephen Jay Gould, Ph.D., is reprinted by permission of Dr. Gould. Copyright © 1985 by Stephen Jay Gould.

The excerpt from *Illness as Metaphor* by Susan Sontag, copyright © 1977, 1978 by Susan Sontag, is reprinted by permission of Farrar, Straus & Giroux, Inc.

"The Far Side" cartoon by Gary Larson is reprinted by permission of Chronicle Features, San Francisco, California.

Figures on pp. 12, 17, 18, 20, 24–25, and 28 are used with permission of the American Cancer Society.

The poem "Cure" by Wendy Podwalny is reprinted by permission of Patricia Fobair, editor, *Surviving!*. Copyright © 1988 by Stanford University Hospital.

CHAPTER 2

The quotation from "Lessons from Living with Cancer" by Robert Mack, *New England Journal of Medicine* 311 (1984): 1640, is reprinted with the permission of the *New England Journal of Medicine*.

The quotation from "Live with Pain, Learn the Hope: A Beginner's Guide to Cancer Counseling" by William Keeling is reprinted by permission of the American Association for Counseling and Development, © 1976.

The poem "Perspective" by Brenda Neal is reprinted by permission of Brenda Neal. Copyright © 1987 by Brenda Neal.

The quotation from *How Could I Not Be Among You?* by Ted Rosenthal, copyright © 1973 by Ted Rosenthal, is reprinted by permission of Persea Books, Inc.

The quotations from *The Outsider* by Colin Wilson, copyright © 1982 by Colin Wilson, Jeremy P. Tarcher Inc., Los Angeles. Reprinted by permission of St. Martin's Press, New York.

CHAPTER 3

The Cancer Survivors' Bill of Rights is used with permission of the American Cancer Society.

Excerpt from *Vital Signs: A Young Doctor's Struggle with Cancer* by Fitzhugh Mullan, copyright © 1975, 1982 by Fitzhugh Mullan, is reprinted by permission of Farrar, Straus & Giroux, Inc.

Sample consent form is reprinted with the permission of the American Medical Association, © 1982.

The poem "They Don't Want Me to Sleep" by Helen Webster is reprinted by permission of Elisavietta Ritchie. Copyright © 1980 by Helen Webster.

CHAPTER 5

The quotation from *Surviving!* is reprinted with permission of Patricia Fobair, editor, *Surviving!*. Copyright © October/November 1988 by Stanford University Hospital.

CHAPTER 6

The quotation from *Heading Home* by Paul Tsongas is reprinted with permission of Alfred A. Knopf, Inc., © 1984.

The quotation from "The Psychological Status of Survivors of Childhood/Adolescent Hodgkin's Disease" by Abby Wasserman, M.D., et al., *American Journal of Diseases of Children* 141 (June 1987), copyright © 1987. Reprinted with permission.

The quotation of Dr. Sidney Wolfe is reprinted from *Medical Records: Getting Yours* with the permission of the Public Citizen's Health Research Group, 2000 P Street, N.W., Suite 708, Washington, D.C. 20036. (Available from the Health Research Group for $5.00.)

The worksheet on p. 128 is reprinted with the permission of the People's Medical Society, 462 Walnut Street, Allentown, PA 18102.

The chart on p. 131 is reprinted with the permission of the American Medical Records Association.

The quotation from "Lessons from Living with Cancer" by Robert Mack, *New England Journal of Medicine* 311 (1984): 1640, reprinted with permission of the *New England Journal of Medicine*.

The quotation from "Of Dragons and Garden Peas: A Cancer Patient Talks to Doctors" by Alice Trillin, *New England Journal of Medicine* 304 (1981): 701, is reprinted with the permission of the *New England Journal of Medicine*.

CHAPTER 7

The quotations from *By Myself* by Lauren Bacall are reprinted with permission of Alfred A. Knopf, Inc., © 1979.

The poems "To My Son" and "To My Daughter" by Claire Henze are reprinted by permission of Claire Henze. Copyright © 1981 by Claire Henze.

APPENDIX A

The list of state enforcement agencies handling handicap-discrimination complaints, pp. 182–91, from *Fair Employment Practices Manual*, pp. 451: 201–207, copyright © 1990 by The Bureau of National Affairs, Inc. Reprinted by permission.

Contents

ACKNOWLEDGMENTS ix

INTRODUCTION **Survivorship: An Idea for Everyone** 1

1. Abolishing the Myths: The Facts About Cancer 7

   Living With and Beyond a Cancer Diagnosis 7
   Cancer Treatment and Prevention 11
   The Physical Impact of Cancer and Its Treatment 21
   Medical Problems of Long-Term Survivors 29

2. Mind and Body: Harnessing Your Inner Resources 31

   The Complex Relationship Between Mind and Body 31
   The Inner Battle 32
   The Social Impact of Cancer 36
   Gaining Control over Stress 38
   Transformation—New Potential for the Cancer Survivor 41

3. The Cancer Survivor as Consumer 47

   Patients and Doctors 47
   Communications—The Two-Way Street 52
   The Hospital: A World unto Itself 58
   Caveat Emptor—Unconventional Treatments 62

4. Helping Therapies and Support Services 71

   The Roles of Helping Professionals 71
   Which Professional Should I Call? 74

5. Survivors Helping Survivors: Peer-Support Networking 79

   Peer-Support Networking 79
   Finding Peer Support 86
   Organizing Peer Support 88
   Role Models—Examples of Four Mutual-Aid Groups 92

6. **Taking Care of Business: Employment, Insurance, and Money Matters** 97

  Your Job and the Law 97
  Medical Malpractice 113
  Confidentiality of Medical Records 115
  Insurance Issues 118
  Money Matters 134

7. **Cancer and the Family** 145

  Dealing with the Shock of Diagnosis 146
  Family Involvement in Treatment 150
  When Mommy or Daddy Has Cancer—The Special Needs of Young Children 152
  Family Involvement over the Long Haul 154

POSTSCRIPT 160

APPENDIX A. CANCER SURVIVORSHIP RESOURCES 163

APPENDIX B. COMMON CANCERS 194

BIBLIOGRAPHY 203

ABOUT THE NATIONAL COALITION FOR CANCER SURVIVORSHIP 213

ABOUT THE EDITORS 215

ABOUT THE AUTHORS 216

ABOUT THE ARTWORK 217

INDEX 219

Acknowledgments

This book was made possible in part through funding from the National Cancer Care Foundation, a voluntary and independent nonprofit agency that has long recognized the complex issues related to cancer survivorship. The National Cancer Care Foundation, through its service arm, Cancer Care, offers professional social-work counseling, educational programs, and financial assistance to help cancer patients and their families cope with the emotional, financial, and social impact of cancer. Cancer Care conducts programs of professional consultation and education, community education and awareness, social research, and public affairs on a local and national basis.

The Department of Veterans Affairs Extended Educational Leave Program and the American Cancer Society Eleanor Roosevelt International Cancer Fellowship provided financial support for chapter 1, "Abolishing the Myths: The Facts About Cancer," and for Appendix B, "Common Cancers."

The editors wish to extend their special thanks to Natalie Chapman, Christopher Kuppig, Roslyn Siegel, and Sarah Uman of Consumer Reports Books; Rhoda Karpatkin, Executive Director of Consumers Union; and Philip Spitzer, our literary agent, for their faith in this project.

Finally, the editors and authors express our appreciation to our families for their patience, support, energy, and insight.

This almanac would not be a reality without the contributions of thousands of cancer survivors and health professionals who have shared their experiences with us. We specifically wish to thank for their time, energy, wisdom, and guidance Betsey Arey; Diane Blum, Executive Director of Cancer Care, Inc.; Donna Bocco of the American Cancer Society/New Jersey Division; Thomasina Borkman, Ph.D.; Murray Bowen, M.D.; Devra Breslow; Ann Bunting; Irene Card of Medical Insurance Claims, Inc.; Barbara J. Carter, Ph.D.; Ronn Dunden; Joanne Frankfurt, J.D., of the Legal Aid Society of San Francisco; Helen Gelband of the Office of Technology Assessment; Barbara Gratwick; Carol Halsted; Meredith Higgins; Edith Lenneberg; Fran Marcus Lewis, Ph.D., of the University of Washington at

Seattle; John J. Lynch, M.D., and Jeff Liebman of the Cancer Institute at Washington Hospital Center; Edward J. Madara of the New Jersey Self-Help Clearinghouse; Edith Marks of Memorial Sloan-Kettering Cancer Center's Post Treatment Resource Program; Grace Monaco, J.D., of the Candlelighters Childhood Cancer Foundation; Harvey Newman, former Executive Director of Cancer Care, Inc.; Julia Ostrowsky of the Office of Technology Assessment; Leonard Reinert of The Society for the Right to Die; Mary-Ellen Summerville of Cancer Care, Inc.; Lydia Temoshok, Ph.D., of Walter Reed Army Hospital; The Wildcat Ladies of Washington, D.C.; and Sara Rank Wolfe of the QuaLife Wellness Community.

Charting the Journey

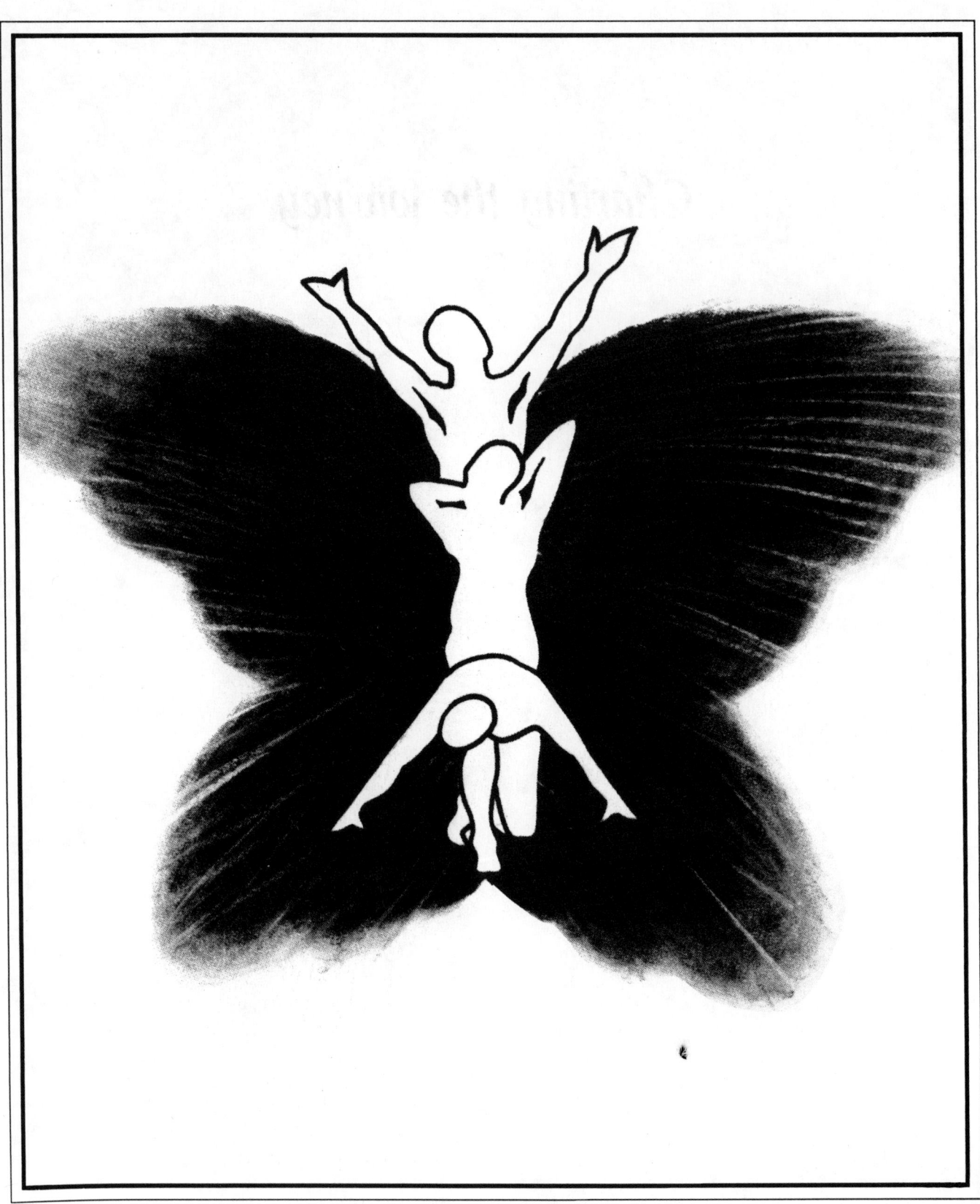

Wendy Traber
Metamorphosis

INTRODUCTION

Survivorship: An Idea for Everyone

Fitzhugh Mullan, M.D.

Survivorship is reason for celebration. It is the act of battling adversity, hanging tough despite bad luck and difficult circumstances. It is living with a constant challenge in life that sets desire to live against the possibility of death. Survivorship *is* victory, because it is the act of living on, no matter what happens.

Survivorship is the challenge faced daily by millions of Americans who are battling cancer. They are engaged in a defiance of disease and an affirmation of life. No matter how troubling the symptoms and the treatments, survival from day to day, week to week, and year to year constitutes an enormous personal and human triumph over what might have been.

Survivorship, in fact, is an especially important concept in relation to cancer, because improvements in diagnosis and treatment, as well as the growth of the overall population, have led to a vastly expanded community of people who are now living with a history of cancer. Current estimates suggest that more than 6 million Americans or 2 percent of our population are cancer survivors. A significant change, though, is taking place in the way many people think about cancer, giving the term "survivorship" even greater power. To many the very diagnosis of cancer initiates survivorship—a survivorship that is not determined by the number of months since treatment or the passing of a two- or a five- or a ten-year point. Survival, quite simply, begins when you are told you have cancer . . . and continues for the rest of your life.

Survivorship, viewed in this way, is a practical and accurate replacement for the judgmental term "cancer victim" and the passive one "cancer patient." Survivorship is a dynamic concept that avoids erecting unnecessary and inaccurate boundaries in the lives of people with cancer. A survivor experiences a continuum of events that are influenced by cancer from the time of diagnosis onward. A 60-year-old woman who is receiving radiation following a recent mastectomy is just as much a survivor as her husband who underwent treatment for colon cancer a decade earlier. His life includes sharing her worries as well as caring

> "The worst thing in your life may contain the seeds of the best."
>
> —Joe Kogel, melanoma survivor, writer, and actor

for his ostomy and dealing with his own fears about recurrence. A law student who overcame leukemia in elementary school is a survivor, as is his roommate who has just been diagnosed with a testicular cancer. The latter is scheduled for exploratory surgery while the former has been denied life and health insurance because of "a history of cancer."

Obviously, the prominence of cancer in the life of an individual depends upon the illness itself, its treatment, its progression or resolution. Survivorship, though, can be divided into three stages that have been called the "seasons of survival."

■ **Acute Survival.** This is the initial phase, dominated by diagnostic and therapeutic efforts to stop the disease. Doctors, nurses, and hospitals take an active role during the acute phase, providing support systems that may be less available later on. Dealing with one's own mortality and the possibility of death is an important characteristic of this time.

■ **Extended Survival.** This phase begins with the remission of the cancer or the termination of the rigorous course of treatment. It is a period of recovery and re-entry marked by uncertainty about the course of the cancer and the future. It is often a time when diminished strength and physical compromise make it difficult to resume old activities and responsibilities. The support systems that were so prominent in the acute period are much less available during this stage.

■ **Permanent Survival.** This phase corresponds to what is often called "cure"—a term that is misleading because it does not acknowledge the many changes in life (bad and good) that result from having experienced cancer. In addition to long-term difficulties (such as barriers to employment and insurance, and troublesome medical problems), cancer also tends to reward its survivors with a gusto for life that many consider a mark of distinction.

The principal message embodied in the idea that survivorship is forever and, indeed, in this almanac itself, is that people with cancer—even in the most acute stages—can live vital, contributory, and gratifying lives.

That idea is a powerful one—one that has spawned an entire movement. Chartered in 1986 and based on these principles, the National Coalition for Cancer Survivorship is dedicated to the development of a network of people and organizations concerned with cancer care. The NCCS is committed to providing a voice, undertaking advocacy, and stimulating research in the area of survivorship.

The NCCS, in turn, launched the almanac. The presence of the NCCS focused attention on the absence of a comprehensive resource book that addressed the needs of cancer survivors. What was needed, we jested, was a *Whole Earth Catalogue* for surviving cancer. As the idea developed, it became a serious undertaking. We envisioned an almanac rich in information concerned (as traditional almanacs are) with the future, that could be consulted on an as-needed basis to help with decisions and actions. The network of friends and colleagues that clustered around the NCCS provided the marvelous mix of people whose personal experiences, professional insights, and literary talents have been tapped to write and edit the almanac.

> "Survival, however, was not one condition but many. It was desperate days of nausea and depression. It was elation at the birth of a daughter in the midst of the treatment. It was the anxiety of waiting for my monthly chest film to be taken and lying awake nights feeling for lymph nodes. It was the joy of eating Chinese food for the first time after battling radiation burns of the esophagus for four months. These reflections and many others are a jumble of memories of a purgatory that was touched by sickness in all its aspects but was neither death nor cure. It was survival—an absolutely predictable condition that all cancer patients pass through as they struggle with their illness."
>
> —Fitzhugh Mullan, M.D.

The almanac, in fact, embodies what has emerged as a guiding principle of the survivorship movement—the systematic transmission of the wisdom of seasoned cancer patients and health care providers to newly diagnosed individuals and families. It is, simply, the veteran helping the rookie. This potent concept underlies teaching, training, and coaching of all sorts in our society but is largely and unfortunately absent from our system of medical care. Not only does the rookie gain unique, tested, front-line knowledge from this interchange, but the veteran has the opportunity to put hard-won, sometimes painfully won, insight to use in a way that is intensely gratifying.

Underlying this principle of shared knowledge is the clear premise that information is strength and that the survivor should be as involved as possible in medical, social, and vocational decision making. Rather than downgrading the importance of traditional medical care, which is essential to survival, our program is supplemental and cooperative. It advocates a broadened and more active role for the survivor in the multitude of decisions that will follow the initial diagnosis. Gathering information is medical consumerism of a very basic sort. Most consumers do some research before they make major purchases such as cars or refrigerators. Yet, until recently, few cancer survivors knew how to make comparably informed decisions about their health care and related issues such as treatment options, insurance benefits, and employment rights. The almanac, therefore, is written to help empower survivors with the knowledge necessary for them to participate in their care in an informed and active way and to affect the medical, social, and economic consequences of their illness.

It is important to emphasize, though, that neither the almanac nor the NCCS prescribes a right or wrong way to be a survivor or advocates specific treatments or choices. Every cancer experience is different, and what people bring to the experience is as variable as they are. Many current issues are hotly debated in the survivorship community, such as the utility of self-imaging and the role of clinical trials. In developing the almanac, the editors have chosen broad topics encountered by most survivors that, taken as a whole, cover the terrain of survivorship. Inevitably, this terrain will shift as cancer treatment improves and as the survivorship movement grows. This volume,

> "The reds all got redder...."
>
> "Celebrate the journey. Stop worrying about the potholes in the road and celebrate the journey!"
>
> —Comments of two cancer survivors about life after diagnosis

> "The bottom line was simply this: an appreciation of the preciousness of life could be a means of living more gracefully; and, as a natural course of things, dying more gracefully whenever that time comes, be it as a result of cancer or the Number 52 bus running over you in the middle of an otherwise harmless Thursday afternoon."
>
> —Joe Kogel

therefore, should be seen as a living document that we intend to update in future years. Please make note of suggestions and additions that occur to you as you read it and send them to us care of the NCCS, 323 Eighth Street S.W., Albuquerque, New Mexico 87102.

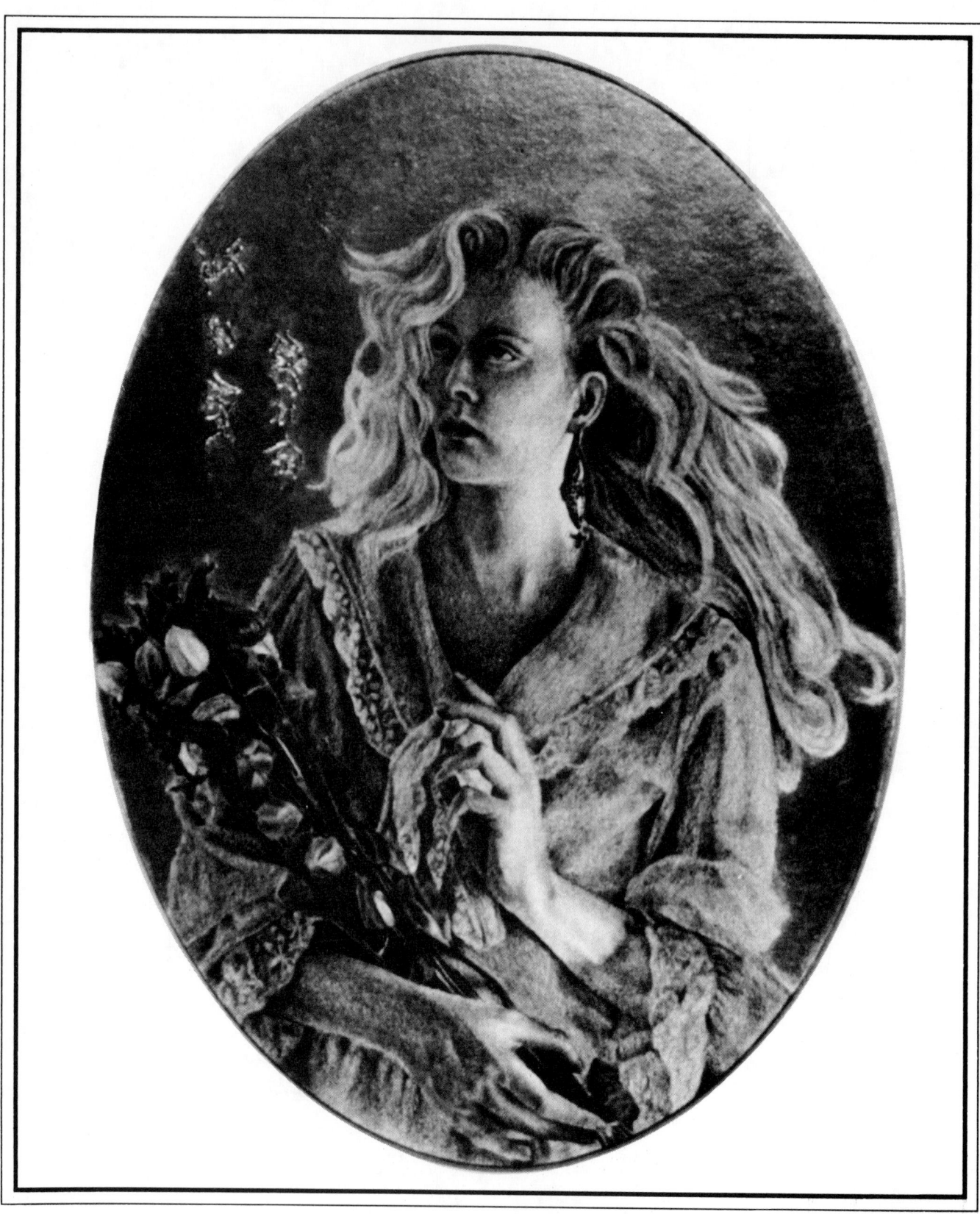

Megan Hart Jones
Soul Portrait
Mixed media
19″ × 14″

1

Abolishing the Myths: The Facts About Cancer

Patricia A. Ganz, M.D.

Living With and Beyond a Cancer Diagnosis

Fifty years ago there was little audience for a book about surviving with and beyond a cancer diagnosis. In the 1930s fewer than one in five cancer patients were alive five years after treatment. A diagnosis of cancer was then, for all practical purposes, a death sentence.

The prevalence of cancer (cancer strikes three out of four families) and the sparsity of successful treatments fanned the flames of cancer paranoia and supported the "cancer = death" equation. Until the identification of AIDS in the 1980s, cancer was for decades the most feared illness. Doctors did not tell their patients details about their diagnoses for fear of upsetting them. The fear and shame of having cancer were so strong that even mentioning the name seemed to be intolerable, and the disease was often referred to as "the big C." Daily obituaries read "died of a long illness" instead of "cancer." "Terminally ill cancer patient" was considered a redundancy, not a clarification.

Patients who knew the nature of their diagnoses seldom discussed it with anyone other than their doctor and immediate family. Shame, embarrassment, guilt, and fear of ostracism caused most to wrestle with their cancer experiences in solitude.

Public officials especially were compelled to conceal their diagnoses. In 1893, President Grover Cleveland had secret surgery to remove malignant tissue from the roof of his mouth. The surgery was performed on a yacht in New York's East River to mislead the press, which was told that the President needed dental work. President Cleveland successfully kept his illness a secret, hoping to avoid further economic chaos during the great financial panic of 1893. He fully recovered and died 15 years later from a gastrointestinal attack.

Medical statistics have improved more rapidly than social attitudes toward cancer. In the 1960s, one in three people diagnosed with cancer lived at least five years after treatment. Of the more than one million

> "There is, in the moment you hear the news, an awareness you are mortal. If you are courageous enough, that feeling lasts forever."
>
> —Joe Kogel

Americans who will be diagnosed in 1990, approximately one-half will win their medical battle against cancer. Survival rates are even higher for individuals under the age of 55.

Despite better public education, medical gains, and a growing population of cancer survivors, myths about cancer still persist, affecting not only how family, co-workers, friends, and strangers react but how survivors perceive themselves. Three cancer myths in particular have a significant impact on survivors' quality of life.

The most common myth is that cancer is a death sentence. In word-association games, "death" is the first word people say in response to the word "cancer." Although some types of cancer, such as esophageal and pancreatic, still offer a poor prognosis, many other types of cancer, especially when diagnosed in early stages, are successfully treated. Approximately 90 percent of those diagnosed with early-stage cancer of the breast, uterus, bladder, and testis will be symptom-free five years after diagnosis. Treatment for other types of cancer, such as prostate cancer, acute lymphocytic leukemia, and Hodgkin's disease have shown dramatic improvements since the 1960s. Six million cancer survivors in the United States, 3 million of whom have lived five years past treatment, are living testament that cancer is no longer an automatic death sentence.

A second myth is that cancer is contagious. One clerical worker in Michigan returned to her job after having a laryngectomy only to find that a co-worker had saturated her work area with Lysol for fear of catching her cancer. Although professionals agree that none of the scores of medical conditions defined as "cancer" is contagious, an estimated 15 million Americans still think cancer is contagious, and another 20 million do not know whether it is or is not.

A third myth is that cancer survivors are mere shadows of their former selves. As a group, survivors are often presumed to be physically or mentally handicapped, unable to hold a job, unqualified to adopt a child, and undesirable as social acquaintances. Well-known survivors, like former First Lady Betty Ford, Olympic gold-medal winner Jeff Blatnick, and author-comedian Steve Allen, exemplify the baselessness of these assumptions. Millions of cancer survivors in the United States have excelled in their chosen fields despite their diagnoses. They include political leaders, doctors, lawyers, businesspeople, clerical workers, union members, performers, authors, and professional athletes.

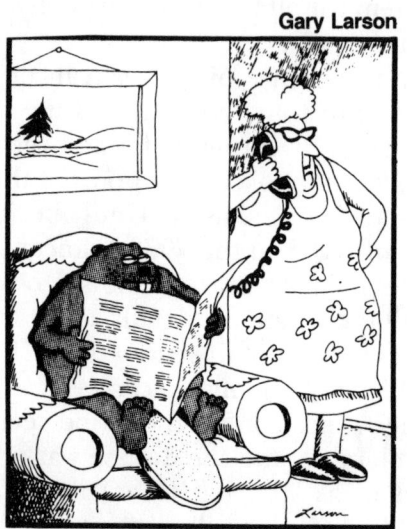

Gary Larson

"No, he's not busy—in fact, that whole thing is just a myth."

THE TEN MOST COMMON CANCERS DURING THE 1980s

Source: National Cancer Institute

Age-adjusted incidence and mortality rates and five-year relative survival rates by site, race, sex, and time period.

White Males

	INCD.	MORT.	SURV.
Prostate	83.5	22.9	73.4
Lung	82.4	65.3	11.7
Colon	42.2	20.7	55.0
Bladder	30.9	6.4	78.7
Rectum	19.1	4.0	51.4
Lymphomas	18.4	8.4	55.9
Skin*	14.9	4.4	68.5
Leukemias	13.5	8.8	34.4
Kidney	11.2	4.7	52.7
Pancreas	10.9	10.0	2.7

White Females

	INCD.	MORT.	SURV.
Breast	99.5	27.8	76.3
Lung	35.1	25.7	15.7
Colon	32.3	15.2	55.3
Corpus	23.4	2.1	83.4
Ovary	14.1	8.2	38.4
Lymphomas	13.1	5.6	57.7
Rectum	11.6	2.2	54.6
Skin*	9.6	1.9	86.4
Pancreas	8.1	7.5	2.6
Cervix	7.9	2.4	66.9

Black Males

	INCD.	MORT.	SURV.
Lung	129.0	98.8	10.4
Prostate	128.9	45.8	62.8
Colon	42.8	23.2	46.9
Stomach	20.0	15.6	18.1
Esophagus	19.5	15.0	4.7
Pancreas	16.9	15.5	3.6
Bladder	15.8	4.9	59.6
Rectum	13.7	3.9	35.9
Lymphomas	12.5	5.7	47.6
Larynx	12.4	4.9	53.2

Black Females

	INCD.	MORT.	SURV.
Breast	86.2	31.2	63.5
Lung	37.9	28.0	14.7
Colon	36.3	17.8	48.6
Cervix	16.3	6.6	59.3
Corpus	14.2	3.2	52.0
Pancreas	12.4	10.6	6.2
Rectum	10.4	2.5	42.9
Ovary	10.1	5.8	38.3
Stomach	8.8	5.8	19.8
Lymphomas	8.3	3.4	55.8

Incidence: the incidence rate per 100,000 people in the United States of new diagnoses each year from 1982 to 1986.

Mortality: the number of people in the United States per 100,000 who died each year from 1982 to 1986.

Survival: the number of people in the United States per 100,000 who were diagnosed from 1980 to 1985 and had not died from their cancer within five years of diagnosis.

*Excluding basal- and squamous-cell skin cancers.

Like people who have heart disease or any other chronic illness, some cancer survivors will be disabled by their disease. Myth overshadows fact when people assume that cancer automatically and permanently disables everyone who is diagnosed with the disease.

Since the 1930s, life for many during and beyond cancer treatment has improved dramatically. More people are surviving cancer, living longer and healthier lives. Cancer treatment often involves a team of specialists who will work with you to heal your body and maintain your normal life-style as closely as possible. Although the side effects of surgery, chemotherapy, and radiation can still be quite harsh, cancer treatment is now designed not only to eliminate the disease but also to mitigate short- and long-term side effects. Surgery has been refined from general cuts by scalpel to microscopic

> "In July 1982, I learned that I was suffering from abdominal mesothelioma, a rare and serious cancer usually associated with exposure to asbestos.... The literature couldn't have been more brutally clear: Mesothelioma is incurable, with a median mortality of only eight months after discovery....
>
> "The problem may be briefly stated: What does 'median mortality of eight months' signify in our vernacular? I suspect that most people, without training in statistics, would read such a statement as 'I will probably be dead in eight months'—the very conclusion that must be avoided, since it isn't so, and since attitude matters so much....
>
> "When I learned about the eight-month median, my first intellectual reaction was: fine, half the people will live longer; now what are my chances of being in that half?"
>
> —Stephen Jay Gould, Ph.D., "The Median Isn't the Message," *Discover*, June 1985

incisions by laser. Body parts can be saved or replaced. Malignant cells can be targeted while healthy cells are protected. Quality of life, and not just life itself, is now an obtainable goal.

PUBLIC-OPINION POLL QUESTION: "DO YOU THINK CANCER IS CONTAGIOUS?"

	Yes	No	Do Not Know
1939	20%	59%	21% (Gallup)
1950	14%	66%	20% (Gallup)
1985	6%	87%	8% (Cambridge Reports)

Because of gains in treatment and early detection, cancer survivors now have more opportunities to participate in and benefit from choices that affect their futures, as well as their quality of life.

For most individuals, cancer is a chronic disease. It will not disappear after a first session with their medical team. They will need to understand as much about their treatments as possible so they can complete them successfully and adapt to any side effects. Lifelong follow-up will be necessary for monitoring recurrence, potential long-term side effects from treatment, and other cancer- or treatment-related problems.

Well-informed survivors and their families are the physician's best partner in this process. Your doctor should provide you with the information you need to ensure the success of this partnership, and it is your responsibility to tell your doctor about new symptoms or side effects. Studies of patients with other chronic illnesses (diabetes and high blood pressure) have demonstrated that, when patients have more understanding about their disease and its treatment, their medical condition objectively improves. Similar studies of cancer patients are under way.

When cancer is first diagnosed, many consulting physicians may be asked to evaluate your medical situation, or you may be

> "[C]ancer will be partly demythicized; and it may then be possible to compare something to a cancer without implying either a fatalistic diagnosis or a rousing call to fight by any means whatever a lethal, insidious enemy."
>
> —Susan Sontag, *Illness as Metaphor*

referred to consultants at a specialized cancer-treatment facility. This may be very confusing for you and your family, and you may not be sure who is in charge of your medical care. Under these circumstances, it is best to identify one physician who will be the captain of your team. That can be your family doctor, internist, pediatrician, or gynecologist at first. After your team develops a cancer-treatment plan, one of the consulting specialists will probably function as the primary care-provider.

Cancer Treatment and Prevention

Cancer is the general term for a large group of diseases that are all characterized by the uncontrolled growth of cells. Cancer cells at first grow locally, but eventually invade and destroy the surrounding tissues. The cancer cells also have a propensity to spread to other parts of the body (metastasis) through the lymph system or bloodstream. Your doctor is the best person to consult regarding the details of your own illness and treatment. For additional information about the different types of cancer, see appendixes A and B.

Principles of Cancer Treatment

After the diagnosis of cancer has been made, a treatment plan will be developed for your unique medical situation based on all of the information that has been gathered through blood tests, radiologic studies, surgery, and microscopic and biochemical evaluation of your cancer. The treatment plan that your doctors develop will have a specific goal. In general, the possibilities include cure, long-term control of the cancer, or symptomatic relief only.

Cure. Cure is the goal for a wide range of cancer today, and over half of newly diagnosed cancer patients will be cured of their disease. Cure, from the medical point of view, means that all of the cancer can be successfully removed with surgery, or completely eliminated from the body by medication or radiation treatments. Cure also implies that once such treatment has been given, the likelihood of the cancer's reappearance at a later date—either in the same local area or in a distant organ—is extremely low. "Curative-intent" treatment means that the initial treatment plan is chosen with the expectation that the person will be cured.

Although some people have focused on five years of disease-free survival as the equivalent of cure, there may be a very high likelihood of long-term cure after as few as two years for some, and others may still be at risk for recurrent cancer for much longer than five years. Curative intent treatment focuses on the ultimate goal of becoming cancer-free, and not on an arbitrary length of time in which cure is anticipated.

12   Abolishing the Myths

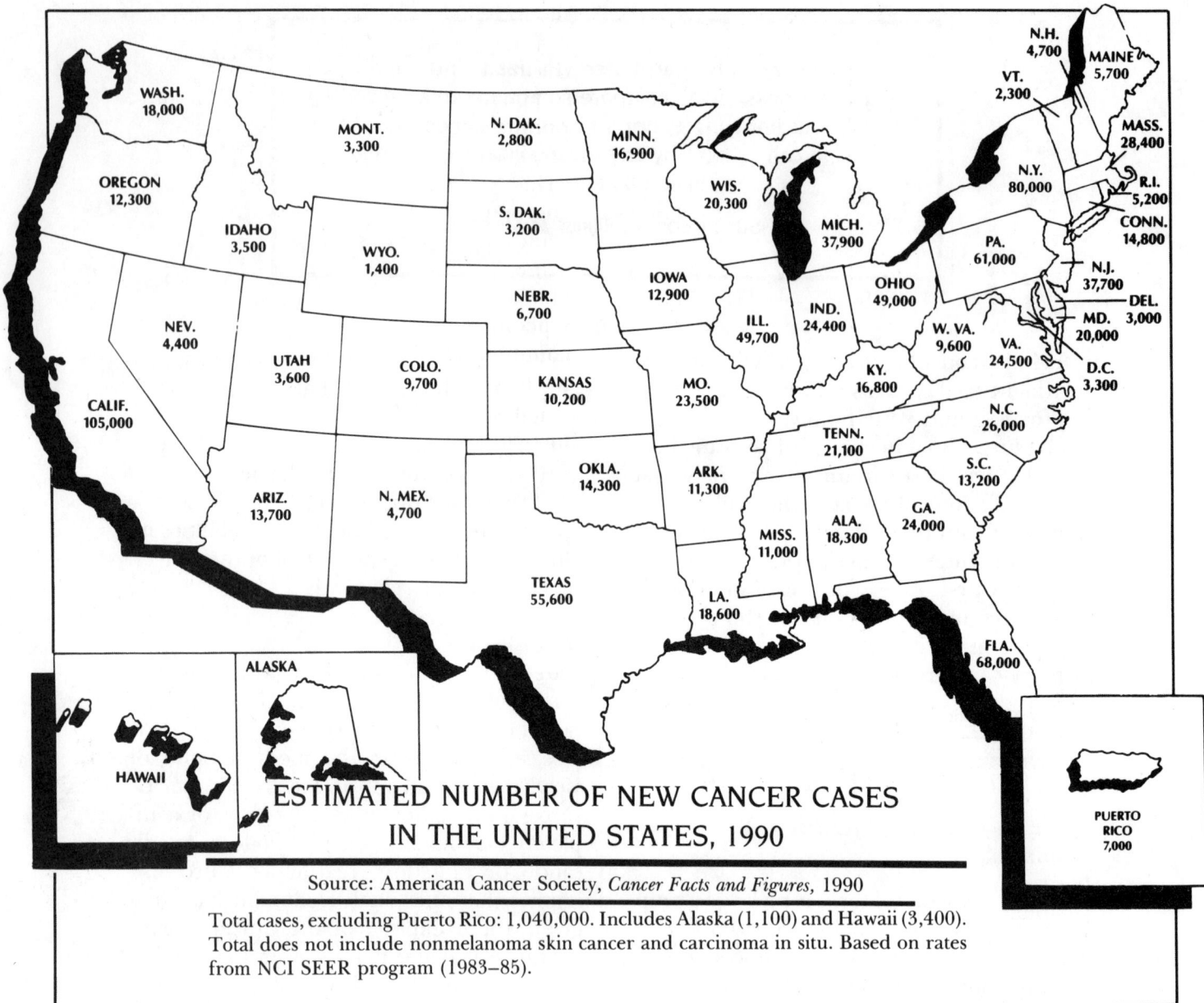

ESTIMATED NUMBER OF NEW CANCER CASES
IN THE UNITED STATES, 1990

Source: American Cancer Society, *Cancer Facts and Figures*, 1990

Total cases, excluding Puerto Rico: 1,040,000. Includes Alaska (1,100) and Hawaii (3,400). Total does not include nonmelanoma skin cancer and carcinoma in situ. Based on rates from NCI SEER program (1983–85).

Long-term control. Long-term control of cancer is the treatment goal for a substantial number of cancer patients. This means that treatment is aimed at modifying the course of the disease, usually by temporarily eliminating the cancer, slowing its growth, and controlling its symptoms; however, it is expected that eventually the cancer will become resistant to the treatment and return, to cause symptoms and ultimately death. Chronic leukemias, myeloma, and some non-Hodgkin's lymphomas are examples of cancers for which treatment provides long-term control. Although treatment for these diseases sometimes may control the cancer for a decade or longer, eventually almost all people with these cancers will succumb to the disease.

Symptom relief. Symptom relief only (palliation) is the treatment goal for most patients with advanced cancers. These cancers, in general, demonstrate only a minor response to treatment with chemotherapy or radiation, and are too extensive to be removed with surgery. However, chemotherapy and radiation are frequently used for symptom

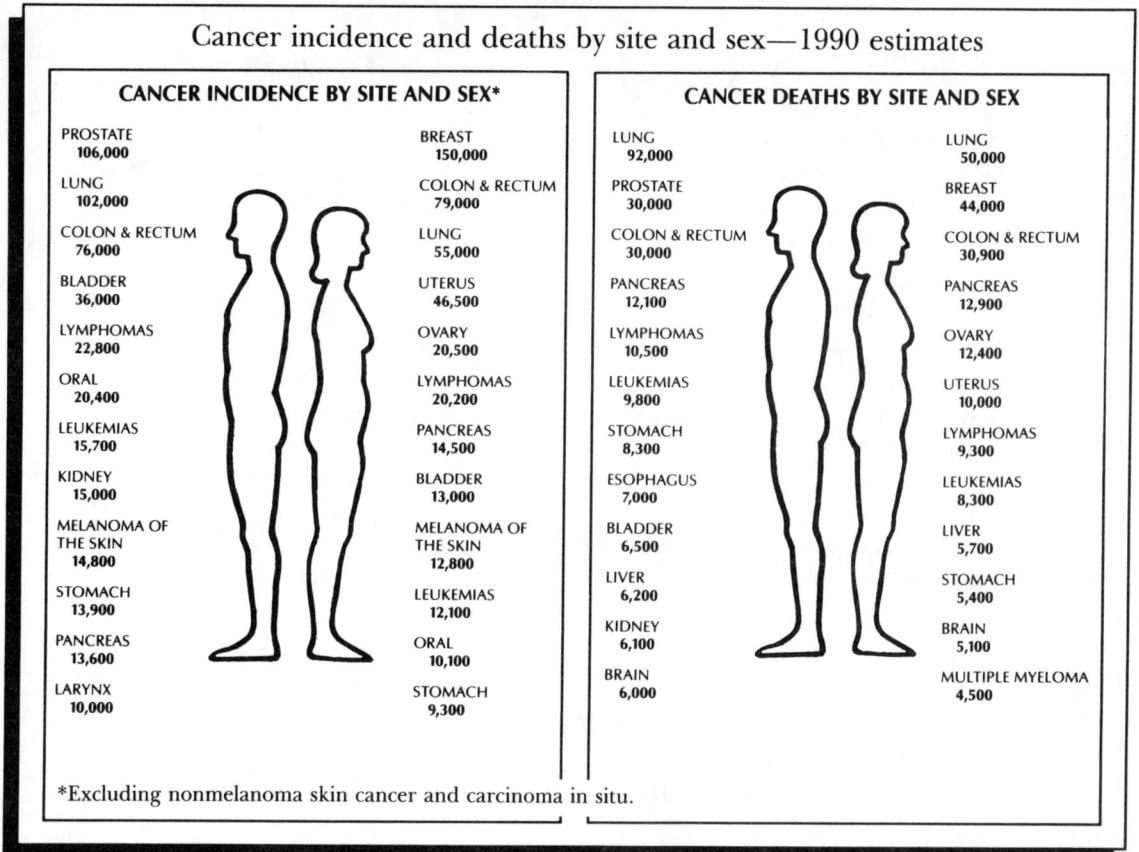

relief. Cancers treated with symptom relief as the major goal include pancreatic cancer, esophageal cancer, and metastatic melanoma. Measures other than anticancer treatment will usually be included in the treatment plan, such as pain relief, and medication for depression, anxiety, and any other symptoms caused by the cancer.

Phases of treatment. Several distinct phases of treatment will occur as you live through your own cancer experience. The first, the diagnostic phase, is experienced by everyone. This phase includes your first encounter with the doctor to report new symptoms or undergo tests, including a biopsy of the cancer (removal of a small piece of tissue for microscopic examination). The next phase usually involves consultation with a number of experts in order to establish the initial treatment plan. For most cancers, a delay of a few weeks to complete various diagnostic tests and consultations should be expected, because this is often the best time to define a treatment plan that will give the best chance of cure or long-term survival. On rare occasions, treatment will be started immediately.

For some cancers, there may be a maintenance phase, during which treatment is continued but usually on a less intensive schedule. For example, maintenance therapy is commonly given to children with acute lymphocytic leukemia (ALL). For some kinds of cancer, this may include a consolidation or late-intensification treatment, where high doses of chemotherapy are given as a final booster before discontinuing treatments.

The follow-up care phase is the time after completion of surgery, radiation therapy, chemotherapy, or a combination of treatments when it is thought that the cancer has

CURE

The vinca*
in my garden
grows wild and disorderly
Along the stone steps
Crowds innocent growth
Unfairly

The vinca rosea
Picked, ground and liquefied
A chemical warfare
against the most dreaded disease
Injected into a vein
Spreads rapidly
through my bloodstream
A raging fire
Wretched violent poison

The vinca
in my garden
a constant reminder
of my dark past
The year of lying perfectly still
in a dark room

Threads of light
monumental irritants
Agonizing sounds—
a neighbor mowing his lawn
Cheerful coos of my baby

The vinca
with each blast
permeates and terrorizes
each cell
Then slowly and methodically
mutated cells die
Healthy cells rally
Reproduce

The vinca
in my garden
trails gracefully
along the stone steps
Glossy green leaves
Tiny periwinkle petal
that healed and restored
the harmony of my body

—Wendy Podwalny, Hodgkin's disease survivor, *Surviving!* (October/November 1988)

*Vinca rosea (the Madagascar periwinkle plant) contains many alkaloids, including vincristine and vinblastine, which are used in chemotherapy.

---

been completely eradicated. During this phase you will be recovering from the effects of treatment and begin to resume a normal life, with less frequent visits to the doctor. Initially you may see your doctor every one or two months, and then only three or four times a year. During these visits the doctor will usually perform a careful interview and physical examination, with emphasis on possible symptoms related to the cancer and any residual side effects from your treatments. You will also have regular blood tests and other studies to monitor your condition. As time passes, your visits with the doctor will be even less frequent, but you will nevertheless need lifelong follow-up, because of possible problems that occur secondary to cancer treatment, the risk of new cancers, or recurrence.

If the cancer recurs, it may occur in the same part of the body where it was originally, a local recurrence, or it may reappear in a more distant part of the body, which is called a "metastasis." In either case, a new treatment plan must be designed, and diagnostic tests will have to be done again to determine the extent of the cancer. The type of treatment that is used at the time of the recurrence will depend on the type of cancer, its extent, and what previous therapy was given. Some recurrent cancers can still be cured, although the chance for cure

> "As a skill for coping with the emotional impact of baldness resulting from chemotherapy, if I saw a really good-looking girl, I would imagine her bald."
>
> —Barbara Smith, Canadian psychologist and breast-cancer survivor

is usually lower than for the first incidence.

Some people will have advanced and incurable cancer from the time of diagnosis, and others will reach this phase after many years of treatment and follow-up care. In either case, the usual goal of treatment for this phase of cancer is symptom relief. Some patients, however, may want to participate in research trials of new experimental treatments (see pp. 62–64).

Surgery, radiation, and chemotherapy. Traditionally, cancer has been treated with surgery, radiation, chemotherapy, or a combination of the three.

1. *Surgery* can be performed under local or general anesthesia, and may be limited to a biopsy or be very extensive. A number of cancers (for example, colorectal and lung cancers) are treated with surgery, and can be cured by the surgical procedure alone. In other forms of cancer treatment, surgery will be combined with radiation and/or chemotherapy in order to limit the extent of the surgery and improve the chance for cure. This approach is called "combined-modality therapy."

2. *Radiation* therapy is the treatment of cancer with high-energy radiation. These treatments are usually given to defined or limited parts of the body. Radiation therapy is sometimes used alone to cure cancers (for example, cancer of the cervix and larynx), thereby avoiding major surgery. More often, it is used to reduce the size of a cancer before surgery or to destroy any remaining cancer cells after surgery. Radiation therapy is also used for the treatment of many patients with advanced cancer who require symptom relief—the radiation will be used to shrink local areas of the cancer that are causing pain or other symptoms.

3. *Chemotherapy* is a general term for treatment with drugs. Hormone medications are also broadly included in this approach to treatment. Chemotherapy is usually given by injection or infusion into a vein, but can also be given by injection into the muscle or skin, or be taken by mouth. These treatments may be used alone to cure a number of cancers (for example, Hodgkin's disease, non-Hodgkin's lymphoma, and testicular cancer), but more often it is used in combination with radiation and surgery. Chemotherapy treatments have the advantage of traveling in the bloodstream to almost all parts of the body, and thus are able to eradicate cancer cells that are out of reach of the scalpel or radiation beam. They are also used to provide long-term control for some cancers, and to relieve symptoms in patients with advanced cancer.

New Approaches

As mentioned previously, surgery, radiation therapy, and chemotherapy have been the mainstay of cancer treatment for several decades. However, new approaches to cancer treatment have met with success in the past few years.

1. *Adjuvant therapy* is an extra treatment that is added to the primary treatment in order to prevent a recurrence of the cancer

16 *Abolishing the Myths*

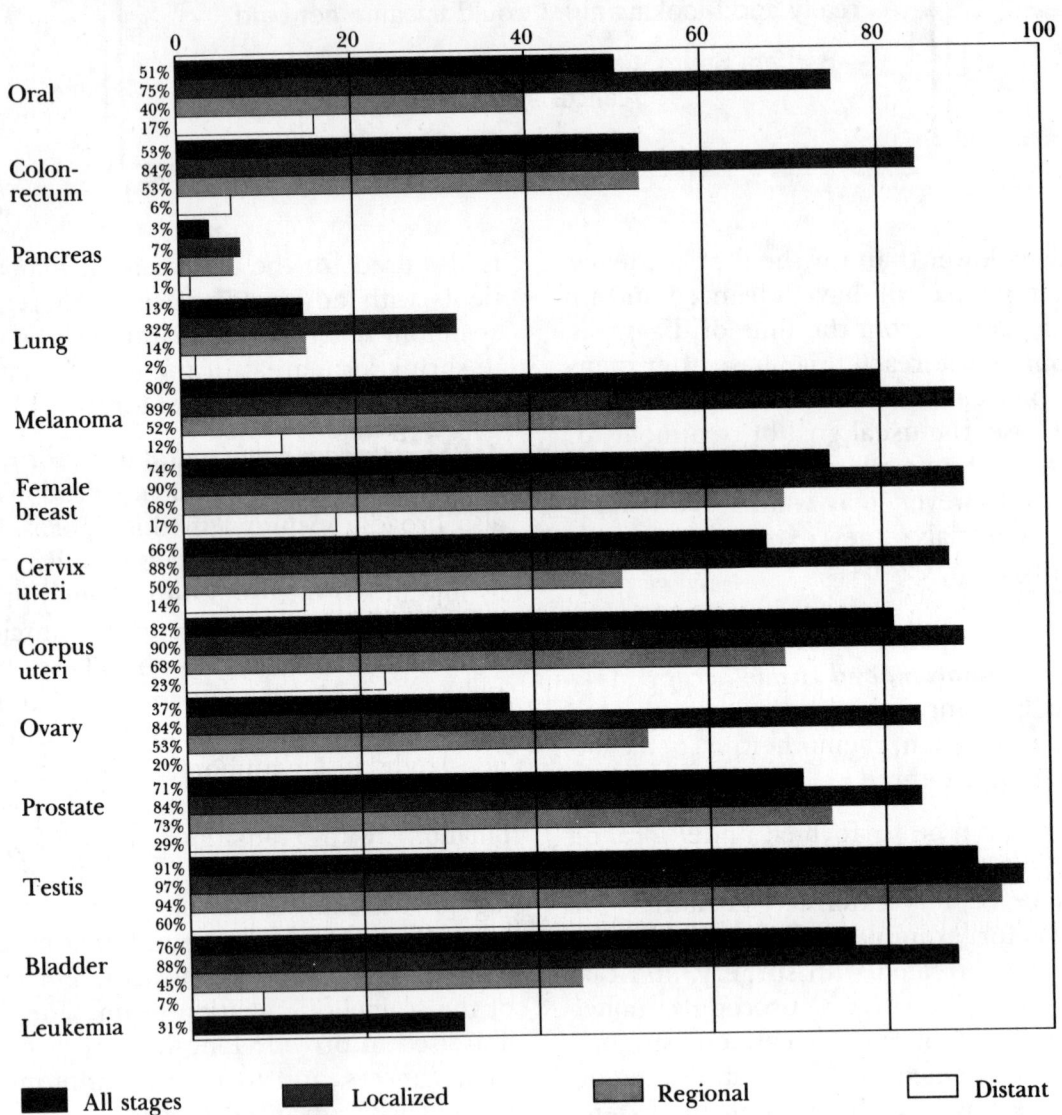

and prolong survival. Distant or local microscopic deposits of cancer may not be detected at the time the original cancer is diagnosed and treated, but may show up several years later as recurrent cancer, more difficult to eradicate. Therefore, for some cancers (for example, breast cancer), early treatment with drugs (chemotherapy, hormones) may eradicate these cells and prevent their regrowth. For some cancers, chemotherapy treatments are given before the cancer is removed. The term "neo-adjuvant" therapy has been used for this situation.

2. Bone-marrow transplantation is a treatment for patients who are given extremely high doses of radiation and chemotherapy in order to eliminate the cancer cells in the body. This would ordinarily cause death, because of its effects on blood counts; however, through the use of bone-marrow transplants, the patient is rescued from the toxic and potentially lethal effects of the

HOW TO ESTIMATE CANCER STATISTICS LOCALLY

Source: American Cancer Society, *Cancer Facts and Figures,* 1989

Community Population	Estimated No. Who Are Alive, Saved from Cancer	Estimated No. Cancer Cases Under Medical Care in 1989	Estimated No. Who Will Die of Cancer in 1989	Estimated No. of New Cases in 1989	Estimated No. Who Will Be Saved from Cancer in 1989	Estimated No. Who Will Eventually Develop Cancer	Estimated No. Who Will Die of Cancer if Present Rates Continue
1,000	10	5	1	3	1	280	180
2,000	20	11	4	7	3	560	360
3,000	30	16	5	10	4	840	540
4,000	40	21	7	13	5	1,120	720
5,000	50	26	9	16	6	1,400	900
10,000	100	52	18	33	12	2,800	1,800
25,000	250	131	45	79	30	7,000	4,500
50,000	500	262	90	158	59	14,000	9,000
100,000	1,000	525	180	325	122	28,000	18,000
200,000	2,000	1,050	360	650	244	56,000	36,000
500,000	5,000	2,625	900	1,575	590	140,000	90,000

Note: The figures can only be the roughest approximation of actual data for your community and should be used with caution. It is suggested that every effort be made to obtain actual data from a state tumor-registry office.

treatment. The procedure is accomplished by removal (under general anesthesia) of about a half-liter of bone marrow from a healthy donor who is genetically identical or extremely well matched to the recipient (allogeneic transplantation). The cells from the donated marrow are then processed and subsequently infused by vein into the recipient, after the chemotherapy and radiation treatments have been given. The bone-marrow transplantation procedure (receipt of high-dose chemotherapy and radiation) has many side effects and is only performed at specialized centers. In general, it is not performed in persons over the age of 40, whose results are poorer and who suffer more side effects. There are a number of cancers for which bone-marrow transplantation has become a standard treatment (for example, acute leukemia). Recently, more research has been done with very high dose chemotherapy and rescue of the patients with their own bone marrow, which they have previously donated and stored in the event of a recurrence. This approach to treatment (autologous bone-marrow transplantation) is not yet routine, but is actively being studied.

3. Modification of the immunologic system (the body's regulatory system to resist disease or invasion by foreign substances, such as cancer cells) is another type of therapy being used in cancer treatment. For several decades, researchers have been studying ways to boost the body's own natural defenses against cancer. Until recently, most of these results have met with limited success. Innovative technologies have permitted the large-scale production of new agents, broadly classified as biologic response modifiers, which are derived from the body's own natural products. Interferon, interleukin-2, and tumor necrosis factor are a few substances undergoing active study. Some of these agents have already found a place in cancer treatment. We can expect to see more research in this area in the years ahead, and many new experimental studies to evaluate how best to use these biologic response modifiers.

4. Hyperthermia treatment, the use of heat to kill cancer cells, is another form of treatment under active investigation. Scientists have known for decades that high temper-

TRENDS IN SURVIVAL BY SITE OF CANCER, BY RACE

Source: American Cancer Society, *Facts and Figures*, 1989,
taken from Surveillance and Operations Branch, National Cancer Institute

	White					Black				
	RELATIVE FIVE-YEAR SURVIVAL					RELATIVE FIVE-YEAR SURVIVAL				
SITE	1960–63[1]	1970–73[1]	1974–76[2]	1977–78[2]	1979–84[2]	1960–63[1]	1970–73[1]	1974–76[2]	1977–78[2]	1979–84[2]
All sites	39%	43%	50%	50%	50%	27%	31%	38%	38%	37%
Oral cavity and pharynx	45	43	54	53	54	—	—	35	35	31
Esophagus	4	4	5	6	7	1	4	4	2	5
Stomach	11	13	14	15	16[3]	8	13	15	16	17
Colon	48	49	50	52	54[3]	34	37	45	44	49
Rectum	38	45	48	50	52[3]	27	30	40	40	34
Liver	2	3	4	3	3	—	—	1	1	5
Pancreas	1	2	3	2	3	1	2	2	3	5
Larynx	53	62	66	69	66	—	—	58	59	55
Lung and bronchus	8	10	12	13	13[3]	5	7	11	10	11
Melanoma of skin	60	68	78	81	80[3]	—	—	62[5]	—	61[4]
Breast (females)	63	68	74	75	75[3]	46	51	62	62	62
Cervix uteri	58	64	69	69	67	47	61	61	63	59
Corpus uteri	73	81	89	87	83[3]	31	44	61	58	52[3]
Ovary	32	36	36	37	37[3]	32	32	41	40	36
Prostate gland	50	63	67	70	73[3]	35	55	56	64	60[3]
Testis	63	72	78	86	91[3]	—	—	77[4]	—	82[4]
Urinary bladder	53	61	73	75	77[3]	24	36	47	53	57[3]
Kidney and renal pelvis	37	46	51	50	51	38	44	49	54	53
Brain and nervous system	18	20	22	23	23	19	19	27	24	31
Thyroid gland	83	86	92	92	93	—	—	88	92	95
Hodgkin's disease	40	67	71	73	74[3]	—	—	67[4]	79[4]	69
Non-Hodgkin's lymphoma	31	41	47	48	49[3]	—	—	47	46	49
Multiple myeloma	12	19	24	24	24	—	—	28	30	29
Leukemia	14	22	34	37	32	—	—	30	31	27

[1] Rates are based on End Results Group data from a series of hospital registries and one population-based registry.
[2] Rates are from the SEER Program. They are based on data from population-based registries in Connecticut, New Mexico, Utah, Iowa, Hawaii, Atlanta, Detroit, Seattle–Puget Sound, and San Francisco–Oakland. Rates are based on follow-up of patients through 1985.
[3] The difference in rates between 1974–76 and 1979–84 is statistically significant (p<.05).
[4] The standard error of the survival rate is between 5 and 10 percentage points.
[5] The standard error of the survival rate is greater than 10 percentage points.
—Valid survival rate could not be calculated.

atures could arrest the growth of cancer cells. Many years ago, patients were given bacterial toxins to induce fever as a means of treating their cancers. We now have more sophisticated ways of applying heat locally, only to the cancer, and can eliminate exposing the whole body to the side effects from the high temperatures. Hyperthermia treatment is still being studied, but is sometimes integrated into the standard treatment of cancer.

Standard and Experimental Treatments

There is a "standard treatment approach" for most cancers, which means that the majority of physicians and researchers have agreed on the way the cancer should be treated based on years of systematic study and research. For some cancers, there may be several equally effective treatments, and doctors may have different opinions about which to choose. Under these circumstances, seeking a second opinion is helpful in order to learn about all your alternatives.

Research is being conducted with new experimental treatments and with new ways of using standard treatments. In general, this research is being conducted at cancer-treatment centers affiliated with universities, but many community cancer specialists participate in these research studies as well. These research studies, called "clinical trials," test the effectiveness of a new treatment, usually in comparison with the best available standard treatment. If a treatment has not been accepted as one of the standard treatments, it is called "experimental" or "investigational." Because of the experimental nature of the treatment, you will be monitored especially carefully for side effects as well as benefits if you participate. You must give your informed consent to participate in such research before it is administered (see chapter 3). Unfortunately, very few patients treated in the United States today are given the opportunity to participate in clinical trials, a situation the National Cancer Institute is trying to rectify.

There are several reasons you may want to participate in a clinical trial. It may give you the chance to receive treatment that is more effective or less toxic than the standard treatment. In addition, your participation in this research effort contributes to a more rapid accumulation of knowledge that will potentially help others. The clinical-trial process is a prerequisite for making progress in cancer treatment.

Cancer Prevention

Although cancer-survival rates are improving every year, it would be best to prevent the disease from occurring at all. Because, however, only some of the causes of cancer are known, and prevention itself is not an exact science (no cancer vaccine exists), preventive steps can only decrease the chances of being stricken. Life-style changes that lower the risk of cancer include:

Eliminating the use of tobacco. Tobacco kills approximately 25 percent of those who use it. Approximately 390,000 Americans and 2.5 million people in other countries die each year from tobacco-induced diseases, including cancer of the lung, head and neck, esophagus, bladder, and pancreas. Roughly half of the cancer deaths each year in the United States are causally related to tobacco use. Many Americans have heeded the warnings of the medical profession and decreased their use of cigarettes, pipes, cigars, and chewing tobacco. Between 1965, when the federal government first required a warning on cigarette packs that smoking causes cancer, and 1987, the smoking rate among adults in the United States decreased from 40 to 29 percent.

Eating a well-balanced diet. During the 1980s, many Americans began to change their diets significantly to reduce the risk of cancer and heart disease. Morning eggs and ham gave way to oat-bran muffins, while fast-food chains promoted salad bars and chicken sandwiches. Although scientists do not agree on the full impact of diet on cancer, they do agree that dietary changes can affect the chances of getting certain types of cancer. For example, high-fat diets increase the risk of colon, breast, and uterine cancer. High-fiber diets decrease the risk of colon cancer.

A well-balanced diet, low in fat and high in fresh fruits and vegetables, is the most prudent cancer-prevention diet. People who do not overeat and maintain a balanced diet do not need extra vitamins and other supplements, which can be harmful in large quantities. Beware of dietary supplements that claim to prevent cancer. No diet can prevent cancer; it can only reduce the risk of some types of cancer.

Avoiding excessive radiation. Cosmetic and pharmaceutical manufacturers are responding to the evidence that overexposure to the sun is the major cause of skin cancers by selling a wide variety of sunscreens. During the 1980s, a dark suntan began to lose

CANCER DEATH RATES IN 20 COUNTRIES, ALL SITES

Source: *World Health Statistics Annual 1979–80*, as adapted by American Cancer Society, 1983

Cancer occurs throughout the world; no country, no population is free of it. Cancer does not, however, occur with the same frequency in all countries; there are wide variations in total cancer death rates from country to country. There are also wide variations among different countries in the death rates for specific cancers. The bar graphs that follow show some of these variations.

The cancer death rates displayed in these graphs were derived from the number of cancer deaths per 100,000 population in each country for the years 1976–77. The 20 countries were chosen because all have major populations with good, nationwide reporting systems, and each of the countries reports to the World Health Organization. To make meaningful comparisons between countries, the rates were all age-adjusted to a standard age distribution. Cancer deaths occur most often in older age groups, but not all countries have the same age proportions. Age-adjusting corrects for these differences.

Cancer death rates indicate only the number of persons who die from cancer in a given year; they do not necessarily coincide with the incidence of new cases of cancer in that year. But tumor registries are needed to monitor cancer incidence, and not all countries have them. Most countries do have systems for reporting vital statistics. Cancer death rates thus provide a way to make international comparisons. (The U.S. cancer death rates in these charts are for all races.)

Death rates per 100,000 population for all cancers in 20 countries, 1976–77, age-adjusted to U.S. standard 1970 population.

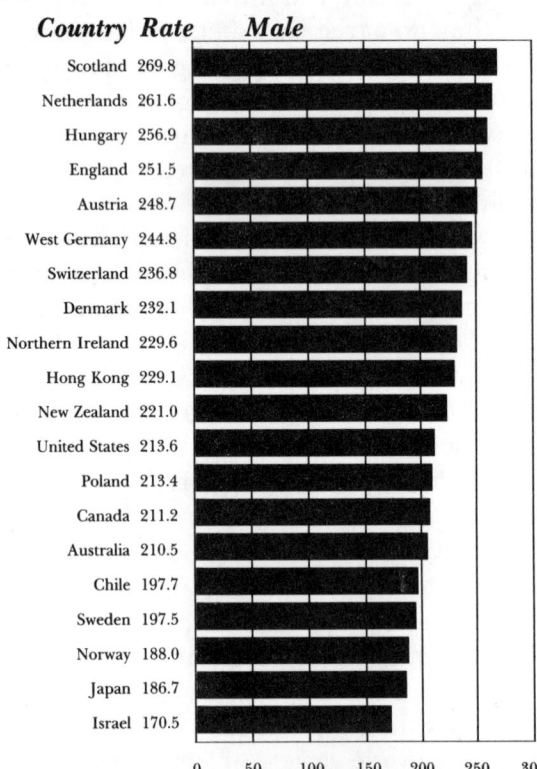
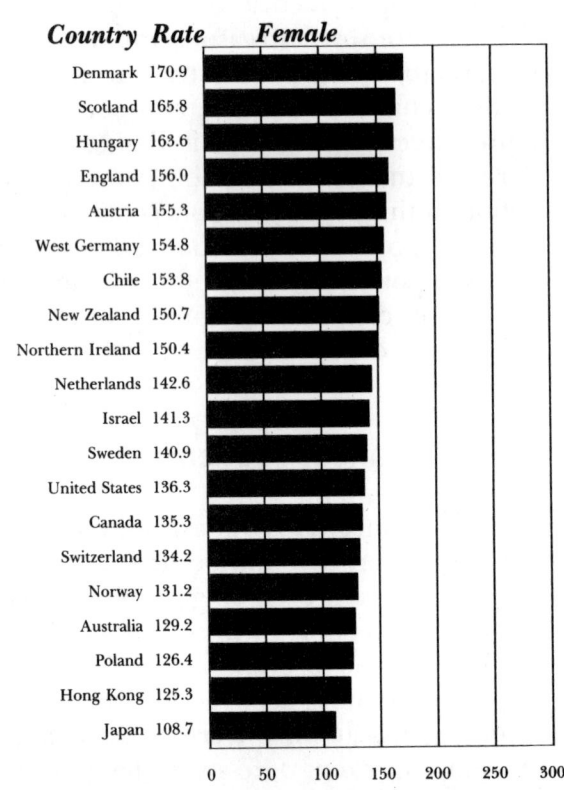

its value as a status symbol as many Americans avoided the sun during midday and protected their skin with clothing and sunscreen.

Radon is another source of radiation to be avoided. A natural, odorless, radioactive gas that in high concentrations increases the risk of lung cancer, radon is found in the ground and can become trapped in buildings with inadequate ventilation. A simple, inexpensive test can measure the amount of radon in a building. Many people in areas with high levels of radon, such as parts of Pennsylvania, New Jersey, and New York, have improved their ventilation systems to decrease the radon levels in their homes and offices.

Decreasing alcohol consumption. Alcohol consumption increases the risk of oral cancers, especially when combined with tobacco use. Heavy drinking also increases the risk of liver cancer.

Regulating sexual activity. The risk of getting cervical cancer can be affected by sexual activity. Women can take several steps to decrease the risk of cervical cancer:

- Avoid sexual activity as a young adolescent.
- Avoid having multiple sexual partners.
- Use barrier contraceptives, such as condoms or diaphragms.
- Avoid intercourse with men who have numerous sexual partners.

Reporting warning signs to your doctor. Although early diagnosis does not decrease the risk of getting cancer, it can dramatically improve the effectiveness of your treatment.

- Report to your doctor any symptoms that may be warning signals of cancer as defined by the American Cancer Society:

1. **C**hange in bowel or bladder habits
2. **A** sore that does not heal
3. **U**nusual bleeding or discharge
4. **T**hickening or lump in breast or elsewhere
5. **I**ndigestion or difficulty in swallowing
6. **O**bvious change in wart or mole
7. **N**agging cough or hoarseness

- Conduct monthly self-examinations of your skin, breasts (women), and testicles (men). The American Cancer Society and National Cancer Institute have booklets that describe how to perform a self-exam.
- See your doctor for routine physicals, which include screening for breast, cervical, and colon cancer.

The Physical Impact of Cancer and Its Treatment

Chemotherapy, radiation, and surgery often cause physical problems that add to the burden of surviving cancer. In most cases, with your doctor's guidance, you can mitigate the effects of the physical impact of cancer and its treatment.

Pain

Pain is the most feared aspect of cancer, even though not every cancer patient experiences pain. Most people equate cancer with pain, and are often surprised to find that their cancer was not painful at the time of diagnosis. Pain is, however, commonly associated with advanced cancer and some treatments. Although treatment to mitigate pain may be a simple matter, survivors are sometimes reluctant to admit they are experiencing pain, because they erroneously believe:

Abolishing the Myths

- Pain associated with cancer is to be expected.
- Pain is unimportant when life is at stake.
- Pain is a sign that the illness is progressing.
- Pain medications are addictive.
- People become immune to pain medications if they start taking drugs in early stages of pain.

Uncontrolled pain can unnecessarily interfere with daily life. You are the best judge of your own pain, and you should not hesitate to give your doctor a detailed description of your pain symptoms. If pain becomes an ongoing problem for you, keep a "pain diary" to chart when the pain began and what helped to relieve it. You need not accept pain as a necessary evil in cancer treatment.

The general principle underlying the use of pain relievers is to control the pain and prevent it from returning. This can be accomplished by taking pain medication on a regular schedule whether or not you are in pain, and to take small additional doses between the scheduled doses should the pain become worse. Taking pain medication on a regular schedule leads to more effective pain relief and to a lower total dose of medication than if it is taken only when the pain is severe. Ninety percent of all cancer patients can have their pain effectively controlled if they take their medications appropriately. Addiction is extremely rare unless the individual has a past history of substance abuse.

Acute pain (of sudden onset and relatively short in duration) is usually related to the cancer's pressing on adjacent tissues or the stretching of the organ in which it is located. With successful cancer treatment, usually all of the pain disappears. If the cancer remains and continues to grow in the same place, the pain often becomes chronic (sustained and enduring).

Some survivors develop chronic pain as a consequence of treatment. This usually occurs in a part of the body where surgery and radiation have been used together, leading to the development of scar tissue, which entraps and injures the adjacent nerves.

Efforts to control pain should be made at all phases of the disease, but it is of paramount importance that pain be controlled in the advanced cancer patient. Different treatments are used to control pain from different sources.

- Medication is the most common form of pain treatment. Nonprescription analgesics, such as aspirin, acetaminophen, and ibuprofen, are effective in relieving mild pain. If your pain is moderate to severe, your doctor may prescribe a narcotic for you to take by mouth. For extremely intense pain, you may be given narcotics by injection, sometimes continuously, using a portable infusion pump.
- Radiation or surgery to anesthetize pain fibers may be used to control pain that is localized in one area, such as a bone.
- Skin stimulation excites nerve endings in the skin and may lessen or block the recognition of pain. Different types of skin stimulation include massage, pressure, vibration, heat, cold, menthol preparations, and transcutaneous electric nerve stimulations (TENS).
- Radiation or chemotherapy may be used to shrink tumors that are causing pain.
- The relaxation techniques discussed in chapter 2 may help eliminate or mitigate pain.
- Other types of pain relief that are usually used in combination with more traditional pain relief include biofeedback, acupuncture, and hypnosis.
- You may find other solutions at a pain clinic.

Fatigue

Fatigue is one of the most common physical problems reported by cancer patients. This can occur as a specific symptom from the cancer, especially in persons with advanced cancer, but also results from radiation and chemotherapy, which may leave a patient tired for weeks or months. For some, energy levels never return to pretreatment levels.

- Fatigue is a warning sign that the body needs more rest, and the best response is to heed the warning.
- Pace your activities according to your energy level, especially during and soon after treatment.
- If possible, exercise routinely to maintain stamina.
- Unless your physician prescribes against it, drink plenty of fluids, at least eight glasses of water per day.

Nutrition and Weight Maintenance

Cancer survivors experience nutritional and weight problems for a variety of reasons. Cancers occurring in the abdomen can cause problems when they invade or compress digestive organs such as the stomach. Some patients experience nausea and vomiting; others feel too bloated to eat. Most dietary problems experienced by survivors are caused, in part, by cancer treatment.

Although most problems involve weight and appetite loss, some patients, especially those receiving adjuvant therapy for breast cancer, may suffer from too much weight gain, possibly because of decreased physical activity and increased food intake. Because weight gain and a high-fat diet may be risk factors for breast cancer, these women are usually encouraged to maintain or lose weight if they are overweight.

Of the seven most common nutritional problems, nausea and vomiting caused by chemotherapy and radiation can be the most physically exhausting. Chemotherapy-associated nausea and vomiting usually begin about four to six hours after an intravenous injection or within an hour after taking some oral medications. The intensity of these side effects varies with the particular drug. Many drugs cause no or minimal nausea, whereas others cause fairly severe nausea followed by frequent vomiting.

To prevent or mitigate nausea, your doctor may give you several medications, usually by vein. In addition, you may be given pills to take at home, usually for the first 24 to 48 hours after treatment. The preventive medications can cause sedation or drowsiness as a side effect, and you will usually need someone to drive you home from your treatment. Sometimes you might be hospitalized, because the treatment and preventive medications are so complex that you need to have more frequent nursing care. If the preventive treatments do not work, tell your doctor or nurse immediately, so alternative approaches can be tried.

With effective prevention of postchemotherapy nausea and vomiting, fewer patients develop "anticipatory nausea and vomiting." This is a problem in which you are conditioned, like the dogs in Pavlov's experiments, to associate many of the aspects of your treatment with the nausea and vomiting that occur after treatment. Patients who have anticipatory nausea and vomiting usually start to feel anxious and nauseous the day before their treatment, with increasing symptoms as they approach the doctor's office. They will often have nausea as they enter the chemotherapy treatment room or have a needle inserted in their vein. These responses are not effectively treated with antinausea medications. Instead, behavioral treatments, which involve relaxation or self-hypnosis, are usually helpful to decondition the response.

Hair Loss

Hair loss can result from head and neck radiation and certain types of chemotherapy. Chemotherapy and radiation result in atrophy of the hair follicle; the hair becomes weak and brittle, and either breaks off at the surface of the scalp or falls out from the follicle. The amount of hair loss depends on the type of treatment you receive, the dose, and the duration. Before you begin treatments, ask your doctor whether you are likely to experience some hair loss.

PROBLEMS RELATED TO NUTRITION AND EATING

Source: American Cancer Society, *Caring for the Person with Cancer at Home: A Family Caregiver's Manual*, 1985

Problem	Cause	What will help
Loss of appetite	May be caused by illness, anticancer drugs, loss of sleep, depression, or fatigue.	■ Light exercise to increase appetite. ■ A glass of beer or wine before meals (with doctor's OK). ■ Plan meals with favorite foods, small appetizing meals in pleasant surroundings. ■ Speak with doctor or dietician for suggestions. ■ Keep nutritious snacks around; offer a snack before bedtime (ice cream with ginger ale, a milk shake, or yogurt). ■ Use seasonings like basil, oregano, tarragon, and lemon.
Weight loss	Maintenance of normal weight is indicative of sufficient caloric intake. Weight loss may be part of the disease process, or a result of anorexia.	■ Keep record of foods each day. Offer between-meal snacks high in calories and protein (i.e., add ¼ cup nonfat dried milk to 8 ounces whole milk, and add this milk to sauces, soups, and gravies). ■ Use cream, not milk, in cereals. Extra calories may be added with a dietary supplement.
Nausea and vomiting	May be a result of anticancer drugs or a consequence of the cancer itself.	■ Small, frequent meals with no liquid during meals. Liquids one hour before meals to prevent large volume of fluid in the stomach. ■ Overly sweet foods may cause discomfort. ■ Greasy, fried foods can cause nausea; try dry foods like toast and crackers (especially in the morning). ■ May need to try several antinausea medications to find the one that works. Check with doctor and keep a record of when symptoms start and how long they last.
Taste	Anticancer drugs may change the way food tastes; e.g., sweet foods taste too sweet. Radiation to the head and neck area can cause a metallic taste.	■ For overly sweet taste, force fluids. Serve protein at room temperature (cheese, chicken). Some foods may taste better with salt or sugar. Marinate meats in wine (sweet) or fruit juices. Salt may need to be restricted if heart disease also exists.
Halitosis (bad breath)	Can occur with anticancer drugs and is caused by breakdown of cells that line the gastrointestinal tract.	■ Use frequent mouthwashes (except where there are sores in mouth) and antacids (check with doctor). Sucking on hard candy can be helpful.
Stomatitis (inflammation of the mouth)	Both anticancer drugs and sometimes the illness itself can leave a person subject to mouth sores and "furry tongue" indicative of fungal overgrowth.	■ A soft, bland diet or favorite foods blenderized. Avoid spicy, hot, or acid (orange juice) foods and coarse vegetables or fruit. Cold drinks are soothing. ■ Use a straw for easier drinking. ■ Remove dentures except when needed for chewing. ■ Mouth care 3 times a day after meals. ■ Saltwater gargles if mouth sores occur. ■ Call doctor if sores don't get better after 3 days. ■ Soft-bristle brush or toothette if mouth sores occur. ■ Doctor may order topical anesthesia. ■ Do not use mouthwash that contains alcohol.

Problem	Cause	What will help
Dry mouth	Radiation to head and neck area. Pain medication.	■ Sips of water frequently. ■ Lubricate lips. ■ Artificial saliva may help. ■ Lemon drops may stimulate saliva.

Note: Each patient is an individual and may or may not have any of these problems. No problem is too insignificant to deserve an answer. Call the doctor if you are concerned!

You may lose hair not only from your scalp but from other parts of your body, such as eyebrows and arms. Most hair loss is temporary. Your hair may return as before, or may grow in in a different texture and color.

You can take several steps to minimize hair loss.

■ Cut your hair in an easy-to-manage style before treatment begins.
■ Avoid excessive shampooing, rinse thoroughly, and gently pat your hair dry.
■ Avoid heat, such as hair dryers and hot curlers.
■ Avoid excess tugging on your hair by brushing only when necessary, using a wide-tooth comb, and avoiding hair clips and elastic bands.
■ Ask your doctor about scalp cooling. Your doctor may encourage you to wear a cold compress ("ice turban") during chemotherapy. This decreases the metabolic rate of the hair follicles and the uptake of chemotherapy drugs from the bloodstream into the hair roots. Hair follicles are exposed to a small amount of chemotherapy and have less chance of having their growth disturbed.

You can take several steps to prepare for expected hair loss.

■ Choose a wig before losing your hair so that you can match it to your natural hair color and texture. Some insurance policies will cover the costs of a wig.
■ If you do not want to wear a wig, consider a hat, scarf, or turban.
■ You may choose to shave off any remaining hair and not cover your head. However, keep your head protected from strong sunlight to prevent sunburn, and covered in the winter to prevent heat loss.
■ At home, consider wearing a hairnet to minimize shedding on your clothes or sheets.

Low Blood Counts

The majority of patients receiving chemotherapy and some receiving radiation will experience low blood counts, because treatment often slows the growth of cells in the bone marrow, which produce red cells, white cells, and platelets. White cells are needed to fight infections. When the white count falls below a certain level, it is unsafe to give additional treatments that slow the production of white cells. If you are receiving chemotherapy or radiation therapy and develop a fever, you should call your doctor immediately. A fever might be the first sign of a low white blood count and an associated infection.

If your blood counts are too low, your treatments will usually be postponed for several days or even weeks, until the counts improve. Although you may feel frustrated when treatment is delayed, the best response is to get adequate rest so that your body can recover.

Skin Changes

Skin problems in the treatment area can result from both radiation and chemotherapy.

Changes can range from a minor reddening to blistering and peeling. Itchy skin (pruritus) is a common side effect of some cancers and treatment.

Your doctor may prescribe antihistamines or corticosteroid creams for itching. There are also several steps you can take to heal dry, itchy, or burned skin.

- Avoid sunlight exposure, which can cause additional burning.
- Lubricate your skin with a water-based, rather than oil-based, moisturizer.
- Drink at least eight glasses of water or other fluids each day.
- Protect your skin from extreme temperatures and wind. Keep indoor temperatures cool.
- Bathe in cool or lukewarm water. Cornstarch, baking soda, oatmeal, or soybean powder added to the bath may be soothing.
- Wear loose-fitting, lightweight clothing.

Neurotoxicity

Injury to the nerves (neurotoxicity) is a side effect of some treatments. Usually this is first noticed as some numbness or tingling in the hands or feet, and rarely as complete weakness in an extremity. Some drugs can cause hearing loss or ringing in the ears. If you are having any of these problems, you should immediately bring them to your doctor's attention so your medications can be altered to modify the side effects.

Loss of Concentration

Many patients report difficulty in concentrating, remembering, and thinking clearly while they are receiving cancer treatments. This may be caused by several factors: direct effects of the chemotherapy and radiation treatments on the brain, side effects from the medications used to prevent nausea and vomiting, and the increased fatigue associated with the disease and its treatment. It is important to eat and sleep well, get enough rest, and do your best to maintain your physical condition and stamina. Usually the greatest loss of concentration will be associated with the treatments themselves (the day of treatment and the first few days thereafter), with return of concentration in between treatments. Try to avoid activities that demand your concentration immediately following treatment.

Respiratory Problems

Lung-cancer and other cancer patients may experience shortness of breath, which can be caused by the cancer itself, chemotherapy, anemia, malnutrition, and other factors. You can improve your breathing in a number of ways.

- Inhale through your nose and exhale slowly through your mouth with your lips pursed as if blowing out a candle. Use your abdominal muscles, rather than your chest muscles, to pull air in and push it out.
- Rest in a comfortable position when experiencing shortness of breath. For example, you will find it easier to sit up in bed than to lie down.
- Move around as much as possible to help your circulation. Even if you are confined to bed, you may be able to do simple arm or leg exercises. A respiratory or physical therapist can suggest the best exercises for you.
- Aid circulation in your feet by not sitting in one position too long or crossing your legs.
- Drink at least eight glasses of water a day to help mucous membranes clear your lungs of secretions.
- Cough deeply from within your chest to help clear your lungs.
- Use a humidifier to keep the air in your house from becoming too dry. Be sure to clean the humidifier and change the water daily to prevent multiplication of bacteria.

MALE SEXUAL PROBLEMS CAUSED BY CANCER TREATMENT

Source: Leslie Schover, *Sexuality and Cancer: For the Man Who Has Cancer, and His Partner* (Atlanta: American Cancer Society, 1988)

Treatment	Low Sexual Desire	Erection Problems	Lack of Orgasm	Dry Orgasm	Weaker Orgasm	Infertility
Chemotherapy	Sometimes	Rarely	Rarely	Rarely	Rarely	Often
Pelvic radiation therapy	Rarely	Sometimes	Rarely	Rarely	Sometimes	Often
Retroperitoneal lymph-node dissection	Rarely	Rarely	Rarely	Often	Sometimes	Often
Abdominoperineal (A-P) resection	Rarely	Often	Rarely	Often	Sometimes	Sometimes*
Radical prostatectomy	Rarely	Often	Rarely	Always	Sometimes	Always
Radical cystectomy	Rarely	Often	Rarely	Always	Sometimes	Always
Total pelvic exenteration	Rarely	Often	Rarely	Always	Sometimes	Always
Partial penectomy	Rarely	Rarely	Rarely	Never	Rarely	Never
Total penectomy	Rarely	Always	Sometimes	Never	Sometimes	Usually*
Orchiectomy (removal of one testicle)	Rarely	Rarely	Never	Never	Never	Rarely†
Orchiectomy (removal of both testicles)	Often	Often	Sometimes	Sometimes	Sometimes	Always
Hormone therapy for prostate cancer	Often	Often	Sometimes	Sometimes	Sometimes	Always

*Artificial insemination of a spouse with the man's own semen may be possible.
†Infertile only if remaining testicle is not normal.

Sexual Function

A number of sexual problems are associated with cancer and its treatment. Even in healthy people, fatigue leads to a loss of interest in sexual activity. In addition, certain treatments lead to specific physical problems that affect sexual function.

Different sexual problems require different personal responses. Your physician, nurse, social worker, or sex therapist can offer specific suggestions for coping with the physical and emotional consequences of decreased sexual function. For example:

- Reconstructive surgery may help repair a physical loss.
- Use of water-based gels may help provide vaginal lubrication.
- Hormonal therapy may alleviate symptoms of premature menopause.
- Penile prostheses may help provide an erection.

Contraception and Sterility

Cancer and its treatment can affect fertility and fetal development. If you are sexually

FEMALE SEXUAL PROBLEMS CAUSED BY CANCER TREATMENT

Source: Leslie Schover, *Sexuality and Cancer: For the Woman Who Has Cancer, and Her Partner* (Atlanta: American Cancer Society, 1988)

Treatment	Low Sexual Desire	Less Vaginal Moisture	Reduced Vaginal Size	Painful Intercourse	Trouble Reaching Orgasm	Infertility
Chemotherapy	Sometimes	Often	Sometimes	Often	Rarely	Often
Pelvic radiation therapy	Rarely	Often	Often	Often	Rarely	Often
Radical hysterectomy	Rarely	Often*	Often	Rarely	Rarely	Always
Radical cystectomy	Rarely	Often*	Always	Sometimes	Rarely	Always
Abdominoperineal (A-P) resection	Rarely	Often*	Sometimes	Sometimes	Rarely	Sometimes
Total pelvic exenteration with vaginal reconstruction	Sometimes	Always	Sometimes	Sometimes	Sometimes	Always
Radical vulvectomy	Rarely	Never	Sometimes	Often	Sometimes	Never
Conization of the cervix	Never	Never	Never	Rarely	Never	Rarely
Oophorectomy (removal of one tube & ovary)	Rarely	Never*	Never*	Rarely	Never	Rarely
Oophorectomy (removal of both tubes & ovaries)	Rarely	Often*	Sometimes*	Sometimes*	Rarely	Always
Mastectomy or radiation to the breast	Rarely	Never	Never	Never	Rarely	Never
Antiestrogen therapy for breast or uterine cancer	Sometimes	Often	Sometimes	Sometimes	Rarely	Always
Androgen therapy	Never	Never	Never	Never	Never	Uncertain

*Vaginal dryness and size changes should not occur if one ovary is left in or if hormone replacement therapy is given.

active during cancer treatment, you should use contraceptives. Both radiation and chemotherapy can lead to malformations or injury to the developing fetus, and conception can occur even if you are receiving treatment. If you wish to have a child, speak with your doctor before trying to conceive. You may be advised to wait several years after your treatments to reduce the risk of a problem pregnancy.

A parallel concern is the risk of permanent sterility from chemotherapy or radiation treatments. Radiation will cause permanent sterility if the testes or ovaries receive direct radiation. For this reason, these organs are usually shielded by lead barriers. Sometimes the ovaries are surgically pinned out of the way so they will not be in a radiation treatment field. When such protective measures are used, subsequent fertility is preserved. It is, however, more difficult to protect these organs from the effects of chemotherapy. Not all chemotherapy treatments cause a decrease in fertility, but some will.

If you have concerns about the effect of cancer treatments on your fertility:

- Discuss your questions with your doctor *before* you begin treatment, so that your treatment can be modified, if possible, to minimize effects on your fertility. Sometimes there will be a choice of two equally effective treatment programs, one of which has a high rate of infertility and the other of which does not.
- Men should consider preserving their sperm in a sperm bank before treatment. If your sperm have not been impaired by the cancer itself, sperm banking may increase your chances of having a child after treatments.

Medical Problems of Long-Term Survivors

Fortunately, there is an expanding community of long-term cancer survivors who have gotten past the early and often complex initial phase of cancer treatment. If you are among them, you will find that, as time passes and you are further removed from the early phase of treatment, you will have a tendency to distance yourself physically and psychologically from the professionals who were involved in your cancer treatment. Although this is natural, you should maintain some form of regular medical follow-up with a physician who knows the details of your previous cancer treatment and its potential long-term side effects. A patient who has had the spleen removed for staging of Hodgkin's disease, for example, is at lifelong risk of serious infections. In these individuals, fever must be treated promptly with antibiotics.

Information about the long-term effects of cancer treatment on important organs such as the heart and lungs is just starting to become available. Chemotherapy and radiation treatments received many years earlier may lead to premature aging of these vital organs. As the number of survivors expands, there will be additional information about these problems, which will help to modify the type and intensity of treatment for current patients.

All cancer survivors need monitoring to detect any recurrence of the cancer. It is important that even minor symptoms be brought to your doctor's attention. In addition, some cancer survivors are at increased risk for the development of acute leukemia or other bone-marrow disorders that are the result of past treatments.

In order to get the best follow-up care, you should have the detailed records of your cancer treatment forwarded to your current family physician, internist, or pediatrician. These records should be carefully reviewed by your doctor.

Childhood-cancer survivors are an important and rapidly growing segment of the survivor population. It is estimated that in the 1990s one in 1,000 young adults aged 20 will have been cured of childhood cancer. The special problems of childhood-cancer survivors are now being actively studied, and more information on this special group should be available in the next few years. We do know that some children experience growth retardation secondary to curative treatment (especially if it involves radiation to growing bones), and this can lead to some long-term physical limitations and changes in body image. Most survivors of childhood cancer have gone on to have normal fertility and healthy offspring; however, some are unable to have children, and others have had permanent learning disabilities as a result of treatments on the brain. Treatment programs are now being designed to minimize all of these long-term problems, but there are currently many survivors of childhood cancer who may be experiencing them. Cancer centers that specialize in the treatment of children, and the Candlelighters Childhood Cancer Foundation, are the best sources of information and guidance about these problems.

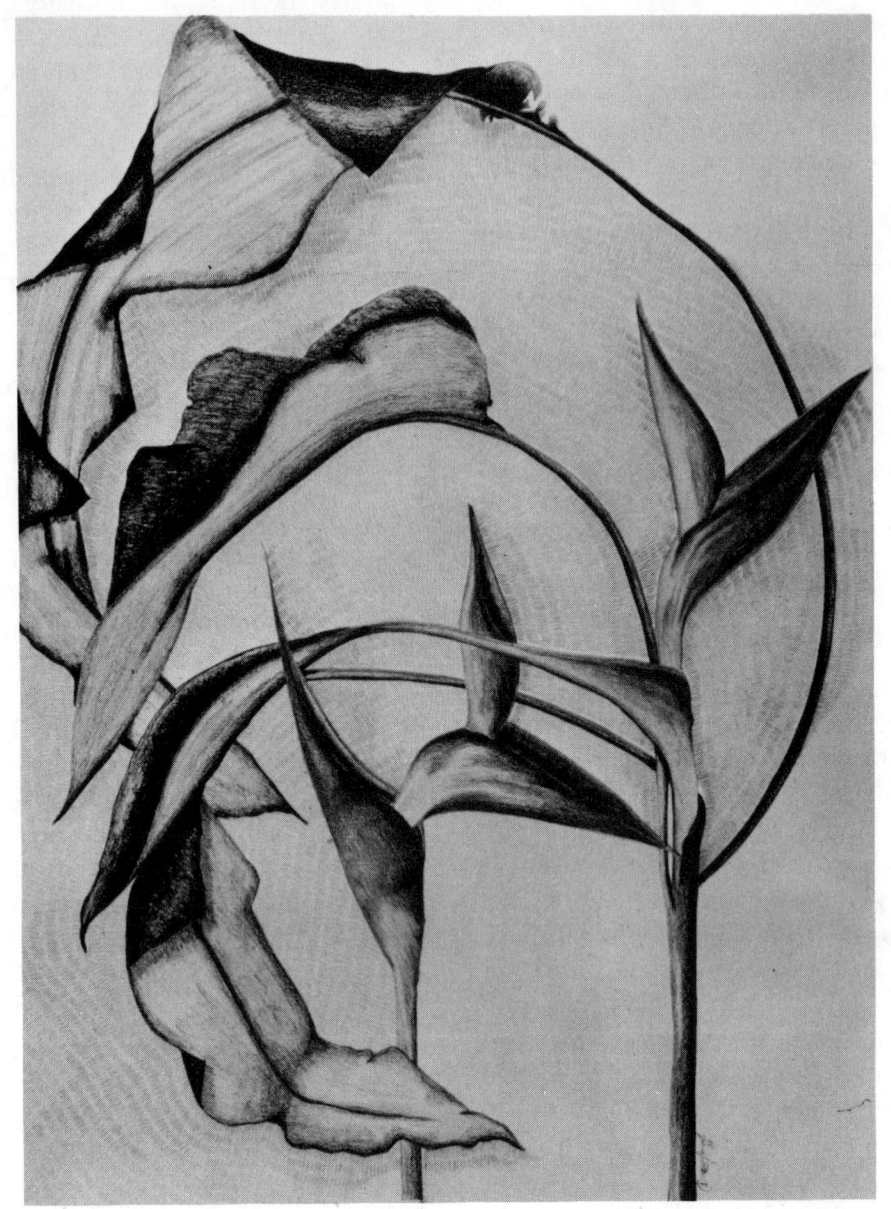

Jan Crawford
Centering
Drawing
25" x 19"

2

Mind and Body: Harnessing Your Inner Resources

Neil Fiore, Ph.D.

The Complex Relationship Between Mind and Body

Fighting cancer involves more than excising a tumor and focusing our latest weapons on the metastases. It must include a recognition, by both the medical profession and the survivor, that the patient's mind and body are powerful factors in his or her fight for survival. To be effective, cancer therapy must support the healthy portion of the survivor's body and psyche as well as combat the diseased cells.

An awareness of psychosocial needs is crucial to regarding a survivor as more than his or her disease. Physicians agree that the mind, the emotions, and supportive relationships play essential roles in adapting to, and recovering from, disease. As a survivor, you must realize that you are more than the host of a serious illness. Less than 1 percent of you has cancer. The rest of you—your mental and emotional resources and the strength of the healthy portion of your body—can work in cooperation with your medical treatment to combat cancer.

Medical providers affirm that there is a relationship between physical and mental health. Although the extent of this relationship—especially whether a positive attitude can enhance physical healing—continues to be debated by professionals, almost all agree that:

- Cancer is not a punishment for wrong thinking, a weak will to live, or a loser mentality.
- Negative emotions and experiences can have a deleterious effect on health and can complicate medical treatment.
- Because human beings are not able to exercise control over all of their biological and disease processes, changes in mental attitude cannot substitute for adequate medical care. You cannot will yourself to have cancer any more than you can will it away.

Psychosocial factors in cancer survival are more complex than simply a positive attitude and a strong will to live. You cannot

> "I have faced the imminence of death and have been permitted to let death pass by. I have ceased to feel that death is a dreadful something that I need to fear. Instead, it will ultimately appear as a peaceful act of letting go when the time comes and I am ready. We are all dying; the difference between persons is only in the length and quality of the time that is left. Death ceases to be the failure; the failure is in not being willing to make the effort to grow and change."
>
> —Robert M. Mack, M.D., lung-cancer survivor, "Lessons from Living with Cancer," *New England Journal of Medicine*, December 20, 1984

cure yourself simply by changing your attitude or trying harder. You can, however, improve the quality of your physical and mental health by coping constructively with your emotional reactions to your cancer experience.

The Inner Battle

Fighting your own personal battle against cancer is, in many ways, like any other fight for survival. It requires a toughness of mind, an intense focus on the task, and a refusal to be deterred by the enemy or your own thoughts and fears.

In the course of coping with cancer, you will need to learn to push away negativism, whether it is generated by yourself or others. You will want to recognize irrational and counterproductive thoughts, and replace them with constructive attitudes supportive of your body's fight against cancer. Learning to fight the inner battle will help you to:

- cope with stress and emotions and adapt to your cancer therapies
- lessen feelings of depression and helplessness
- formulate positive challenges to counteract negative beliefs
- maintain a sense of worth and self-respect throughout your cancer experience.

Many diseases are more severe, traumatic, and fatal than cancer. Yet the stigma attached to this disease makes the diagnosis disproportionately terrifying. The meaning of the word "cancer" is very different for the doctor, who deals with it every day, than it is for the patient hearing the diagnosis for the first time or a family that has heard it before.

When the diagnosis is first presented, the emotional stress can be so great that survivors seek to attribute the diagnosis to some understandable cause in order to assume a feeling of control over the situation. They may prefer blame and guilt to the discomfort of lack of control and the acceptance of unknown causes and random victims. Uncertainty about the causes of many cancers leaves us vulnerable to potentially harmful speculation about connections between our health habits, mental activity (thoughts, images, and beliefs), and cancer. Young children in particular often blame themselves for problems that occur in their families.

Discovering Your Beliefs

In the long run, self-blame as a means to explain uncontrollable events is damaging

An Exercise to Address Your Reactions to Your Diagnosis

This exercise can help you to identify the troublesome beliefs that persist from your initial diagnosis, unnecessarily taxing your energy and clouding your thoughts. Developed at the University of California Medical Center, San Francisco, the following exercise may be helpful in sharpening your awareness of initial reactions to cancer and in giving you an opportunity to share these reactions, often for the first time, with those close to you.

In preparation for this exercise, read through it, setting aside 15 to 30 minutes to experience the exercise and talk about it with your family. If you do it by yourself, leave time to write down your reactions.

Begin by finding a comfortable position, perhaps sitting in a chair with your feet flat on the floor. Take three slow, deep breaths, holding your breath briefly, and then exhaling slowly and completely. As you drift down in the chair, letting the chair support your body, you can let go of your muscles. You can allow the relaxation to flow. There is no need for you to hold those muscles. Just allow the chair to support your body, and the floor to support your feet and legs.

Now simply drift back to that time and place when you first were told of the diagnosis. Imagine being in that place: Re-create for yourself that room, the furniture, the colors and lighting, and the sounds and voices. Just be there and allow your mind to present what it will. Just let it happen. Once you are there, back in that place, at that time, focus your attention on three areas within you.

■ Become aware of what you are feeling physically—your muscles, your breathing, your pulse and heartbeat, and anything that makes itself physically evident.
■ Become aware of what thoughts and images are going through your mind, of what you are saying to yourself—what your attitude is.
■ Become aware of what you are feeling emotionally. Notice that you can shift from one area of focus to another, thus taking control of your attention and feelings.

When rethinking what happened at the time of the diagnosis, many people find that their first reaction was to assume that they would soon die, revealing an underlying belief that cancer automatically meant death. Others became aware of anger—at the diagnosis, at the doctors, at God—and some even experienced relief at finally knowing what was wrong.

All reactions are legitimate, and, whatever your reactions were, *simply note them*. Do not judge them. You coped as well as you could under the circumstances given your needs and the information you had at the time.

Now your job is to re-examine those beliefs and attitudes to see if they still serve you. If they only cause more stress, identify them and try to replace them with new ways of thinking that will help you to adjust to your illness and make positive changes in your life.

---

to one's ability to cope with cancer. It can result in feelings of depression that contribute to a delay in seeking medical treatment, inhibitions about discussing concerns, and a diminished ability to form helpful relationships with doctors, social workers, and family members. Moreover, realistic information about cancer and its causes can help you to adjust to the unpleasant realities of a tough situation and to do something about it.

The psychological stress of cancer may put your religious and spiritual beliefs to the test. If your spiritual beliefs serve as a source of comfort and strength in your hour of need, however, your stress can be minimized. Any beliefs that lead you to think of cancer as punishment from God should be carefully examined with the help of your clergyman. An acceptance of all of life as natural—its suffering and its joy, death and birth—can lead to a constructive adaptation to your illness. With acceptance, your spiritual beliefs may more readily support you through your current experience.

Replacing Negative Reactions

Examining your reactions to your diagnosis and your underlying beliefs is the first crucial step toward learning a new view of cancer and discovering alternative ways of coping. Here are some common negative reactions to cancer and some suggestions for useful responses to them.

> *Negative Reaction:* Why me? Why now? I feel pitiful.
> *Response:* Now that it *has* happened and that it *is* me, what can I do about it? As unwanted as it is, what can I do to better my chances of beating it?

> *Negative Reaction:* Cancer is powerful and my body is weak. Cancer means death.
> *Response:* Cancer cells are, in fact, abnormal cells that are weak. My body routinely identifies and eliminates malformed cells. My body can cooperate with radiation and chemotherapy in destroyng the cancer.

> *Negative Reaction:* If I had lived life differently, I wouldn't have cancer. I wish I could do it over again.
> *Response:* My past is behind me and I have no control over it now. Brooding on it will only make me feel weaker. I do have a say about the future, about my choices and my attitude now. That is where I will make my stand.

Coping with Strong Emotions

If you have ever felt the ground shake beneath your feet from an earthquake, lived through a war or a near-fatal accident, you know how quickly feelings of tranquillity can change to overwhelming anxiety. The emotional response of cancer survivors to their diagnosis is just as legitimate as the shock, anger, and depression expected in those who survive accidents and wars, and recovery involves similar steps of emotional and physical rehabilitation.

Worry about recurrence and fears about an uncertain future make the task of getting back to normal a complex one for any cancer survivor. Over time, it is not so much the strong emotions themselves that cause difficulties as it is the fear of expressing them. With understanding and patience, physicians, family members, and the survivors themselves can find helpful avenues for release of legitimate feelings.

Anxiety. Anxiety can be common during any part of the cancer experience, but survivors have ranked the time of diagnosis as the most upsetting. During this time, thoughts about life and death predominate and survivors are most vulnerable to psychosocial problems. This is a period of monumental adjustment to:

- the shocking news that your life is in danger
- the consideration of treatments that may be more severe than any of your cancer symptoms
- the loss of your physical integrity
- rapid changes in your work and relationships
- the possibility of a long period of rehabilitation

During this initial period, especially, expressions of anxiety, sadness, and anger are quite natural and potentially healing. Some studies suggest that survivors who were more expressive of their anger and

> "You see, some things you get ready for gradually. Like an apple. It slowly ripens, then it's picked, then it's taken to the supermarket. You buy it, you take it home and put it in your fruit basket for a couple of days, then finally you take it out and you eat it. Then there's the mango. The mango is an incredibly stupid fruit. It takes ten years to ripen. It's ripe for about seven minutes, then it goes bad. So I'm coasting along in my life, thinking I'm an apple. I'm ripening at a reasonable rate, then suddenly a lab report tells me I'm not an apple. I'm a mango. I've got seven minutes left to live."
>
> —Joe Kogel

sadness in the initial period fared better than those who were less so. This does not mean that survivors should force themselves to be emotional but that it is better if they do not repress their natural feelings. Other studies indicate that survivors who maintain a support network of friends and family are more likely to weather this difficult time with fewer psychological problems. The first months of cancer therapy are intense for most, but some comfort can be gathered from knowing that the second 100 days will probably be less stressful, as they adjust to their medical treatment and the process of healing.

Once the initial shock of the diagnosis is past, the next task will be to become familiar with the treatment steps and options—what can be done medically and what survivors can do for themselves. At that time, the disbelief and anxiety about having cancer will generally give way to the tasks of living and adapting to life after cancer.

Depression. Depression, a common reaction among cancer survivors and their supporters, is often regarded as a negative emotion, when in fact it may be a natural way to cope with shock by conserving energy and providing a time to think about ways of adjusting to change. Cancer survivors, says Dr. Jimmie Holland, chief of New York's Memorial Sloan-Kettering's Psychiatry Service, are no more depressed than people with other severe medical conditions. The depression of most cancer survivors differs from that of patients suffering from chronic mental depression. Survivor depression is a result of a dramatic external event that has deeply upset the patient. The Psychiatry Service of Memorial Sloan-Kettering reports that half of the cancer patients they see have suffered from acute stress and "reactive" (as opposed to "chronic") depression.

The relatively short-term, reactive depression that often accompanies the stress of a cancer diagnosis and treatment can be handled more easily if it is accepted as natural and a "mourning" process is allowed. Recovery from the depression of cancer is helped by experiencing a grieving period that focuses on the loss—loss of control, loss of a body part, and loss of self-image. But, as with any other loss, the mourning phase must give way to thoughts of the present and the future. Sometimes, however, this psychic healing is inhibited by the passivity of the "sick role." The regimentation of a hospital encourages dependence, adding to the sense of hopelessness, and reinforcing the negative image of the "cancer victim."

Hopelessness can be dangerous medically, because it can cause patients to rebel against traditional treatment. A National Cancer Institute study demonstrated that the majority of those patients who turned to laetrile and other unconventional therapies had been told by their physicians that they had a "terminal disease" and that "nothing else can be done." These patients felt abandoned and powerless, and turned to treatments that offered them some active role, encouraging them to alter their lifestyles and get involved.

In order to lessen depression and hopelessness, you can try to accept some level of depression as normal, let go of your need to control everything, mourn your losses, and avoid assuming a passive role in your treatment. You can also talk to your doctor about what can be done to reduce treatment side effects that might be adding to depression, and try to find counselors or support groups to help with the emotional components of surviving cancer.

Once you have acknowledged that you are in a distressing situation and must face many hard choices, you can direct your thoughts toward the future by asking yourself, "Where do I go from here?" The initial shock of the cancer diagnosis will soften as you become more familiar with the steps in your treatment—with what can be done for you and what *you* can do to improve your health. Most likely, you will find that your cancer experience will be different from your initial beliefs and fears.

By understanding how cancer affects your emotions and relationships, you will prepare yourself to master the skills of coping with trauma, transition, and survival. Concerns about life-and-death issues, while never totally dismissed from the thoughts of any cancer survivor, can then give way to the challenges and joys of daily life.

The Social Impact of Cancer

Even though the shock of a cancer diagnosis is primarily physical, a major portion of the impact is emotional and social. It affects how you perceive yourself and how others react to you.

If the diagnosis of cancer is your first experience of the vulnerability associated with serious illness, its influence on your self-image can be especially traumatic. You feel that the very cells of your body have turned against you. You no longer have confidence in your own body. In a very concrete way you realize that you are human and mortal, that life does end, and that your time is limited.

A dramatic change in self-image is most evident in teenagers with cancer. It makes them quite different from their carefree playmates, who seldom believe that the threat of death or even serious illness applies to them. They have not yet had to face the body's gradual decline that adults begin to experience. Usually they have not seen illness and death strike their peers, so they are quite unprepared for a life-threatening illness. It shocks them and makes them doubt their underlying assumptions about the world. But this rapid change in perception can take place in people in their 60s who are accustomed to good health and energy. Some people maintain a teenager's sense of invulnerability and immortality well beyond the age of 60. For these older people whose self-image has been stable for decades, the cancer diagnosis can be dramatically inconsistent with their view of life.

The experience of facing a life-threatening event unites survivors with the human courage to face a new view of the world. It also separates survivors from those who cannot appreciate the cancer experience. Physicians will treat your physical losses, but you, your friends and family, and your psychosocial counselors will need to deal with the emotional and psychological changes.

You can improve your self-image by accepting mortality and vulnerability as facts for all human beings rather than as signs of weakness or failure. A more robust and realistic self-image will enhance your ability to fight for life. It will equip you with a better understanding of the social impact of cancer and prepare you to cope.

Affirmations for a Positive Self-Image

Cancer survivors often find personal affirmations helpful in making the transition to a new, robust self-image and greater strength to cope with changing relationships. These affirmations are a way of being there for yourself despite the events in your life. Affirmations can be like Ivan's credo in Dostoyevsky's *The Brothers Karamazov:* ". . . [i]f I lost faith in the order of things, if I were convinced that everything is a disorderly, damnable, devil-ridden chaos, if I were struck by every horror of man's disillusion—still I should want to live . . ." The following are suggested affirmations for cancer survivors.

- Regardless of what happens in life, I am worthwhile.
- Regardless of how my body is scarred by the experiences of life and survival, I will remain compassionate toward myself.
- Regardless of whether I win or lose, I deserve love, pleasure, and freedom from self-criticism.
- Regardless of what I can or cannot do, I am always worthwhile. My worth is not based on what I do, but on who I am.
- Regardless of what happens to me, I deserve to be treated with human dignity and respect. I always respect myself.
- Regardless of who stays or who goes, I am on my side. I will never abandon myself.
- Regardless of how healthy or ill I become, I appreciate my body's effort, wisdom, and protection.
- Regardless of how negative or intense my emotions become, I acknowledge their validity for me.
- Regardless of how uncomfortable others are with me, my feelings, my body, or my illness, I will always remain at peace with myself.

As a cancer survivor you may feel quite isolated at times, as if no one could possibly understand your shock and agony. In "Live with Pain, Learn the Hope: A Beginner's Guide to Cancer Counseling," from the *Personnel and Guidance Journal* of the American Association for Counseling and Development, survivor William Keeling expressed his reactions to his diagnosis as follows:

> Self-doubts begin to play tricks with your head, like, "Does anybody give a damn whether I live or die?" You begin to see and hear evidence that nobody does. No one else seems panicky, just you. The doctor seems cool, scientific. Your spouse and parents are cool, sad-looking. Your boss is cool and has a few sad, sympathetic words that sound like "have a nice trip" (to wherever).

This young man felt that everyone was indifferent toward him, but some survivors feel they have to repress their own fears and needs to protect others around them who seem too demonstrative. They may even think that their doctors or spouses are too emotional about the diagnosis to consider the feelings and needs of the patient. Sometimes survivors find themselves comforting distraught family members while wondering, "Who's going to listen to my feelings? I'm the one with cancer!"

Others in the survivor's community may attempt to help by offering a new "miracle cure" they have read about, or by giving religious advice. Some may need to avoid the cancer survivor, because cancer for them is an uncomfortable reminder of their own mortality and vulnerability. Even doctors and nurses, at times, may have difficulty working with survivors with whom they identify.

Although a social stigma is attached to having cancer, there is a new openness about it in the media and society in general. Some people may shy away during times of crisis, but you may also be pleasantly surprised by offers of help from unexpected sources. During the course of cancer treatment, you may need someone to provide transportation, buy groceries, clean the house, and listen to your concerns. Accepting this help from people can ease your own burdens and reduce the feelings of inadequacy others may have concerning their inability to help. Prepare yourself for a variety of social reactions to cancer, and try to accept the humanity and good intentions behind most people's actions.

A job or some form of employment for cancer survivors can be a stabilizing influence. It gives you the opportunity to focus your attention on something other than cancer and to experience yourself as more than someone with a dread disease. When work expands the roles you play in life, it can have a healthy effect on your self-image.

With some cancer treatments the disruption of the work schedule and the impact on co-workers is minimal. Many cancer treatments, however, do require lengthy periods of recuperation and rehabilitation. Survivors frequently encounter prejudice on returning to work, and reactions from co-workers and employers have ranged from hostility to solicitude. The fear of cancer among colleagues and co-workers can result in additional feelings of isolation for the cancer survivor.

Conventional misconceptions about the severity of various cancers and their cure rates may cause some people to wonder if and when you are going to die, while others may be shocked that you look so healthy. Statements such as "You don't look like you're dying" and "Just my luck, I finally get some help in this department and he gets cancer" are not uncommon. Most people will not be that blunt or insensitive, but colleagues and employers may—even with good intentions—treat you as if you are preparing to die rather than fighting to stay alive.

Others may simply wonder about your ability to handle your share of the work load, whether they will need to hire someone new, and if you will be a financial burden on the company. Such concerns can lead to overt and covert job discrimination and isolation from fellow workers who fear cancer (see chapter 6).

Throughout the course of your treatment, you will probably experience significant changes in your relationships. Some may become deeper, some more superficial, and some may end. When your treatment causes you to appear weak or sick, even some old friends may avoid you, resuming the relationship when you appear healthier. Whatever relationships remain will be intensified and strengthened during this challenging period of your life.

A healthy relationship should be a major source of support, not something that drains you emotionally. This is a time when your first priority must be to yourself and your health. *You* may need to change those relationships, even your most intimate ones, which are not supportive of your commitment to survival.

Sex becomes a low priority during times of stress and preoccupation with survival. For most survivors, as physical energy and feelings of vitality return, so will the sense of attractiveness and interest in sex. The psychological component of sexuality is strongly influenced, however, by a person's feelings of personal value and security. This adjustment may require more than just the return of physical energy and health. Counseling may be required to restore self-esteem and provide training to overcome sexual dysfunction when illness or medical treatment has affected performance.

Reassurance from one's mate is a great asset for self-confidence, self-esteem, and the return of sexual desire. Ultimately, however, it is up to the survivor to accept him- or herself as lovable and capable of loving. As one survivor, after months of adjusting to a new sense of self, put it: "I want to grasp every moment as it presents itself to me as I am now, without fretting over how I should be, should feel, or should think."

Gaining Control over Stress

The stress caused by cancer and its treatment is psychological and emotional, as well as physical. Usual coping strategies for events that are not life-threatening may prove inadequate in coping with the stress of cancer survival.

The ability to manage stress, however, can be learned. Stress management techniques can be used for: (1) *physical control* over a body whose very cells seem to have gone awry; (2) *cognitive control* over the flood of distressing and counterproductive thoughts and images; and (3) *assertiveness* to maintain control and a sense of worth. These skills provide a level of personal satisfaction and self-nurturance essential to stress management.

Because illness is often experienced as a loss of control over one's body, the restoration of even minimal control over anxiety and pain can be revitalizing. The ability to relax deeply, to experience the release of tension, and to feel that one's body can still provide pleasure is a powerful sign of hope to any person facing a life-threatening illness. Relaxation itself is physically recuperative and can lead to a decrease in the need for some types of medication.

There are a number of methods for relaxing that provide varying degrees of comfort for different individuals: listening to music, warm baths, massage, exercise, yoga, meditation, autogenic training, self-hypnosis, and biofeedback. Your personal comfort will determine which selection is best for you.

Your thoughts, beliefs, and attitudes determine your emotional reactions. Panicky thoughts can cause extreme emotions, which make you feel out of control. Focusing your attention on the thoughts, feelings, and behaviors that are the most beneficial, however, will help you to control your emotions. Just as you can frighten yourself by viewing a horror film and soothe yourself by watching nature scenes, so too can you affect your feelings by choosing the thoughts you allow in the theater of your mind.

You can learn mastery over your internal physical, mental, and emotional states. But to be effective in controlling external pressures, you will need to communicate your wishes in a forthright, assertive manner. Being assertive does not guarantee that you will always get what you want, but you will at the least receive the satisfaction that comes from standing up for yourself. Moreover, communicating to your doctor and family your fears and your preferences regarding your medical care may well lead to changes that will alleviate fear and worry.

Coping Through Imagery

Most survivors experience some negative images of their body as a helpless victim of a virulent disease. Healthy imagery combats these negative images and provides a way of reducing stress and enhancing one's sense of well-being. The image of the "spread of cancer," for example, can be supplanted by the more accurate image of the body's trapping deformed cells in the lymph nodes and the lungs' filtering mechanisms. Though it is not necessary to engage in healthy imagery to survive cancer, such imagery can provide emotional comfort. Imagery exercises are an easy, beneficial technique for relaxing the body in order to improve mental and physical functioning.

Healthy imagery emphasizes reduction of stress by encouraging survivors to allow the body to work naturally without conscious direction. For example, during a stressful medical treatment, a survivor might say to himself or herself: "I can relax my will and allow the superior wisdom of my body to do what it knows best. There's nothing much for the conscious *me* to do, except to be receptive to the flow of relaxation, recuperation, and remission. And it's nice to know that there is a part of me that knows more than *I* know."

There are three types of imagery that are particularly useful for cancer survivors—autogenics, centering, and healthy imagining.

Autogenics is a method of controlling or influencing bodily functions, such as blood

Autogenic Exercise

"Autogenics" means "self-control of your body." This particular exercise is directed toward warming your hands and relaxing your entire body. You can only achieve this by letting go of conscious attempts at control, and by allowing the automatic part of your nervous system to do its job.

In this exercise, you will be dilating the blood vessels and capillaries in your hands and fingers. You cannot accomplish this by commanding it to happen, the way you might if you wanted to open your hand. It can only be accomplished by relaxing fully and cooperating with your unconscious mind.

Start by sitting erect with your feet flat on the floor, with your hands on your thighs. Breathe deeply, hold your breath for a moment, and then exhale slowly and completely. Do this three times, counting each time you exhale. Let each exhalation be a symbol of released tensions. Now allow your eyelids to close softly. You can try to keep them open, but you will find that it is much more comfortable to allow them to float down over your eyes. Now allow that relaxation to flow down over your entire body.

Now you can focus your attention on the chair. Let it support you, and let yourself float down into the chair. Shift your attention to the floor, and let it support your feet. You can now let go of those muscles. As you let go, continue to exhale away any remaining tension.

Quietly let the change from tension to relaxation happen, using your body's natural tendency to cooperate. Now you can be comfortable. Continue to breathe deeply and slowly and repeat quietly to yourself the following:

- "I feel quiet. I am beginning to feel quite relaxed—my feet feel quiet and relaxed. My ankles, my knees, and my hips feel light, calm, and comfortable. My stomach and the entire center of my body feel light, calm, and comfortable."
- "My entire body feels quiet, calm, and comfortable. My arms and my hands feel quiet and warm. My entire body *feels* quiet and warm."
- "I feel calm and relaxed. My hands feel calm, relaxed, and warm. My hands *are* relaxed. My hands *are* warm. My hands are slowly becoming warmer and warmer as I continue to breathe deeply and slowly."
- "My entire body is quiet, calm, and comfortable. My mind is quiet. I withdraw myself from my surroundings and feel serene and still. My thoughts are turning inward. I feel at ease. Within myself I can visualize and experience myself as quiet, calm, and comfortable. In an easy, quiet, inward-turned way, I am quietly alert. My mind is calm and quiet. I feel an inward quietness."

Continue these thoughts for exactly two minutes and then open your eyes. You will feel quietly alert, completely relaxed, comfortable, and better than before.

Discover how deeply relaxed you can become in such a short time. Even a few minutes allows the unconscious mind to dream, to problem-solve, and to experience deep relaxation and recuperation.

---

flow leading to the warming of your hands, by using a language through which your body and mind can cooperate. Through autogenics you learn to use "passive volition" in communicating with yourself. Words and images can produce relaxation, and recovery from fatigue, by dilating the blood vessels and affecting the flow of blood to different parts of the body. In this first stage of gaining physical control through relaxation, you can achieve satisfactory levels of relaxation, with increasingly improved re-

> ## Centering Exercise
>
> Begin by taking three slow breaths just to float down into your chair or bed. Let go of muscle tension. With your next three breaths, exhale away all thoughts and images of work or concern about the past. Clear your mind and your body of all concerns about what "should have" or "shouldn't have" happened in the past. Just let them go. With your next three breaths, let go of all images and thoughts about what you think may happen in the future—all the "what if"s. Clear your mind and body of all concern about what you expect to happen. And with your next three breaths, choose to be in the present, where there is nothing much for you to do now. Just allow the natural processes of your body to provide you with deep relaxation, recuperation, and remission. Avoid focusing on any particular time—just be here now, where it does not take much effort to breathe deeply and to make more energy available for healing and recuperation.

sults within a week or two of daily practice of 10 to 15 minutes.

Centering is a rapid, two-minute procedure that brings your mind back from ruminating about the past and future into the present, where your body must be. This helps you clear your mind of past or future problems that cannot be addressed now. As you withdraw your thoughts from these problems, you also release their accompanying guilt and stress, and experience a stress-free moment in the present. You automatically practice centering whenever you experience moments of joyful abandonment or intense concentration.

Healthy imagining centers around the concept of the "inner healer." Use it when you are ready to replace negative images about cancer and treatment with more relaxing, positive images. If you are new to imagery, you might start with the autogenic exercise, the centering exercise, or your own meditation or prayer. Use any of these methods to become relaxed and to experience the way your body responds to your words and images.

As you practice these relaxation and imagery exercises, your control over stressful images will improve, and you may find that you can enhance your sense of well-being.

Transformation—New Potential for the Cancer Survivor

During the course of coping with the cancer diagnosis, treatment decisions, and adjustments to side effects, it is difficult to imagine any benefit coming from the experience of cancer. Yet those who have written and spoken of their survival often tell of the positive changes that have taken place in their outlook and character as a result of facing the challenges of cancer.

For many survivors, cancer calls forth a transformation in attitude, health habits, and self-image. They learn to replace ineffective and limited ways of coping with healthier methods of dealing with work and social challenges. In this sense, any crisis offers an opportunity for positive change. Facing a life-threatening experience stretches your abilities beyond previous limits and gives you a chance to achieve your greatest potential.

Healthy Imagining Exercise

Focus your attention on any part of your body about which you are concerned. Take a deep breath and exhale through that area, releasing any tension you may be holding there. As you let go, allow your muscles to relax, your blood vessels to dilate, and your circulation to improve the flow of oxygen and potential healing elements to that area. By exhaling and relaxing your willpower—letting go of concern—you are helping your body's ability to heal itself. You might say to yourself:

"Ninety-nine percent of me is healthy and working for the removal of the weak, confused cancer cells. Even now, as I am sitting here, breathing easily, and reading, I am making thousands and thousands of healthy new blood cells every minute . . . and I don't even know how *I* do it. But my mind and body do know how, and they do it for me, for my protection, and for my healing and recuperation even while I sleep.

"I imagine my body bathed in sunlight and clear water, washing and dissolving cancer cells out of my body while coating and protecting the healthy cells. I see and feel chemotherapy as a powerful cleanser, and radiation as bullets of light removing cancer cells from my body while doing little harm to my healthy cells. My body is robust and can rapidly heal and recover from surgery, chemotherapy, or radiation. My body welcomes the help of my medical treatment team and works with them to free me of cancer."

Most cancer survivors are forced to develop their latent skills, to refine their strengths, and to drop negative patterns of behavior. There are survivors who stop worrying about money and begin traveling around the world. Others leave destructive relationships and unsatisfying jobs. Some just take life a little less seriously.

The experience of cancer will not give you more power over nature, the economy, world events, or other people. But it can show you the power you have over your own thoughts and attitudes, and how those attitudes affect the events of your life.

Life-threatening experiences remind people that life is a precious and limited resource. The impact of cancer and survivorship will tend to change people's self-perception, their ability to withstand hardship, and their perception of time. For some, the possibility of death can bring about unexpected feelings of calm and power. For others, the return of health and energy—whether temporary or permanent—gives them a second chance at life and mobilizes them to do things differently.

Some survivors have noted that they never had so much power with their family and within themselves as when they had cancer. Even the shy find it easier to express their wishes, feeling as if they have nothing to lose and, therefore, nothing to fear. The taste of power and effectiveness can have a significant impact on a survivor's personality and behavior.

In short, the cancer experience holds the possibility of making one's life more meaningful. Learning to control stress, worry, and social pressures can prepare survivors for the burdens imposed by cancer as well as energize them for a fuller life.

> **PERSPECTIVE**
>
> In a fragment of eternity
> I went from
> victim to visionary.
> No longer content
> to wallow in the past,
> I live on the edge of tomorrow
> with my feet squarely planted
> in the timeless NOW.
>
> —Brenda Neal, non-Hodgkin's lymphoma survivor,
> *Living Through Cancer Journal*, Jan./Feb. 1987

> "The whole experience [of cancer] made me reorder my priorities. I'm not so attuned to working long hours and making more money. I'm more tuned in to relationships with people. It's just more satisfying."
>
> —Charlene Williams, young-adult cancer survivor,
> *Washington Post*, September 7, 1989

> "I realized I wasn't frightened at all.
>
> "I realized in fact that I felt really good for the first time in my life. Not just a flash of good feeling like twenty minutes of good feeling, but a sustained feeling that I had nothing, and having nothing I had nothing to lose, and having nothing to lose I could be anything. I didn't have a self-image to worry about. And not having a self-image to worry about meant that I had no definition. I had nothing I had to be, nothing I had to care about. And I felt free. I felt as if I could leap out the window, not out of despair or fear, but just for the hell of it, just for the fun of it."
>
> —Ted Rosenthal, diagnosed at thirty with acute leukemia, *How Could I Not Be Among You?*

> "There is a margin of the human mind that can be stimulated by pain or inconvenience, but which is indifferent to pleasure.... It is the recognition that man's moments of freedom tend to come under crisis or challenge, and that when things are going well, he tends to allow his grip on life to slacken."
>
> —Colin Wilson, *The Outsider*

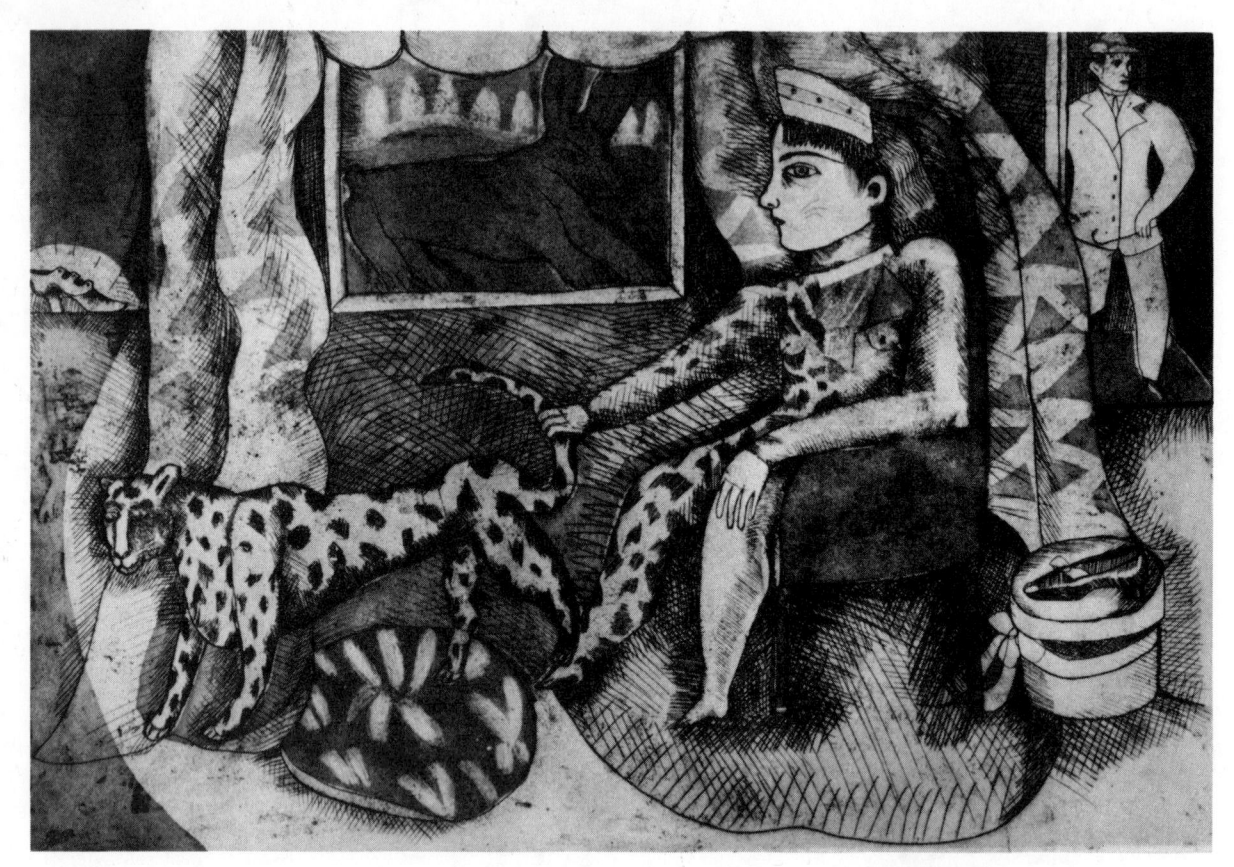

Barbara Leventhal-Stern
You Can't Keep It Under the Rug
Etching
18" x 22"

3

The Cancer Survivor as Consumer

Natalie Davis Spingarn

Patients and Doctors

We are all consumers, or users of goods and services, yet there is no other area of life where we know so little about the choices we must make as in the field of health care.

You and Your Doctor: A Historical Perspective

We investigate prospective schools and colleges carefully before enrolling our children in them, asking detailed questions about facilities and particularly about faculty—its credentials or its record. Whether we buy a big item like a house or a car, or a small one like a vacuum cleaner, we probably shop around for weeks, even months, comparing quality and price to see which is the best buy.

But, like most cancer survivors, you probably did not shop in the same way for the services of one of the people who influence your life most profoundly—your doctor. You came to him or her because of the recommendation of another doctor, or a friend, or a relative. You probably did not subject your new doctor to rigorous questioning about credentials or practice.

All this is part of a tradition handed down from a simpler time, when patients had one family doctor who took care of them, perhaps their whole life long. Though there was not much these doctors could do for you if your diagnosis was cancer, you trusted them and were not accustomed to challenging their judgment, or that of other health-care givers they recommended.

But in recent decades, as health services have burgeoned and changed, a revolution in attitudes and a growing interest in medical matters and preventive health care have transformed once-passive patients into active participants in their own health care.

The New Approach: The Aware Survivor

When you become a cancer survivor today, you become a consumer in a vast, complex marketplace about which you usually have had no education or training.

In this peculiar marketplace, buyers rarely reach for their wallets, count their bills, and pay for a service directly. Patients sign forms documenting doctor or hospital use, medical offices feed items about patients' care into a computer, and eventually patients receive a bill or reams of incomprehensible computer printouts.

Because buyer and seller seldom face each other at the cash register, both tend to be less sensitive to the price of an operation or a scan than they are to that of a vacation or a television set. Patient-doctor discussions about treatments center on which treatment might prolong life or sustain its quality; they rarely center on cost (the assumption is that if the insurance company does not pay someone else, either the taxpayer or a private charity, will).

What's more, survivor-consumers' approach to those who deliver medical services is far more complex and significant than that of most other consumers. For example, you may be one of those who do not want to conduct in-depth discussions with your health-care providers about the services or the costs of services. Assuming the doctor knows best, you may be more comfortable leaving the tough medical choices and treatment plans completely to him or her, and this is your privilege; some survivors, particularly older ones, agree with you.

But most of us feel better when we are involved in developing a plan for our treatment and recovery. If for some reason we cannot discuss the plan directly with the health-care provider, we can ask someone else (usually a family member or a close friend) to do so for us. Not only are we better able to follow this plan when we understand it completely, but we feel more in control and less afraid of what will happen next. In any event, we are all forced to participate to some extent, because we have to give our "informed consent" to treatments (see p. 53).

To participate in your treatment, you need to train yourself to be a better consumer. You should get in the habit of reading about your diagnosis and the different treatment options available to you, and of tapping the large quantity of information available from government and private organizations, and from survivors who are willing to share their experiences.

Every survivor should know the information number of the National Cancer Institute's Cancer Information Service (see Appendix A). CIS information specialists at 1-800-4-CANCER, usually based at cancer centers and community hospitals around the country, are trained to answer questions about cancer and its treatment. They will provide free publications and answer any cancer-related questions, ranging from how to quit smoking to how to deal with side effects of cancer treatment. What they provide is not medical advice but medical information, as well as facts about community resources.

The CIS staff will use many resources, which are constantly being updated, to answer your questions. One is an important computerized information service (on line since 1983) called PDQ (Physician Data Query). Through PDQ, you can learn about up-to-date treatment options, physicians in your area, major centers offering state-of-the-art treatment, and clinical trials for which you might be eligible (see Appendix A).

Predominant among the private organizations that provide such consumer information are the American Cancer Society, the Candlelighters Childhood Cancer Foundation, and the National Coalition for Cancer Survivorship (see Appendix A). For a discussion of professional support services, see chapter 4. For a discussion of hotlines and other sources of community support, see chapter 5.

Finding the Right Doctor

The doctor you select to treat your cancer will be a significant person in your life, not only during treatment, but for many years of follow-up care, so select him or her carefully. Take the few days required to check out his or her credentials, style of practice, and hospital affiliations. If possible, learn about the experience of those treated by your prospective doctor.

If you do not have names from previous doctors to check out, call your local medical society or PDQ at 1-800-4-CANCER. Other good sources of referral are the chief resident and experienced nurses in the hospital, and peer-support groups composed of seasoned survivors.

Be cautious: doctors and other medical professionals will tell you good news about one another, but seldom will they level with you about the bad news. To put together a list of prospective doctors in your area, it might be a good idea to consult the *Directory of Medical Specialists* or the *American Medical Directory*, which can be found in the reference rooms of many public libraries. Then call the offices of the doctors you are considering for any information you still need.

What everyone seeks in a doctor is competence. You want the best doctor available to you, to help you get well and, if that is not possible, live well as long as possible. The problem is that today the "best doctor" means more than the doctor with the best education. It means a wide variety of things, including the doctor who practices in the finest hospital, uses the most knowledgeable radiologists and other specialists, can tap into such resources as clinical trials, runs the most efficient office with a friendly receptionist and skilled nurses, and can communicate with you in a way that leaves you feeling good about yourself and your treatment.

To make your choice, you will need at least this information:

Basic credentials. Though credentials are not everything, they are still important. Note the quality of the doctor's education, teaching affiliations if any, publications, and PDQ listing.

Board certification. Find out whether or not the doctor is the sort of medical specialist you need (for example, medical oncologist, radiation oncologist, general surgeon). Note that some doctors are self-proclaimed specialists, without having satisfied requirements for certification in a field established by the professional board in the United States supervising that field.

You should check to see whether your prospective physician is *board certified* in his or her specialty or subspecialty. This means passing rigorous peer-administered written and oral examinations in a field and satisfying its residency-training requirements. Some physicians are double-boarded, which means they are certified in more than one field. A few specialty boards require recertification after a certain number of years. Initials starting with "F" (like F.A.C.P.) after a doctor's name means he or she has been honored by election to a specialty "college" fellowship.

Experience. Length of experience is always important. But medical oncology is a relatively new subspecialty (of internal medicine) and has been certified as such only since 1973. So, when you are considering older doctors, check carefully on other factors, such as reputation among support-group members, publications, teaching affiliations, PDQ listing, the study groups to which they belong, and whether they enroll and/or follow patients in clinical trials (or have colleagues who do so).

Type of practice. Ask: *How* do doctors practice? Are they in a group practice, or on their own? If they are with a group, or in a university setting, do they see you themselves each time you have an appointment? Or are you seen by an assortment of associates (and if so, who are these associates and what is the level of their education and training)?

American Cancer Society
The Cancer Survivors' Bill of Rights

A new population lives among us today—a new minority of 6 million people with a history of cancer. Three million of these Americans have lived with their diagnoses for five years or more.

You see these modern survivors in offices and in factories, on bicycles and cruise ships, on tennis courts, beaches, and bowling alleys. You see them in all ages, shapes, sizes, and colors. Usually they are unremarkable in appearance; sometimes they are remarkable for the way they have learned to live with disabilities resulting from cancer or its treatment.

Modern medical advances have returned about half of the nation's cancer patients of all ages (and 59 percent for those under the age of 55) to a normal lifespan. But the larger society has not always kept pace in helping make this lifespan truly "normal": at least, it has felt awkward in dealing with this fledgling group; at most, it has failed fully to accept survivors as functioning members.

The American Cancer Society presents this Survivors' Bill of Rights to call public attention to survivor needs, to enhance cancer care, and to bring greater satisfaction to cancer survivors, as well as to their physicians, employers, families, and friends:

1. Survivors have the right to assurance of lifelong medical care, as needed. The physicians and other professionals involved in their care should continue their constant efforts to be:

- sensitive to the cancer survivors' life-style choices and their need for self-esteem and dignity
- careful, no matter how long they have survived, to have symptoms taken seriously, and not have aches and pains dismissed, for fear of recurrence is a normal part of survivorship
- informative and open, providing survivors with as much or as little candid medical information as they wish, and encouraging their informed participation in their own care

Office procedure. Ask: When are doctors usually in the office (days and hours of the day)? How can they be reached evenings or weekends? How long, on the average, do patients have to wait to see them? Who "covers" for them when they are away or not available by phone? Who manages the office, answers the phones, and deals with the billing? Do they make house calls? If not, or even if they do, how do they want you to proceed in the event of an emergency?

Hospital affiliation. Find out with what hospitals the doctor is affiliated, which ones he prefers, and why. Also determine in what hospital or clinic he would arrange for you to have radiation therapy, chemotherapy, or any other such special outpatient treatment.

Nursing and paraprofessionals. The nurses and paraprofessionals who work with a doctor may draw your blood and administer your chemotherapy. Find out how many of them are R.N.s (registered nurses), and how many have been tested and awarded the O.C.N. (Oncology Certified Nurse) credential. Factor in the importance of experience, just as you did in choosing the doctor.

- knowledgeable about counseling resources, and willing to refer survivors and their families as appropriate for emotional support and therapy which will improve the quality of individual lives

2. In their personal lives, survivors, like other Americans, have the right to the pursuit of happiness. This means they have the right:

- to talk with their families and friends about their cancer experience if they wish, but to refuse to discuss it if that is their choice and not to be expected to be more upbeat or less blue than anyone else
- to be free of the stigma of cancer as a "dread disease" in all social relations
- to be free of blame for having gotten the disease and of guilt for having survived it

3. In the workplace, survivors have the right to equal job opportunities. This means they have the right:

- to aspire to jobs worthy of their skills, and for which they are trained and experienced, and thus not to have to accept jobs they would not have considered before the cancer experience
- to be hired, promoted, and accepted on return to work, according to their individual abilities and qualifications, and not according to "cancer" or "disability" stereotypes
- to privacy about their medical histories

4. Since health-insurance coverage is an overriding survivorship concern, every effort should be made to assure all survivors adequate health insurance, whether public or private. This means:

- for employers, that survivors have the right to be included in group health coverage, which is usually less expensive, provides better benefits, and covers the employee regardless of health history
- for physicians, counselors, and other professionals concerned, that they keep themselves and their survivor-clients informed and up-to-date on available group or individual health-policy options, noting, for example, what major expenses like hospital costs and medical tests outside the hospital are covered and what amount must be paid before coverage (deductibles)

Rapport with your doctor. Competence to treat you is your first concern. But today medical competence includes personality and management skills that enable you to be comfortable in a medical relationship over the long haul. If you are to be treated successfully, you will need to find a doctor who is sensitive to your needs and your concerns, who understands you as a person as well as a patient with a disease.

To see if you feel comfortable with a doctor, you will have to visit his or her office. Even then it is sometimes difficult in the first interview to determine whether you have chosen wisely; it may take months to find out. But here are a few suggestions about what to watch for and how to proceed at the beginning of your professional relationship:

The atmosphere of the office. Note the manner in which the doctor's staff conducts business. Are they warm and patient with you and with others—on the phone as well as in person? Do they seem efficient and willing to answer your questions, even if these concern such mundane things as your next appointment? Check out how the office looks. Is it comfortable and cheerful, or dark, drab, and cluttered? In one major city, many patients left a practice simply because their chemotherapy was administered in a small, dark, messy room crowded with black chemotherapy chairs. (As one who left put it: "That depressing place makes me feel like death warmed over; why make things worse than they have to be?")

The doctor's manner and style. In the old days, people talked about a physician's "bedside manner." Now, when doctors rarely sit at your bedside, and you are in an office chair more than in a hospital bed, it is more appropriate to check out "chairside manner." Does your prospective doctor seem warm, concerned with you as a person? Talking with you, does he or she sit down or hover at the door? Does this physician take time to answer your questions and, if called away in an emergency, arrange a time when you can have your questions answered? (See p. 57.)

Specific tips. To test a doctor's ability to relate to you, you might show him the Cancer Survivors' Bill of Rights (see pp. 50–51). Ask the doctor how he or she feels about statement number one. Any marked disagreement with statement number one should serve as a warning that you may not have chosen the right doctor. If there are other, compelling reasons why you want to stay in treatment with this doctor, you should discuss the matter frankly with him or her.

If your test results, biopsies, and other indicators of the success of your doctor's treatment plan (including how you feel) do not please you at *any* stage, get a second or even a third opinion. You should probably get a second opinion at the time of diagnosis, when your treatment plan is mapped. Even if you elect to stay with the same doctor, a second opinion approving your treatment plan will make you more comfortable and reinforce your trust. Some insurance policies cover the cost of a second opinion. But if, after all this, you do not have confidence in your doctor, you should look for another.

Technically, your medical records belong to your health-care provider, but you have "a bundle of rights" to your medical records that permits access to them, limits dissemination of information in the records, and assures that the information they contain is correct and is used appropriately. Because patients have these rights, most doctors will forward their records to a successor physician (see pp. 115–18).

Communications—The Two-Way Street

To work successfully with your doctor—both in the office and in the hospital—you must be able to talk frankly with him or her.

Modern medical care can be highly technical, complex, and difficult to understand. Moreover, it is delivered by a team of specialists, including surgeons, radiologists, and a multitude of nurses and technicians. Psychiatrists, gastroenterologists, gynecologists, neurologists, and others may be consulted. Communicating with these specialists, and getting the benefit of their shared views, is an integral part of survivorship.

Barriers to Communication

Doctor-patient communication is a two-way street. The responsibility for it rests, in large measure, with the doctor, but some of it rests with you. In its 1985 pamphlet *Communication: It's Good for Your Health,* the American Society of Internal Medicine reported that, although internists believe that about 70 percent of correct medical diagnoses are made simply through communication between patient and physician, patients often hold back information.

Why is this so? Communicating with your doctor sounds easy. But many survivors report that it is not. They would like to know

> "A good physician is one who sees the patient as a whole person, a complex human being, rather than a series of organ systems in various states of repair. This was not an argument against knowledge or even specialization, but rather a recognition once and for all that good physicians are something more than Midas muffler dealers. Generalist or specialist, family practitioner or plastic surgeon, a good doctor needs to love his patients at least a little bit."
>
> —Fitzhugh Mullan, M.D., *Vital Signs: A Young Doctor's Struggle with Cancer*

more about their various therapies. Or they are not sure just what medicine they are supposed to take when, and why they are supposed to take it. They may be anxious to learn whether new pains are serious or simply unimportant side effects of old treatments. But a variety of attitudes and fears restrain them. These include:

Awe of the doctor. Most survivors stand in awe of their doctors, in whose hands their comfort and even their lives lie. They want these doctors to like them and succeed in making them better, and not to consider them pests or hypochondriacs.

Lack of self-confidence. Survivors are too often afraid to ask the questions they have on their minds, afraid that the doctor might consider these questions "stupid" or "dumb." They ask themselves: Doesn't this busy physician have more important things to do than answer my questions? The answer is NO!

Difficulty of remembering. No matter who they are, or how extensive their education, survivors can grow anxious discussing life-and-death matters with their doctors. Listening to new words and new concepts, they can suffer "information overload." They can have trouble focusing, absorbing abstract ideas, and remembering all but certain emotionally charged buzzwords (like "cure" or "handicap"). It's a common experience to return home from an important medical interview and find you are unable to give your family or friends detailed information as to what the doctor said.

"Iatrogenic" bewilderment. "Iatrogenic," according to *Webster's*, means "induced by a physician." Some doctors may make it difficult for you to understand them. They may use complex medical jargon instead of plain English (i.e., "alopecia" rather than "hair loss"). Or they may act as though they have no time for you, looking at their watch or even hovering near the door.

Informed Consent: Your Right to Choose and Refuse Treatment

Ironically, a patient's right—the right to accept or refuse medical treatment—is another factor that both complicates good doctor-patient communication and makes it even more necessary. Before performing certain nonemergency procedures, your doctor must obtain your agreement for treatment.

> "The first doctor I saw when I was diagnosed with cancer came into my room and asked me how it felt to be dying. I had the presence of mind to say I thought we all were."
>
> —Barbara Lazarus, Ed.D., breast-cancer survivor
>
> "Upon recommending that I have a mastectomy, a male physician told me, 'When you are dressed, no one will know.' That's like telling a man who is about to be castrated, 'When you're dressed, no one will know.'"
>
> —Barbara Smith

This agreement is called "informed consent." State laws vary as to what procedures require your specific consent. They include surgery, internal examinations such as sigmoidoscopy (examination of the colon), and dye injections for a CAT scan.

Informed consent is not just a legal exercise. Doctors who take time to explain the consent form to you are in the process discussing the benefits and side effects of treatment. As a result, they give better care and protect themselves from lawsuits.

The doctor's responsibility. Before starting treatment or a medical procedure, your doctor has a duty to give you enough information to allow you to make an informed decision about whether you want to undergo treatment. He or she does not have to tell you everything about your treatment, just enough to help you make a reasonable choice. You must be told:

- the nature and purpose of the procedure
- the risk and consequence of the procedure
- the medically acceptable alternatives to the procedure
- the risks of not having the procedure

Be certain you understand each of these explanations before you have an operation or any other serious medical procedure. If your doctor has not volunteered adequate information, ask for it. If you do not understand what you have been told, ask for a clearer explanation *before* you sign a form consenting to treatment.

Signing an informed-consent form. When you sign an informed consent form, you state two things:

- That you are an "informed" patient. This means that your doctor has given you the four explanations listed above and that you understand them.
- That you give your "consent" to be treated. This means that you agree to let your doctor perform the procedure described to you, and that you understand a particular result cannot be guaranteed.

Take time to read a consent form carefully. This is important for you and your doctor: some malpractice cases result from patients not asking questions, being confused about treatments, and then blaming physicians, usually inappropriately, for not "informing" them.

If you do not agree with every statement on the consent form, you can make changes. For example, if the form states that you agree to have your operation videotaped for use by medical schools and you do not want to be videotaped, just draw a line through that sentence.

By signing a consent form, you are simply giving your doctor permission to treat you. You do not give up your right to receive professional medical care. You are not prevented from suing your doctor for malpractice should he or she fail to follow professional standards and cause you harm.

When your consent is not needed. Your doctor does not have to obtain your consent if:

- emergency treatment is needed to save your life or to prevent permanent harm
- you have given your consent to one type of surgery, and during that surgery a serious unanticipated condition arises (for example, you gave your consent to having cancerous lymph nodes removed, and during surgery your doctor finds cancer in another organ and therefore removes it too)
- you "waive" your right to consent to each treatment and agree to let your doctor make decisions about your care without consulting you

The right to refuse treatment. A competent adult has the right to refuse medical treatment, even if the result may be death. There are some limits to this right, and they vary from state to state. Some are the subject of current lawsuits. The question of what treatment options a pregnant woman with cancer may choose is now the subject of debate.

Children and informed consent. Under most circumstances, parents have the right to make treatment decisions for their children. (Most states give children the right to choose their own medical treatment at the age of 18.) There are two exceptions to this rule:

- The child is mature and emancipated (married or living away from home).
- A parent's refusal to consent to treatment may cause avoidable harm to the child. In this case, a court may decide that the child is suffering from neglect and appoint a guardian to make medical decisions for the child.

Some Suggestions

There are those who argue that medical competence is more important to patients than communication skills. As one lawyer put it, she would rather see a "bleeding bastard" who would cure her, than a "sweet-talking," less competent physician. But the fact is that there can be no true medical competence in today's world when your doctor is not getting sufficient information from you or relaying important concepts to you.

Here are some practical suggestions about how you might communicate effectively with your doctor:

1. *Speak frankly to your doctor.* Remember, he or she cannot read your mind. Describe your symptoms—not only the obvious aches and pains, but other signs you have observed, such as trouble falling asleep at night, unhealthy eating habits, or overindulgence in alcoholic beverages.

2. *Bring a family member with you.* If you have trouble asserting yourself, bring a family member or friend to speak for you. If there are several people involved, be sure you make clear to the doctor to whom and to what extent they have your permission to discuss your case.

3. *Jot down your questions in a notebook.* Before your visit to the doctor, jot down your questions in a notebook so you cannot forget them. And with the notebook in hand, you can write down your doctor's instructions.

4. *Tape important conversations.* Because most people have trouble absorbing new in-

SAMPLE CONSENT FORM

Reprinted from Medicolegal Forms, with legal analysis from the American Medical Association. Copyright © 1982.

This sample form, prepared by the American Medical Association, outlines a patient's consent to operations, anesthetics, and other medical services.

Date _____ Time _____ A.M. / P.M.

1. I authorize the performance upon _____
   (Myself or name of patient)

of the following operation _____
   (State nature and extent of operation)

to be performed by or under the direction of Dr. _____ .

2. I consent to the performance of operations and procedures in addition to or different from those now contemplated, whether or not arising from presently unforeseen conditions, which the above-named doctor or his associates or assistants may consider necessary or advisable in the course of the operation.

3. I consent to the administration of such anesthetics as may be considered necessary or advisable by the physician responsible for this service, with the exception of _____ .
   (State "none," "spinal anesthesia," etc.)

4. The nature and purpose of the operation, possible alternative methods of treatment, the risks involved, the possible consequences, and the possibility of complications have been explained to me by Dr. _____ and by _____ .

5. I acknowledge that no guarantee or assurance has been given by anyone as to the results that may be obtained.

6. I consent to the photographing or televising of the operations or procedures to be performed, including appropriate portions of my body, for medical, scientific or educational purposes, provided my identity is not revealed by the pictures or by descriptive texts accompanying them.

7. For the purpose of advancing medical education, I consent to the admittance of observers to the operating room.

8. I consent to the disposal by hospital authorities of any tissues or body parts which may be removed.

9. I am aware that sterility may result from this operation. I know that a sterile person is incapable of becoming a parent.

10. I acknowledge that all blank spaces on this document have been either completed or crossed off prior to my signing.

(CROSS OUT ANY PARAGRAPHS ABOVE
WHICH DO NOT APPLY)

Signed _____
(Patient or person authorized
to consent for patient)

Witness _____

---

formation when they are upset, some doctors ask patients to tape important conversations so they can listen to the tape again later in the quiet of their homes and they can review medical explanations and instructions in calmer, more rational moments.

5. Insist on privacy during important interviews. Under no circumstances should such an interview take place in a busy hallway, where anyone can hear what is being said.

6. Give your doctor "cues" about information sharing. It used to be that doctors told patients nothing about cancer, not even that they had it; now they tell patients everything, including their statistical chances for survival. Patients have different coping "styles"; for some it is frightening to know, for others it is frightening not to know. If you feel your doctor is overloading you with facts and statistics that you do not want, simply say so, or offer a hint or "cue" as to how you feel. Try something like "My father's already gathered statistics about my tumor from PDQ" or simply "You know best." Sometimes body language—such as simply turning away and looking down—can help indicate you have had enough. If you want to know more about your disease and its treatment and possible outcome, say so.

7. Ask for interpretations of puzzling medical words or terms. Never be embarrassed if you do not understand a word like "metastasis" or "sarcoma." It is reasonable to insist on a translation into plain English. It is also reasonable to ask your doctor to show you a diagram or medical-text picture of the organs he or she is describing, so you can understand where they are in your body and their relation to one another. Your doctor will most likely respect your need to have your situation described in a way that makes sense to you.

8. Don't forget doctors are people too. Medical professionals respond to you just as you respond to them: pleasantness is usually met with pleasantness, and courteousness with courteousness. Express your appreciation when your doctor sits down to talk with you in the hospital or examining room and gives you complete attention during your limited time together.

If the doctor is called away for an emergency, you should be told when he or she will return. If such a courtesy is not possible, or if it is overlooked, or if the doctor takes nonemergency telephone calls during your consultation, speak up. Say you realize the doctor is busy but you would like to know when you will be able to finish your talk, because you still have unanswered questions.

9. Don't present yourself to your doctor as a disease, but as a person living with a disease. One survivor reported that she made it a rule to tell her doctor one thing about her life on each visit: that she had been to London or had seen a ball game or taken a poetry course. In this way, the doctor learned more about her and could look at her and treat her as a whole person. Another reported she traveled frequently but was anxious about going too far from sophisticated medical care. The physician prepared a special medicine kit for her to take along when she went to underdeveloped countries.

10. Be sure, before you leave the doctor, that you understand your treatment plan. Be sure you understand the tests and medicines that have been prescribed, and how long and when you will be taking them. Ask the doctor to repeat whatever you are not sure of, including the benefits and risks involved in your treatment. Find out where you can call him or her and at what time, in case a new problem occurs.

11. If you are unable to communicate with your doctor, find another one. If you feel hurried as you talk, or think your questions are not being answered satisfactorily, or you are not being given a fair hearing, try discussing this with your doctor. You may be surprised at the results. A support group or a cancer counselor might show you how other patients have handled such problems and how you might do better. If all this fails, you should consider changing physicians.

The Hospital: A World unto Itself

Most cancer survivors do not spend too much time in the hospital nowadays. Hospital beds and expertise are expensive; hospital managers and peer-review committees guard them closely, steering as many prospective patients as possible to outpatient care.

Most survivors, however, do spend some time as inpatients, particularly at the beginning of treatment. Almost always, this is a significant experience that sets the tone for care during the rest of the illness, and perhaps the rest of a life.

The Choice of a Hospital

The hospital experience is one for which people are seldom prepared. Indeed, unless you are an unusually sophisticated consumer of medical services, you did not shop carefully for a hospital, if you shopped at all. Your doctor stipulated the hospital you would enter, which is one where he or she has "privileges." If this doctor works in an HMO (health maintenance organization) or some other form of group practice, he or she sent you to the hospital used by that practice.

One of the first questions you should ask a physician, and particularly a surgeon, is *with what hospital or hospitals he or she is affiliated.* When you have the names of these hospitals, check them out. Here, as in your doctor search, the public library is a good resource; in large cities the main library has the most material. The NCI number 1-800-4-CANCER can also provide information. Recommendations from seasoned survivors and nurses and other health professionals can be more reliable than the local medical society or hospital association, which is beholden to its members.

Here is a checklist for you to use when you are considering specific hospitals:

Type of hospital. Cancer care today is offered in many different settings. Find out exactly what sort of hospital you are considering. Is it a *comprehensive cancer center*—one of 22 so designated by the National Cancer Institute? If so, you can be sure it offers high-quality, up-to-date medical care (researchers here have been involved in many of the most important advances of the last decades). You can also be sure of a wide variety of services, from counseling and rehabilitation to home-care supervision.

In addition to these comprehensive centers, 21 *clinical cancer centers* around the country are funded in part by the National Cancer Institute to carry out research and training programs, as well as patient care. *If an institution purports to be a cancer center, ask its administration officials whether it has been designated as such by the federal government's NCI.* Some *for-profit hospitals* call themselves "cancer centers," or even "comprehensive cancer centers." But, with a few exceptions, if they are freestanding (not affiliated with medical schools) and do not have research or teaching obligations, they may be more attuned to the state of their pocketbooks than state-of-the-art oncology.

Find out if the hospital in question is a teaching hospital, *affiliated with a medical school.* Does a medical school use the hospital for internship and residency programs? The advantages of medical school affiliation (i.e., the availability of the best doctor–faculty members, round-the-clock medical attention, and a broad variety of services) usually outweigh the disadvantages (i.e., being poked and prodded a bit more, especially when the medical team makes its early-morning teaching rounds).

Accreditation. If, for whatever reason, you are considering a *community hospital,* which is not a federally designated cancer center and not affiliated, either directly or indirectly, with a medical school, *be sure it is fully accredited.* The Joint Commission on Accreditation of Healthcare Organizations (JCAHO), formerly the Joint Commission

> "My daughters stayed with me on the first night until visiting hours were over. I hated to see them leave. The hospital room seemed strange and empty, with unfamiliar sounds and smells throughout the night. The nurses kept telling me to rest, but then they would wake me for food, medication, and to take my temperature. On the second day, I asked my daughter to bring me my photographs, some books, and my bathrobe. Seeing my things helped me to feel at home in that hospital bed. I also got to know my primary nurse, who cared for me almost every day during my stay. I got friendly with the medical intern who used to drop by to talk about baseball whenever he had a free moment. Although I was glad to leave the hospital, I knew that I would miss the friends I had made among the staff—and I did."
>
> —70-year-old lung-cancer survivor admitted to the hospital for ten days of tests and chemotherapy

on Accreditation of Hospitals (JCAH), a professionally sponsored group employing physicians, nurses, health-care administrators, and other experts to perform periodic surveys, surveys hospitals carefully before granting them accreditation, holding them to some 1,200 staffing, safety, and quality of practitioner care standards. Some 1,444 of the nation's 6,821 hospitals, the American Hospital Association reported in 1988, were not accredited.

You can ask a hospital's administration officials about the date and results of their last JCAHO survey or you can call the JCAHO in Illinois at (708) 691-5632 for survey results. You can also learn about a hospital's accreditation as well as other information about a hospital's services from the *American Hospital Association Guide to the Health Care Field,* an annual survey of hospitals available in most public libraries (see bibliography).

Usually a hospital's failure to gain accreditation or reaccreditation will be reported in the local press. Some large city magazines at times carry annotated ratings lists of local hospitals caring for federally insured patients. Such lists include information from various sources, both objective and subjective, which can be oversimplified. Though they may be useful, you should not rely on them, or on national consumer books that "rate" hospitals, as foolproof assessments of the best hospital for you.

For example, the government's Health Care Financing Administration (HCFA) publishes a volume of *Hospital Mortality Information* at the end of each year, which measures mortality rates of Medicare patients with 16 different diseases, including cancer. But such mortality rates depend on many factors besides the quality of care: a very fine cancer center, for instance, can have high rates because it cares for many patients with lethal cancers.

Convenience. There are great advantages to going to a hospital close to home, where your friends and family can visit you easily. But if that hospital cannot provide you with the quality of care you need, you should at

> **THEY DON'T WANT ME TO SLEEP**
>
> They don't want me
> to sleep.
> When I do,
> they wake me,
> drip another
> bottle in my vein,
> feed me a pill,
> check my vital signs.
> I'm very clever,
> sleep when they
> least suspect.
> They bring me lunch.
> I say, "thank you,"
> and sleep.
> They ask me
> to watch the bottle
> drip. I promise,
> and sleep.
> Night and day
> the loudspeaker
> outside my room
> broadcasts coded
> messages.
> I know they turn
> it louder when
> I begin to sleep.
> Throughout the night
> they examine me
> to see
> if I'm still alive.
> so far, I surprise
> them.
>
> —Helen Webster, copyright © 1980

least consider another one, even if it is some distance away. A sensible compromise is a consultation at the closest comprehensive cancer center. Usually the experts there can make the diagnosis, map out your treatment plan, and consult with your local doctor and hospital as they carry it out.

Size and source of funding. Size is a questionable variable when you are selecting a hospital. Some big hospitals (500 or more beds) are very good; others are not. The same is true of medium-sized (100–500 beds) and small (fewer than 100 beds) hospitals. Although big hospitals seem more bureaucratic and impersonal, they have more resources and more ability to help you. Moreover, the staff is often more experienced, since it sees a wider variety of cases.

The *source of a hospital's funding* is another variable. Public hospitals (like Department of Veterans Affairs hospitals, county hospitals, and urban hospitals for the needy) can suffer from a poor image, and indeed they at times do lack certain amenities. But amenities are less important than quality care. If it is affiliated with a good teaching hospital, attracting interns and residents eager to care for a variety of patients, a public hospital may give outstanding service.

Services. It is difficult to assess the services of a given hospital until you have experienced them—or the lack of them. But you can check on what services a hospital has to offer, and the quality of these services, through your doctor, the administrative offices of the hospital itself, or other survivors who have used it. If you are going in for surgery, for example, you might ask your surgeon if the hospital has a recovery room or an intensive-care unit. Ask about the reputation of its pathology laboratory and blood bank.

Some community hospitals do not serve enough cancer patients to have a special cancer floor, or unit. Where will you be taken care of? Will the hospital have the high-tech equipment necessary to treat you after surgery—radiation-therapy equipment, for example, or scanning equipment? If not, where will you be given such therapies when they are necessary?

Respiratory and physical therapy are available in hospitals today. Nursing care is of course routine, and, to a lesser extent, so are social-work services. But the size and quality of hospital nursing and social-services staffs, so important to your health and well-being, vary enormously. Some comprehensive cancer centers have competent, experienced registered nurses and a trained social worker on every floor to help you begin your life after cancer. Some other community hospitals are willing to supplement their too-often short staffs with "agency" nurses, but they hire aides without sufficient training to help keep your tubes in place after surgery. Their social-work services can be limited to a single business office, dealing largely with discharge arrangements.

The Hospital Experience

Try to arrange to be admitted to the hospital on a Sunday or a Monday, so you can be ready for treatment early in the week (nothing much goes on there over the weekend, anyway). In many places, a pleasant voice will call from the hospital a few days before you are scheduled for admittance (assuming, of course, that you do not enter through the emergency-room door), to query you at length, particularly about your health insurance. If you cannot produce evidence of coverage, you may be in for a rude financial awakening.

The preadmission process saves some time when you enter the hospital. You usually go through a battery of tests before you ever reach your room: chest X ray, EKG, blood and urine analyses. Here you will get your own first hints as to the atmosphere of the institution you have chosen. You can be passed from hand to hand efficiently and cheerfully and made to feel like a human being instead of a diseased body, or you can be worried by a seemingly disorganized bunch of paraprofessionals, jabbing at your veins, or barking orders at you in front of the X-ray machine.

Once in bed—which may turn out to be in a semiprivate room, even if you asked for a single room and are willing to pay the noninsured difference—you will have plenty of time to contemplate the special hospital culture of which you are now a part. You will want to know something about the schedule—visiting hours, lights-out, and meal times. You will want to know where to store your wallet and other worldly belongings.

For the hospital is a world unto itself, a world you will have to learn and master. The bad news is that an impersonal staff wedded to sometimes mindless institutional routines can make you feel dehumanized—waking you up to give you a sleeping pill in the evening, for instance. The good news is that in this same world you can feel hopeful, even ennobled by the marvelous care the modern hospital with its trained staff is able to offer you. And there is a growing awareness in health-care circles that too much has been lost to specialization; more effort today is made to look at you as a whole person, rather than a lung or a breast or a set of bones.

"Primary-care nursing," in effect in many hospitals, for example, emphasizes this approach. Primary nurses are each assigned four to six patients. They are in charge of your care throughout your hospital stay, not only performing everyday routine tasks, such as dispensing medicines and emptying bedpans, but visiting you in the recovery room after surgery or taking your phone calls after you are discharged.

Surviving in the Hospital

Seasoned survivors have found that their attitude—the way they respond to the hospital culture—has a lot to do with their success in taking advantage of the good that hospitals offer and learning to deal competently with the not-so-good. Here are some hints for developing such an attitude and negotiating the system:

Be assertive. If your common sense tells you something is wrong, learn to act, not aggressively or rudely, but *assertively.* This means that, if someone wakes you up for no good reason or jabs at your veins until your arm is speckled black and blue, you ask politely but firmly for an explanation and a remedy.

Empathize with others. Make an effort to treat hospital staff (and your fellow patients) as you would like to be treated, with respect for them and for yourself. Tactfully "stroke" the nurse who forgets to fill your water pitcher, or turns up the television when you are trying to read. This means telling her (and nurses today are still most often females) dispassionately that you know how busy she is, how much she is doing for others in the hospital, but that you are not feeling too well and you would appreciate fresh water and a little quiet.

Do not take yourself too seriously, though you take your situation seriously. Try to keep your sense of humor, and your ability to laugh and joke—even if you are being quizzed about things that do not seem to have much to do with your cancer—your work, your education, your "perception" of your disease.

Ask questions. Many people are fearful of hospital authority. An extreme example is the patient handed a pill he or she is sure is the wrong pill but afraid to ask questions lest doctors and nurses think he or she is being uncooperative or dumb. But it is better for your care givers as well as yourself if you tell them what's bothering you, and what information you need to be more comfortable (and so a "better" patient).

As a last resort, complain. When you have exhausted your new assertiveness, and things still do not seem to be going your way, by all means complain—to your doctor; the nursing supervisor on your floor, director of nursing, or head nurse; or hospital administrator. If your hospital has a "patient representative," he or she is a good resource. Present the facts quietly and clearly, and ask for attention to your problem.

Going Home, Re-Entry

Some patients enjoy the postsurgery part of hospital life. Free of the cares of job and household, they savor their visitors, the plants they bring, the ministrations of the staff, and the companionship of other patients—particularly when the prognosis is good. But most people find their hospital stay more stressful than the time spent at home after their release.

Everyone looks forward to going home. Most hospitals help you plan to assure that your re-entry into the real world of self-care and responsibilities is accomplished smoothly. In the discharge-planning process, a nurse, a social worker, or some other designated professional will work with you to make sure you have the proper setup during your convalescence (see chapter 4).

Caveat Emptor—Unconventional Treatments

One of the most challenging and worrisome questions for many survivor-consumers is whether or not to try unconventional (or unproven or questionable) treatments—either in addition to or in place of conventional medical care. Call them what you will, these treatments come to the attention of cancer survivors at every stage of their illness.

Well-meaning friends, even magazine articles, relay the message that there is something out there in addition to standard medical treatment that might cure your cancer. Contrary to the "cutting, burning, poisoning" conventional therapies, it is a natural treatment—relaxing, peaceful, and gentle—which you may be able to administer yourself. The medical establishment, they say, only disapproves of these treatments for selfish financial reasons.

How do you judge the claims made for unconventional treatments, whether they have to do with diet, mind control, detoxification, or some combination thereof? How can you separate the good they might offer from the bad? These thorny questions are part of today's survivor culture.

Something Natural, Easy, Hopeful...

If you are like most survivors, the notion of doing something about your own bodily health appeals to you. Tired of protracted, harsh treatments, depressed by the knowledge that, after many years of trying, the researchers have still not come up with a sure cure for cancer, you may ask yourself: "Why not try something more natural, like 'imaging' my good cells, designed to keep me well, eating up the bad cancer cells? Or eating a restorative grain, or purifying and cleansing my system with coffee enemas or colonics?"

The establishment itself seems to favor this "natural" approach. The National Cancer Institute points to the virtues of eating broccoli; the American Cancer Society advertises the advantages of cooking up the right foods in your kitchen and even talks about "behavioral approaches."

In this atmosphere, you are likely to be curious about one of the currently popular unconventional treatments, developed and offered by practitioners who have chosen to work outside the mainstream. In virtually all cases, this also means outside mainstream research, with its animal studies and formal clinical trials, as well as outside mainstream practice. The problem for the patient, even if a treatment seems effective, is the lack of objective evidence to distinguish the potentially helpful remedy from the useless—or, worse, harmful—ones. Most fall into one or more of the following categories:

Diet treatments. Most popular is a "macrobiotic" diet, consisting primarily of whole grains and vegetables and avoiding dairy products, based on the Eastern yin-yang philosophy, which aims to "balance" food intake to counteract bodily dysfunction. In Mexico, Charlotte Gerson Straus uses another popular treatment founded by her father, Max Gerson, M.D. It is based on an elaborate dietary regimen and detoxification program (including baby calves' liver, raw fruit juices, and coffee enemas).

Vitamin and mineral supplements. High doses of different vitamins and minerals—i.e., vitamin C, betacarotene, and selenium—are taken to strengthen the body's ability to destroy malignant cancer cells.

Mental guided imagery applied for antitumor effect (see pp. 41–42). This means using your brain to work through your nervous system in an effort to bolster your body's immune defenses. Some call this "psychoneuroimmunology" or "psychoimmunology"—hundred-dollar words for a mind-over-matter concept in which the patient visualizes or imagines the conquest of malignant cells by "good" T cells, and so tries to reverse the malignant process. This type of treatment has been popularized by Dr. Carl and Stephanie Simonton and advocated by Dr. Bernie Siegel and others.

Metabolic treatments. These combinations of treatments employ enemas (especially coffee enemas) and colonic cleansing; special diets, enzymes, vitamins and minerals, laetrile, and DMSO (a solvent).

Pharmacological and biologic treatments. These include Burzynski's "antineoplastons" (synthesized urine proteins), Burton's "immuno-augmentative therapy" (IAT or blood therapy), ozone, hydrogen peroxide, cell therapy, or the herbal treatments (i.e., Hoxsey's tonic treatment, Livingston-Wheeler's autogenous vaccine, Revici's "biologically guided chemotherapy").

Spiritual or faith healing. This ranges from the laying on of hands to New Age crystal healing and psychic surgery.

A Different Picture

The consensus used to be that survivors turned to unconventional treatments when standard medical treatment had become ineffective in controlling their disease. Medical scientists also felt that people who sought such treatments were rare and somehow marginal—at the most, emotionally immature and lacking in courage; at the least, poorly educated and at the end of their ropes.

Now we are beginning to see a different picture: the use of treatments varies in different parts of the country, but most are common. Many mainstream patients, with college degrees, are trying them (and, if one does not work, shopping around for another). A study of a national sample of 1,000 patients with cancer, done at the University of Pennsylvania Cancer Center in the early 1980s by a group headed by Barrie R. Cassileth, Ph.D., and considered seminal by experts in the field, reports that these "new survivors" are as likely to try the treatments at early as at later stages of their illness (Cassileth et al., "Contemporary Unorthodox Treatments in Cancer Medicine," *Annals of Internal Medicine* 101 [1984]: 105–12).

But it is still true that many survivors, dissatisfied with the cool, detached doctors or clinical groups providing their care, are attracted by unconventional treatments and what seems to be the warmer, more caring world of unconventional treatment.

This is a world of clinics and individual practitioners and sometimes just homes and health-food stores, where herbal teas sit on coffee tables, acupuncture charts adorn the walls, first names and tapes (for relaxation, for sleep, for nervous stomachs) prevail, and the talk is of such remedies as biofeedback, megavitamins, or therapeutic touch. It's a world that can be found both in the United States and outside of it (especially south of the border, in places like Tijuana, Mexico). Finding a treatment in the United States does not guarantee its credibility.

Mixing the Conventional and the Unconventional

Exactly how many cancer patients took unconventional treatments in the United States at the end of the 1980s is not clear; there are no hard data. Estimates range from a low of 15 to a high of 30 or 40 percent; the difference probably reflects how treatment is defined. The Food and Drug Administration's low 15 percent estimate of patients taking "questionable" therapies, for example, classified products as "scientifically acceptable" only if there was a body of scientific evidence to support their effectiveness; the higher estimates may include patients taking nonmainstream treatments that are more loosely defined (Louis Harris and Associates, *Health, Information, and the Use of Questionable Treatments: A Study of the American Public* [Washington, D.C.: Food and Drug Administration, U.S. Department of Health and Human Services, 1987]).

Of particular interest is the fact that unconventional treatments are now used in combination with conventional treatment (surgery, radiation, chemotherapy, and hormone therapy) more than half of the time (Cassileth et al.).

And more of these treatments claim to target not just a specific disease but the body's ability to fight all diseases, and thus to stave off cancer. Generally, patients used to seek out an unconventional treatment directed toward their cancer—like the Hoxsey herbal tonic and paste treatments, the Revici method (a complex chemical formula), Krebiozen (an injection of material derived from horse serum), and of course laetrile (the famed apricot-pit derivative discredited after scientific clinical trials in the 1970s, and much less popular since then).

Krebiozen is no longer in the picture, but the others, in combination with some of the most popular treatments (with vitamins, for instance, or special diets), are used to stimulate the immune system to fight cancer. Some, like Burzynski's "antineoplaston" treatment and Burton's "immuno-augmentative treatment" in the Bahamas, try to attach themselves to the medical model, in that each is a "medicine" or an "antimedicine" for patients to take, though scientific proof of its efficacy is lacking.

Unconventional Issues

Serious questions confront you as a consumer-survivor when you consider unconventional treatments.

1. Most important is *how* you are thinking of using this treatment. If you are going to remain in conventional treatment, under the care of an oncologist, and simply use the treatment as an addition, your chief worry is whether, taken in large doses (certain vitamins, for example, could *make* cells grow), it could be harmful or could interfere with your conventional treatment. But if you are thinking of quitting your conventional treatment, and of pursuing the unconventional treatment as an *alternative* to it, that is quite a different story.

Michael Lerner, Ph.D., president of Commonweal, in Marin County, California, and an advocate of what he calls "complementary" cancer treatments, has reviewed over 30 major unconventional treatments and interviewed several hundred practitioners and over 1,000 patients in an eight-year period (Michael Lerner, *Varieties of Integral Cancer Therapy*. [A Work in Progress]. Seventh edition, updated in February 1990, is available from Commonweal, P.O. Box 316, Bolinas, CA 94924, (415) 868-0970). He agrees with other experts that most of today's cancer patients are using unconventional therapy as an adjunct to conventional treatment. (A fairly common combined regimen of an educated cancer patient seeking to add to his or her medical therapy, he reports, might include gentle stretching [yoga or Tai Chi]; meditation; progressive deep relaxation; imagery; a wholesome balanced vegetarian diet; moderate nutritional supplementation; psychological counseling; spiritual support; and the use of traditional Chinese medicine, including both herbs and acupuncture.)

But there are patients—even some with probably curable cancers—who leave conventional treatment, turn to various unconventional treatments, and suffer setbacks. Indeed, they may suffer not only progression of their cancer, which might have been effectively checked by traditional treatment, but outright harm, ranging from the general weakness caused by a stringent diet, to mild infection resulting from the administration of treatments in unsanitary circumstances, to, in rare cases, outright toxic poisoning.

2. What are your expectations of the unconventional treatment you are considering? If you are expecting a miracle as a result of the therapy—if you think your tumor will melt away as you take it—you may be in for a disappointment. This is particularly true in the area of mind control; at this state of our knowledge, the exact connection between cortical function and immunological response in cancer is largely speculative. Although there are, as Memorial Sloan-Kettering's psychiatric chief Dr. Jimmie Holland puts it, "blips on the screen" reported in the literature that indicate psychological interventions might enhance the immune system, we simply have no hard knowledge now of what they might be, or if they ever make a difference, as far as your cancer is concerned.

If, on the other hand, you simply expect to "feel good" or at least feel better about yourself and your disease, to relax, to get rid of some of the pain and stress that can surround cancer treatment, you have a better chance for success.

Although he found no cure for cancer among the treatments he has followed, and little evidence on which to evaluate most of them, Michael Lerner reported anecdotal evidence that some patients do well while using them. But this might be because of the warmth and optimism of the unconventional caretakers, or simply because you feel better when you perceive that you are doing everything possible to fight your disease. When treatments—particularly mind-control treatments—seem to improve your outlook and mood, you are apt to conclude they work for you (see chapter 2). You may also come to expect too much of them—that they will affect your tumor as well as your quality of life.

3. A more subtle but equally confusing issue confronting survivors using unconventional treatments is that of guilt. Cancer patients, who may already feel severely punished, can feel more so if self-help therapists convince them that their disease is their *fault*. And they can feel more depressed still if the cancer progresses despite their efforts to contain it.

Unconventional mind-control theory is based on the idea that you can influence the course of your disease through psychological means. Long-term unremitting stress can depress the immune system, the argument goes; positive emotions strengthen the immune system, and a strengthened immune system makes the possibility of fighting off cancer and recovering from it (cause and cure) more likely. So if you do not succeed at whatever treatment you have chosen, you have not tried hard enough—you are at fault.

Prominent "psychoneuroimmunological" practitioners insist that they are not pointing the finger at cancer patients for causing or failing to cure their diseases. For example, former surgeon Dr. Bernie Siegel, author of *Love, Medicine & Miracles* and *Peace, Love & Healing*, says he is not blaming the patient when he writes, for example, that women who have unhappy love relationships are especially vulnerable to breast or cervical diseases; he is only trying to empower such patients with a will to resist and achieve a more realistic sense of participation in their treatment.

And Wellness Community leader Harold Benjamin, in his book *From Victim to Victor*, adds that a woman who refused to give up her "immune-depressive" behavior toward the partner who squeezed her out of her business, and subsequently died, should not have blamed herself as she did, because she "can't be to blame for failing to stop something from happening that she didn't know was happening." Nevertheless, the implication of self-blame remains strong in survivors who believe they are responsible for the course of their disease.

4. How much does your unconventional therapy cost? How much does it cost you?

The costs of conventional treatment are often not of primary importance to the insured patient. What is important is whether it will help you get well—or at least achieve a reasonable quality of life. With unconventional treatment, it is a different story. There's a good chance that health-insurance plans will not cover more than an entry office visit and routine blood and similar tests. You will have to pick up the tab even if you are adequately insured.

Therapy (which may include guided imagery) provided by a licensed psychiatrist, psychologist, or social worker is covered by some insurance plans. But the bills for unconventional treatment, which may run into many thousands of dollars, usually have to be picked up by survivors themselves. And they may be more ominous than anticipated, because practitioners reluctant to disclose details of their treatment are often specific about the manner in which you will have to pay, including the amount you have to pay up front. (For an idea of the possible size of unconventional treatment bills, see John M. Fink, *Third Opinion: An International Directory to Alternative Therapy Centers for the Treatment and Prevention of Cancer*, Garden City Park, N.Y.: Avery Publishing Group Inc., 1988.)

As far as costs to the whole community are concerned, the Louis Harris and Associates study for the Food and Drug Administration in 1987 estimated the cost of "questionable" cancer treatments at around $141 million a year. However, the survey authors noted that this projection underestimates the likely cost because, first, it does not take into account multiple product use by the same user, and, second, it assumed no individual spent more than $1,000 for a questionable product.

Suggestions for Survivors

In a co-bylined newspaper article ("Fighting Illness, the Mind Has Both Power and Limits," *Los Angeles Times*, October 3, 1985), University of Pennsylvania Cancer Center psychologist Barrie R. Cassileth and Norman Cousins, adjunct professor at the UCLA School of Medicine, bemoaned the fact that the public had placed them on opposite sides of the controversy over the relationship between emotions and health. In truth, said Cassileth (lead author of an article in the *New England Journal of Medicine* suggesting that positive attitudes had little value for patients with advanced high-risk malignant disease) and Cousins (famed author of *Anatomy of an Illness*, which promoted laughter as a metaphor for positive emotions in curing illness), they both feel emotions and health are closely related—in a complex way.

Negative emotions can have a deleterious effect on health and complicate medical treatment; not so well known is the connection between positive attitudes and the possible enhancement of the body's healing system, Cassileth and Cousins continued. This relationship is now the subject of study at a number of medical centers.

Until all the information is in, and while even renowned experts are forced to clarify and explain themselves, what do you, as a survivor, do? Until there are sure cures for cancer that preclude such arguments (there are no unproven treatments for diseases, like tuberculosis, with proven cures), how do you approach unconventional treatment?

Although there are no hard guidelines, here are some practical suggestions:

■ Be sure you understand your conventional treatment thoroughly (see chapter 1). Take time to gather as much information as you want and need about what your doctors expect surgery, radiation, chemotherapy, and/or hormone therapy to do for you. Understand your options. Weigh the costs and the benefits—the utility of each conventional treatment for the kind of person you are and for your life-style. Are you the sort of person who likes to take radical treatment, getting it over with as fast as possible? Or do you prefer longer-term, less risky treatment?

■ Find out at the very beginning whether any unconventional treatment you are considering can be used in addition to whatever conventional treatment you are undergoing. If the prospective practitioner will give it to you only if you leave conventional treatment, reconsider. Then, if you are still determined to have the treatment, find another practitioner—if there is one (some practitioners—e.g., Burton, Revici, and Burzynski—have a monopoly on their particular treatments).

■ Check out the unconventional practitioner's credentials, and under what conditions he or she practices. Some well-trained nurses, psychologists, and even physicians may give the kind of treatment you are looking for. And they may offer it under optimum professional conditions. Again, quite the opposite may be true.

Try to be objective when you search for

information. Avoid the double standard; if either conventional or unconventional practitioners are unlicensed, are missing degrees, or occupy dirty office space, you should question their competence.

■ Find out everything you can about the track record of any unconventional therapy—if there is such a track record. Normally one would look at the literature practitioners publish about treatment efficacy. Have patients taking it participated in controlled studies? What effect has it had on them? Have they lived longer? Enjoyed a better quality of life? When it comes to unconventional treatments, however, such literature may be nonexistent. And when you can find it, it may be full of unsubstantiated testimonials, claiming that the treatment is safe or effective, but unable to prove to you (through clinical-trial results, etc.) that this is so.

Nonetheless, call the clinic or practitioner and ask for all the available literature about the treatment you are considering. Try going to the library; look at the medical literature, and see if you can find anything written about its efficacy by experts who are not personally involved. There is a developing body of such material about mind-control therapies.

Ask the clinic or practitioner directly what the treatment consists of and what are its claims for your particular cancer, and what evidence supports them. Ask about both positive and negative effects.

If you are told the treatment is experimental, ask how it is being tested. Be cautious; you might believe a treatment is effective if you are told it is being used in a Food and Drug Administration (FDA)–approved clinical trial (i.e., treatment under an Investigational New Drug application process). But times are beginning to change, and the FDA has helped at least one unconventional practitioner get his treatment (which was not considered harmful) studied formally in a small trial for patients with advancing disease and no other options. At this stage, such a treatment would not generally be covered by health insurance.

If you want to call the Food and Drug Administration directly for information about drugs, call (301) 295-8012 (Legislative and Consumer Affairs Branch [HFD-365], Food and Drug Administration, 5600 Fishers Lane, Rockville, Maryland 20857). For information about biologic products, like vaccines or blood products, call (301) 443-7532 (Center for Biologics, Evaluation and Research, Food and Drug Administration, 5600 Fishers Lane [Room 158, Park Building], Rockville, Maryland 20857).

The American Cancer Society's brochure *Unproven Methods of Cancer* provides a brief history of unproven cancer treatments and a list of treatments considered to be so by the American Cancer Society. Additionally, the ACS offers brief policy statements (one to six pages) on individual types of treatment. The brochure and policy statements are available from your local ACS office or by calling 1-800-ACS-2345.

Another eagerly awaited resource is *Unconventional Cancer Treatments*, authored and published in 1990 by the United States Congress Office of Technology Assessment. This several-hundred-page report, the first detailed, dispassionate description of unconventional cancer treatments, is available for a small fee from the United States Superintendent of Documents at (202) 783-3238.

■ When you have answered all these questions to your satisfaction, ask yourself if you are comfortable with the treatment. Do not try something that does not seem to fit in with your style and values. For most of us, whether or not a treatment is offered within the borders of the United States is not as important as whether it is on the ACS's "unproven" list, or whether its practitioner has been sued in a nasty court case by a dissatisfied patient.

What can you do if you have zealously tried to find out about a treatment and have not been successful? Or if you have found conflicting information about it? Or if you have found information about the risks it entails but do not know how to evaluate such risks?

Here a good rapport with your doctor is like money in the bank. If you are able to sit down and talk openly with him or her, you will get valuable help in weighing possible risks and benefits of prospective treatments. Other people you trust in your medical setting—the chief nurse at the clinic, for example, or a very experienced survivor—may be able to give you good advice.

But doctors experienced with cancer patients are most qualified, not only to help you figure out risk-benefit questions (whether or not a coffee enema, for instance, will adversely affect the electrolytes in your body) but to monitor their effects if you do decide to try them.

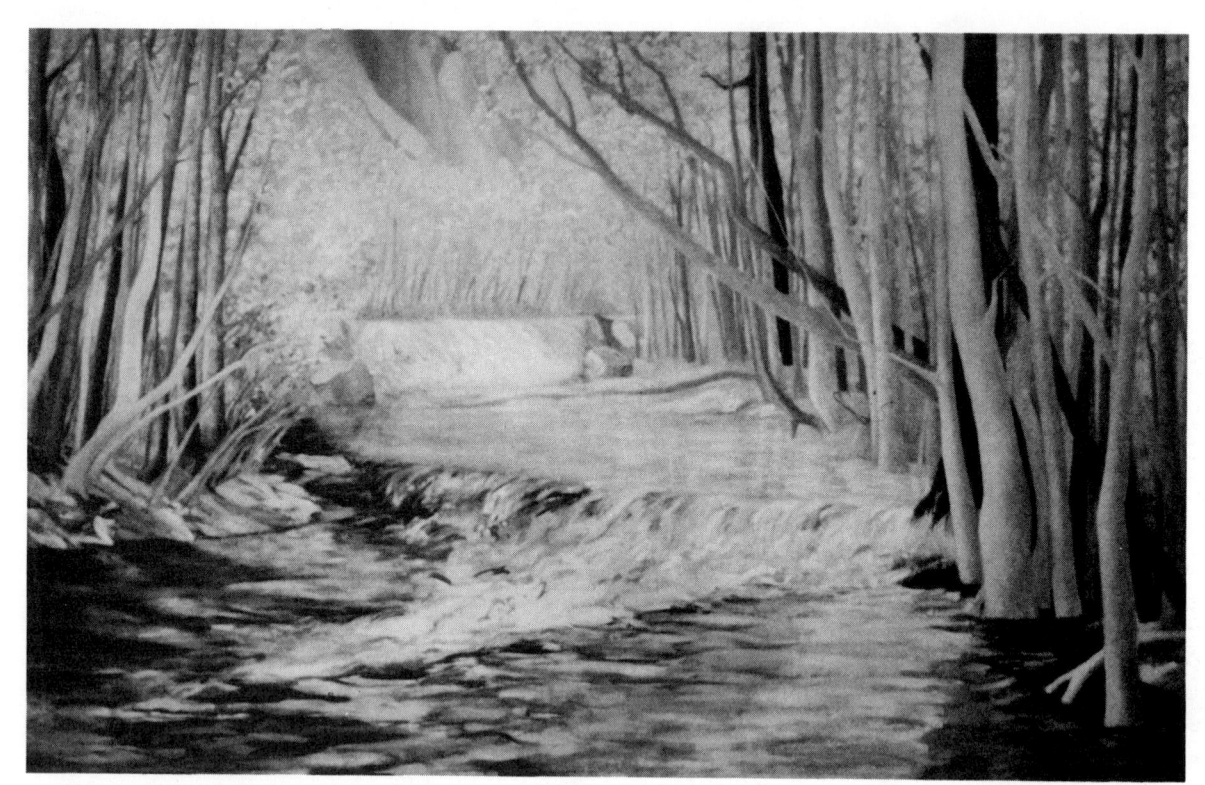

Ellin Chin James
McGee Creek #5
Oil on canvas
60″ x 96″

4

Helping Therapies and Support Services

Myra Glajchen, M.S.W., Ph.D.

Cancer can be a frightening, lonely experience. Coping with it involves more than medical management. It requires attention to your psychological, social, emotional, and practical needs as well. It is natural to experience intense anxiety around the time of diagnosis and treatment, but this distress sometimes becomes overwhelming. When this occurs, it may be time to reach outside your family and social circle for assistance. There are a number of therapists and other professionals who can help you respond to the psychosocial impact of cancer.

Medical and mental-health professionals are available in the hospital and in the community. They are trained to help the cancer survivor's transition from the hospital back to the home. Survivors, family members, and professionals can work together to prevent problems from developing, or to resolve problems as they arise. But in order to select the appropriate professional to deal with your unique set of problems, you need to understand what each has to offer and where services can be obtained.

The Roles of Helping Professionals

The Physician

The primary physician is in charge of coordinating your treatment plan. This doctor will direct your medical care through the diagnosis of cancer and help you evaluate and choose the course of treatment. Any one of the specialists listed below could act as the primary physician, including your family doctor. Because cancer requires a multidisciplinary approach, a team of physicians will generally become involved in diagnosing and treating the disease.

The diagnosis is usually made by one of several physicians—your family doctor, an oncologist, a pathologist, or a surgeon. Treatment can then be administered by one or many physicians. A medical oncologist is a board-certified physician who specializes in treating cancer with chemotherapy. If

> "I think that each person who has cancer or any other life-threatening illness needs to find a sensitive, safe, and nonjudgmental listener—a counselor of some sort who can guide the patient through the tough spots."
>
> —Robert M. Mack, M.D., *New England Journal of Medicine*

surgery is indicated, you will be referred to a surgeon to perform the procedure. A hematologist is a medical specialist who has concentrated on treating cancers of the blood, such as leukemia. For radiation therapy, you will be referred to a radiation oncologist.

Most newly diagnosed people with cancer begin treatment at a cancer center or a large university hospital or medical center. Once the treatment plan is under way, chemotherapy and radiation can be administered in smaller community hospitals or in a doctor's office close to home.

If your treatment begins in a hospital, you may be seen by physicians at various stages of their training. The "attending physician" is a fully qualified specialist who assumes responsibility for your medical care. The "fellow" has completed his or her training as a physician and has chosen to specialize in treating cancer. Recent medical-school graduates are called "residents" (in the second, third, or final year of training) or "interns" (in the first year of post-medical-school training). You may also be observed by medical-school students. If you receive contradictory or confusing information from different doctors, talk to the attending physician in charge of your case.

The Nurse

The nurse plays a vital role as part of the health-care team. Nurses are educated to provide nursing care as well as additional explanation of medical facts. They are responsible for initiating the plan of care ordered by your physician, and are educated to administer medications and to monitor their side effects. You may encounter different types of nurses during the course of your hospital stay and treatment. A registered nurse (R.N.) has received longer and more specialized education than a licensed practical nurse (L.P.N.) or licensed vocational nurse (L.V.N.). Nurse specialists are educated in oncology, chemotherapy, and radiation.

Many medical services can be provided in the home by visiting nurses under the direction of your physician. Homemaker and home-health-aide assistance are also available in most communities. In order to find out more about these services, contact the home-care department or discharge-planning unit in your hospital. Some hospitals offer home care on a short-term basis as part of your treatment plan, and these services may be covered by your medical insurance. Alternately, you can pay for the services of a nurse, home health aide, or homemaker on an hourly fee-for-service basis.

Counselors

Cancer represents a crisis of major proportions for even the strongest of families, and it is sometimes helpful to speak to a professional in order to deal with the practical, emotional, and psychological problems that often arise. "Counseling" is a general term describing help and advice offered by professionals dealing with concerns related to your cancer experience.

Psychotherapy is a type of counseling that focuses on deep-seated personality issues as well as the crisis at hand and can be long-term in nature. Counseling can be provided by a variety of health-care professionals, including a psychiatrist, a psychologist, or a social worker. Each of these professionals has received a different kind of training. Psychiatrists receive medical training, psychologists are trained in counseling as well as psychometric testing, and social workers are trained in counseling and practical assistance. During the early phases of diagnosis and treatment, you may want to select a counselor with expertise in dealing with cancer-related issues. Later, if you decide to remain in counseling to work on longer-term issues, it will be more important to select the expert whose approach best meets your deeper, more clearly defined needs.

The social worker. The medical social worker is specially trained to provide counseling and practical assistance to meet your specific needs. Some social workers have chosen to specialize further in dealing with the unique issues that arise when a person has cancer. During individual counseling, you can discuss your fears and questions related to diagnosis, treatment, side effects, and the impact of these procedures on your life as a whole. Counseling can help you and your family overcome communication problems and tension within the family, and help you put things into perspective so you can make appropriate decisions.

In addition to counseling, social workers are trained to provide practical assistance with home care, transportation, child care, and financial planning. You can request that your doctor or nurse refer you to a social worker while you are in the hospital. The service is often provided free as a part of your treatment plan. When you leave the hospital, you can see a social worker on an outpatient basis at the hospital, through a social-service agency, or in private practice.

Psychiatrists and psychologists. Psychiatrists are physicians trained to provide psychotherapy and prescribe medication. It is natural to experience intense anxiety when faced with the diagnosis of cancer, but this distress sometimes becomes overwhelming and uncontrollable. The psychiatrist can prescribe medication if problems such as depression and sleep disturbances become overpowering. The psychiatrist can also provide counseling to help you deal with the psychological and emotional issues that may arise as a result of your illness. Some psychiatrists are also trained in hypnosis, behavioral intervention, and relaxation techniques that can help reduce and manage anxiety. You can ask to see a psychiatrist through your hospital or through your primary physician.

Psychologists are also trained to provide professional counseling, but they are not physicians and do not prescribe medication. In addition to training in formal psychological testing, many specialize in areas such as marital counseling, sex therapy, or relaxation techniques. Referrals are available through your physician or hospital.

Additional Professional Assistance

There are a number of other hospital- and community-based professionals who play important roles in the care of cancer survivors. Physical therapists are available to assist individuals who have been bedridden or inactive for extended periods in regaining strength and mobility. They can also design specific exercise and range-of-motion programs for long-term rehabilitation. Occupational therapists evaluate an individual's ability to perform the routine activities of daily living and design programs of assistance and retraining where necessary. Speech therapists work with speech impediments, and teach techniques of chewing and swallowing for survivors who have had treatments to the head and neck. Nutritionists and dieticians are available to provide instruction and planning for survivors with special dietary needs. These professionals are on staff at most hospitals and are available to you on referral from your doctor.

Additionally, most cancer centers and larger hospitals have a chaplain on call. These men and women can be of great help to survivors and their families in times of crisis, and can provide links and referrals to ministers, priests, and rabbis in the community.

Which Professional Should I Call?

Depression

Most cancer survivors experience some sadness during their illness, but a few develop severe depression, which is not alleviated by talking things over with family, friends, and the health-care team. Such depression is unlikely to resolve itself spontaneously. In these instances the intervention of a psychiatrist may be warranted.

Common signs of severe depression include:

- loss of appetite (leading to weight loss)
- increase in appetite (leading to weight gain)
- sleep disturbances (insomnia or too much sleep)
- prolonged feelings of sadness, despair, or anxiety
- suicidal thoughts
- inability to meet everyday responsibilities

Your doctor, nurse, or social worker can refer you to a psychiatrist at the hospital, at a mental-health clinic, or in private practice. Most medical insurance will cover at least part of this medical expense. Depending upon the source of the depression, treatment may consist of antidepressant medication, psychotherapy, or a combination of both methods. Seeking the services of a psychiatrist does not mean you are either weak or going crazy. Depression in the face of a life-threatening illness is not the fault of the person with cancer, and may develop for medical—as well as psychological—reasons. The cumulative physiological effects of chemotherapy and radiation can sometimes produce depression. A psychiatrist will evaluate the cause of the depression and recommend an approach to its treatment. Whereas any trained psychotherapist can help you deal with depression, only a psychiatrist is licensed to prescribe medication should this be deemed necessary.

Home Care

Home care is another practical need experienced by cancer survivors who are weak as a result of the illness and its treatment. It is natural to feel somewhat anxious about leaving the security of the hospital team to go home, although people report feeling much better as soon as they are back in their own environment. Before you are discharged from the hospital, it is advisable to review your plan of care with your doctor. He or she can tell you what to expect in the way of side effects from your medication and limitations due to physical weakness, as well as physical problems to anticipate and what to do about them.

The hospital social worker can tell you about home-care services available in your area, some of which may be covered by medical insurance. If necessary, you can have a skilled nurse, a trained home health aide, a physical therapist, a dietician, or a social worker visit you in your home. If you have nonskilled-nursing needs, you may request a home health aide or homemaker to help you with the activities of daily living. These nonskilled services are generally not covered by medical insurance, and must be paid for on a fee-for-service basis. You can also obtain hospital equipment at home, such as a hospital bed, side rails, and a wheelchair.

If you are recovering from surgery, grab bars in the tub, a tub seat, a bedpan, a commode, and an elevated toilet seat are available. This equipment can be obtained through the hospital, your doctor, a nurse, or a social worker. If you need equipment once you are at home, you can find resources listed in the Yellow Pages of your telephone book under "Hospital Equipment and Supplies" or "Pharmacies." Such supplies can be purchased or rented, and are covered by some health-insurance policies.

"Community resources" generally refers to a variety of agencies managed by local groups, churches, synagogues, or voluntary agencies to serve people's needs within their home communities. The hospital social worker or the home-care coordinator can put you in touch with the local community resources in your area. See Appendix A for a list of national resources.

Dealing with Marital and Sexual Problems

A diagnosis of cancer may result in the development of new strains in close relationships or, alternatively, long-standing problems may surface as a result of the stress of having to deal with cancer. Communication patterns can break down if each person tries to withhold fears and worries in an effort to protect the other. Family members may try to project a cheerful attitude for the benefit of the person with cancer, but this approach may make it more difficult for the patient to express his or her needs. Shifts in family responsibilities may occur if one partner is temporarily unable to meet his or her usual obligations. For a spouse suddenly faced with child care, homework, shopping, cooking, laundry, the finances, or decision making, a change in roles can create a great deal of anxiety and resentment.

Many of these problems will be temporary, and the relationship will return to normal once the acute phase of the diagnosis and treatment are over. You and your partner may try to resolve matters through open communication and discussion. But if the difficulties persist, you may decide to seek assistance. Couples therapy, offered by psychiatrists, psychologists, or social workers, can be very helpful in this process. If specific sexual problems are involved, you may want to locate a therapist specializing in sex therapy.

Nutrition

Loss of appetite is a common complaint among cancer survivors. This can occur as a result of the illness, treatment, pain, fatigue, stress, or depression. Taste sensations can change as a result of medication or radiation treatment, which can also lead to a dry or sore mouth. Constipation, diarrhea, bloating, and heartburn are other unwanted side effects associated with treatment that may interfere with digestion. Whatever symptoms you experience, discuss them with your doctor and your nurse. There is generally a simple explanation for each of your symptoms and a way to remedy the problem.

Your doctor or nurse can refer you to a registered dietician early in your treatment. A dietician can suggest food substitutes if your tastes change and you are able to tolerate certain foods better than others. He or she can help you plan a diet suited to your tastes, life-style, and individual needs, and make useful suggestions about food preparation by providing you with educational booklets and cookbooks specifically written for the person undergoing treatment for cancer. The effects of cancer treatment may require you to build adequate amounts of protein, calories, vitamins, and minerals into your daily food intake. In addition, your doctor can prescribe antinausea medication, which will help you stay on your diet.

Spiritual Guidance

Serious illness can lead to questions about the meaning of life as well as questions such as "Why me?" and "Why now?" A cancer survivor may want to explore these concerns with a member of the clergy at any time before, during, or after treatment. It is natural to reconsider your life-style and value system when facing a life-threatening situation. Prayer can be used as a means of providing hope and comfort. Spiritual counseling can help you find renewed meaning in life during a time of disappointment and despair. A compassionate member of the clergy who is trained to provide support through life's major crises can be a valuable asset during this time of upheaval and uncertainty. You can ask your nurse for a referral to the hospital chaplain, or locate a chaplain in your own community.

If Treatment Fails

Today many people facing a diagnosis of cancer can look forward to a lengthy remission or a full recovery, but treatment is not always successful. Hospice services have been established to provide support and care for people in the final stages of a terminal illness so that they can live as fully and comfortably as possible. The hospice philosophy regards dying as a normal process, and stresses a coordinated team approach as well as effective pain control.

Hospice care is generally provided in the patient's home, with inpatient admission being arranged as needed. The hospice team—doctor, nurse, social worker, volunteer, and chaplain—works in conjunction with the patient's family, to educate them in caring for the patient by giving medication, changing dressings, and performing other simple medical tasks. Regular visits from the hospice nurse and other members of the hospice team provide relief and support to the family caring for the patient at home.

Hospice care is appropriate when cancer treatment has proved ineffective and the patient's life expectancy is limited to a few months. But the hospice approach is not suitable for everyone. Bearing the responsibility for the cancer patient's medical care in the terminal stages of an illness can be financially and emotionally exhausting for a family with strained resources. Also, some people with cancer prefer to pursue aggressive treatment approaches until the end of life, and to keep fighting as long as possible.

If you are considering hospice care, discuss a referral with your primary physician. Hospice programs may be hospital-based, community-based, or offered through a visiting-nurse service in your neighborhood.

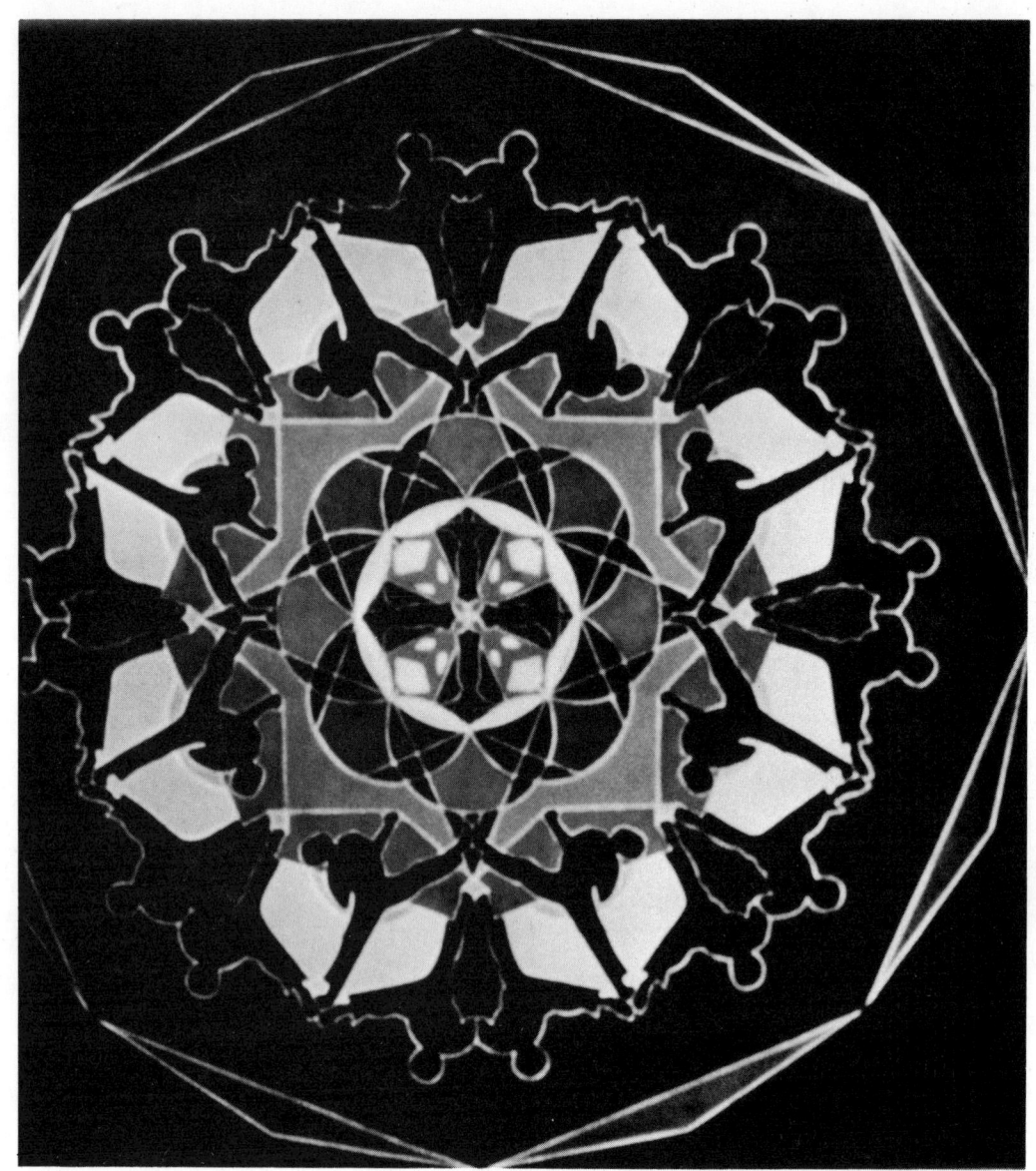

Betty Boltuch
Karate
Oil on canvas
50″ x 50″

5

Survivors Helping Survivors: Peer-Support Networking

Annette Jolles, M.S.W., L.C.S.W.;
Barbara Hoffman, J.D.; and Catherine Logan

Peer-Support Networking

Millions of cancer survivors now enjoy an opportunity for quality living. Survival is no longer measured in the black-and-white terms of death or cure, but in a spectrum of colors that acknowledges the brightness of special moments as well as the darkness of difficult times. Many cancer survivors are now emerging from their experiences to support and encourage one another, and to empower themselves to survive. Everyone who becomes involved in a battle with cancer—whether patient, family, friend, or care giver—learns from living through the cancer experience. These survival experiences create a wealth of information that can assist millions of others who are subsequently confronted with cancer.

Survivors have always provided some level of support for one another. In the past several decades, this support has become more organized, growing from a private moment between friends, to small support groups and community organizations, to national organizations of tens of thousands of constituents. By the 1980s, the needs of a growing population of survivors fueled the growth of a cancer survivorship movement to ensure that the social and emotional as well as the medical concerns of cancer survivors were addressed.

How Peer-Support Networking Can Serve You

Depending upon where you live and receive treatment, you may or may not be offered professional resources for emotional support and counseling. Within the survivorship network, however, experienced help is always available.

Support from professionals and support from experienced cancer survivors are not mutually exclusive. They can offer a flexible combination of valuable aid. In recent years, survivors, often with the aid of professionals, have worked together to create resources designed to lighten the burden of a

> "Self-help organizations are an effective way of dealing with problems, stress, hardship and pain."
>
> —C. Everett Koop, M.D., former United States Public Health Service Surgeon General

cancer experience. Peer-support resources address a wide variety of survivorship concerns, including:

1. Treatment issues
- side effects of treatment
- unconventional treatments
- effective use of medical resources
- relationships with health professionals

2. Social, emotional, and economic issues
- the emotional impact of diagnosis
- "Why me?" questions
- family and social relationships
- depression
- death and dying
- change in personal perspective
- financial, insurance, and employment issues

3. Physical-health issues
- recurrence and fear of recurrence
- questions about the effects of attitude on physical health
- changes in physical appearance and ability
- sexuality
- diet and nutrition

Networking arises from the desire to resolve the isolating effects of cancer. Cancer survivors may isolate themselves because of their own altered perceptions and emotional stress, or may allow themselves to be isolated by the fears and discomfort of others.

Even for survivors who have very supportive families and friends, relationships can be strained and uncomfortable. Reaching out to other survivors can alleviate much of that isolation.

A Brief History of the Cancer Survivorship Movement

Cancer is but one of many experiences that give rise to mutual-aid networks. Historically, individuals who have shared financial, political, social, medical, religious, and other mutual concerns have worked together to create resources to meet their needs. Alcoholics Anonymous is one of the oldest and most established of these peer groups.

The United Ostomy Association is another mutual-aid organization with a long and effective history. In February 1949, five people who had ostomies (surgery to construct an artificial opening in response to colon cancer and other illnesses) met in Philadelphia to share their experiences and knowledge. By 1988, the United Ostomy Association represented 672 chapters in the United States. The association in turn joined the International Ostomy Association, founded in 1975, which represents more than 40 countries.

Although many of the United Ostomy Association's members have ostomies because of cancer surgery, the primary focus of the organization is on the common experience of living with an ostomy. Other peer-support organizations, which concentrated exclusively on cancer issues, began to evolve in the early 1970s. Two of the oldest organizations are Make Today Count and the Candlelighters Childhood Cancer Foundation.

Make Today Count was founded by Orville Kelly in 1974 as a support organization to address the emotional needs of people with cancer and other life-threatening illnesses. It is one of the largest cancer-sup-

> "I was going to say that it's not a journey for the weak—but that's precisely who it is for. It's for the weakness we all feel, for the protection and admission of that weakness. We are here to borrow from each other's strength, for strength is a natural resource we know we *must* share if the great ecosystem is to right itself. We are learning not to hoard ourselves—and discover abundance in the process. We take some of that surplus back with us, to our private ecosystems of health, home, work, and family."
>
> —Joe Kogel

port organizations in the country, providing practical information and emotional support to both survivors and their families. In addition to support groups, Make Today Count provides printed materials. Some chapters also have home-visitation programs and offer advice on how to obtain disability insurance and other benefits.

In April 1970, parents of children who had cancer founded the Candlelighters Childhood Cancer Foundation to address the needs of their families. By 1990, Candlelighters had grown to an international network of more than 200 chapters. On the local level, Candlelighters chapters provide an informal forum where families share experiences and information about caring for the needs of a childhood-cancer survivor and other family members. On a national level, the organization serves as a clearinghouse for information about childhood cancer, develops resources to address their members' concerns, produces comprehensive publications, fights for adequate funding for medical research in pediatric oncology, and advocates for the legal, economic, and social rights of childhood-cancer survivors.

Cancer-related mutual-aid organizations provide support *from* cancer survivors and their families *to* survivors and their families. However, many cancer organizations that offer education, rehabilitation, and psychosocial services have both a professional and a peer-support component. The largest of these organizations is the American Cancer Society.

The American Cancer Society was formed in 1945 from the Society for the Control of Cancer (a group founded in 1913) to disseminate knowledge concerning the symptoms, treatment, and prevention of cancer. In its first three decades, the organization focused primarily on cancer research. In 1944, however, the society began to train lay volunteers to provide information and emotional support to survivors and their families. Additionally, the society began to provide services such as donated medical supplies and transportation to treatment. Over the years, the American Cancer Society has expanded both its professional and its peer-support programs. By 1990, the society had over 2 million health-professional and lay volunteers, many of whom were cancer survivors.

The national office of the American Cancer Society in Atlanta, Georgia, administers the research program, distributes medical grants, and coordinates the work of 58 state divisions. Within each state, the society has local units, which are usually organized by county. Although most people associate the ACS with its comprehensive public and

> "My first meeting with a peer-support group of cancer patients was in a radiologist's office in downtown Washington, D.C., in the 1940s. I was in grade school, the eldest child in my family, and was given the responsibility of accompanying my aunt to her daily treatments. My aunt was a young woman—considered somewhat radical and a bit too outspoken and liberated for her time. Before her illness she had a job which had required traveling around the country often by airplane. How I loved her stories of people she met, her adventures, and the souvenirs from places I knew from pictures in my geography book. Her cancer changed everything. There wasn't much treatment for cancer in the 1940s. There certainly wasn't an acknowledgment that quality living was part of dealing with terminal disease. People died of 'a long illness' the name of which was kept secret from the 'victim' by concerned physicians and loving relatives.
>
> "The place for respite, the sanctuary for patients and their families, became the waiting room of the radiologist's office. I'm sure that everybody knew, on some level, why they were there. I cannot recall the mention of the word 'cancer,' but I can recall people exchanging ideas about dealing with their problems about appetite, weight changes, pain, and discomfort just getting around. Most of all, I remember people laughing, talking about things they enjoyed—music, politics, travel, their jobs, their families. They could feel better by making each other feel better."
>
> —Annette Jolles, oncology social worker

professional education services, the society does operate a number of mutual-aid programs. Some of these programs founded by American Cancer Society volunteers, while others were begun in the community and later became affiliated with the society. Three of its best-known programs are Reach to Recovery, I Can Cope, and CanSurmount.

Reach to Recovery was started in 1952 by Terese Lasser, a New Yorker who had undergone a mastectomy. Ms. Lasser founded Reach to Recovery to provide emotional support and rehabilitation counseling to women who had mastectomies. Reach to Recovery now provides the first step to rehabilitation peer support to women who have had any type of surgery for breast cancer and to their families. Services focus on hospital or home visits after surgery by veteran survivors, literature about breast surgery, and a temporary breast form.

I Can Cope was created in 1978 as a research project at North Memorial Hospital in Minneapolis by two oncology nurses, Judi Johnson and Pat Norby. This professionally

> ## QT Alumni
>
> In 1950, Mount Sinai Hospital in New York City had two wards, Q and T, for patients recovering from life-saving ileostomy surgery. Although surgeons had lately learned how to perform ileostomies successfully, living with them was quite another matter. People living with ileostomies faced a lack of adequate appliances to collect bodily waste and to prevent its corrosive nature from injuring the skin around the ileostomy. Not content to live with appliances that leaked and fell off, patients on both wards began to share ideas about how to improve their quality of life.
>
> Once they returned to their homes, QT Alumni and ostomy patients from other cities kept in touch. Driven by a need to create better appliances, some group members made models of improved appliances in their garages. They shared their discoveries with others as their ideas developed from drawing-board sketches to effective appliances. The QT Alumni were pioneer survivors who had in common practical adversity and, sometimes, social isolation. The drive to find practical solutions to mutual problems led to the first peer-support network for people with ostomies, and laid the foundation for the development of other health-oriented mutual-aid organizations.

designed educational program is divided into eight sessions to help people find a balance between fatalistic acceptance of, and unrealistic resistance to, their disease, and to help them regain control of their lives.

CanSurmount was founded in 1974 by a Denver oncologist, Paul K. Hamilton, and one of his patients, Lynn Ringer, to help survivors deal with their turbulent thoughts and feelings. CanSurmount is a one-on-one, veteran-to-newcomer support program usually based in a hospital setting. Most often a CanSurmount coordinator within the hospital arranges for a trained volunteer to visit someone who has just undergone cancer surgery. The contact is limited to six visits and must be done at the request of a physician.

Current Status of Peer Support

Although cancer survivors have always exchanged mutual aid, the peer-support movement first began to gather national momentum in the 1980s, because more people could look forward to longer, productive lives.

The stigma of cancer has gradually begun to wane and the interest in self-care health maintenance has blossomed. The expanding interest in cancer support and mutual aid has resulted in the development of a diverse and rich variety of groups and survivor networks.

Yet, with all of this development, prior to 1986 no means or structure existed to encourage communication between people involved in survivorship activities or to coordinate the newly evolving groups, activities, and educational materials. As a result, limited resources were quickly consumed, and useful ideas failed to reach the majority of survivors. The National Coalition for Cancer Survivorship was founded to meet these needs.

Because there are 6 million cancer survivors in the United States, and therefore 6 million different cancer experiences, the survivorship movement reflects a wide variety of resources created to address the diversified needs of survivors. By recognizing that cancer survivors' concerns are best addressed by the availability of both mutual aid and professional support, NCCS promotes the growth of a broad spectrum of services from which different survivors can draw support.

The Many Faces of Survivorship Networking

Cancer-related peer-support groups are organized in several different ways. Some are small, local units, often associated with a large organization or a medical institution. Many are neighborhood cancer-support groups that meet in homes, churches, or medical centers. Others have evolved into independent nonprofit organizations with a variety of support and educational services. Health professionals play leadership roles in some groups, while other groups provide exclusively peer support. Services may be organized by type of cancer, age of survivor, and/or type of service. Here are some examples:

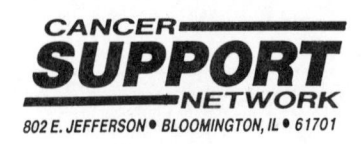

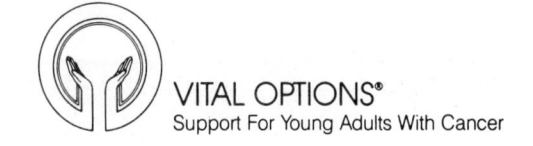

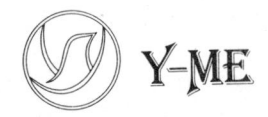

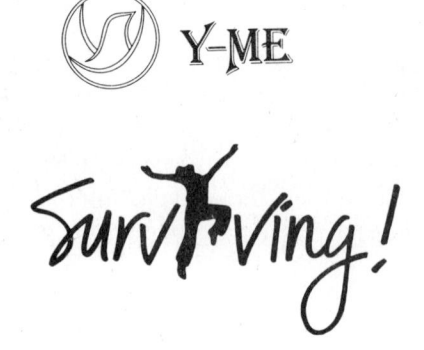

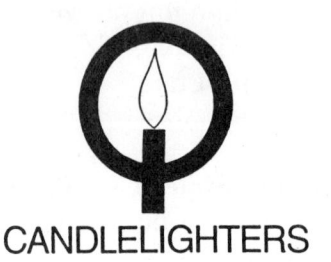

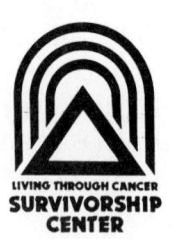

Examples of organizations offering peer support for cancer survivors: Cancer Lifeline, Seattle, Washington; Vital Options, Studio City, California; Living Through Cancer Survivorship Center, Albuquerque, New Mexico; Candlelighters Childhood Cancer Foundation, national; Surviving!, Stanford University Hospital, Palo Alto, California; Y-ME National Organization for Breast Cancer Information & Support, national; Cancer Support Network, Bloomington, Illinois.

Vital Options is a nonprofit organization in southern California for young-adult survivors that operates on a local level. It was founded in 1984 by Selma Schimmel when she was undergoing treatment for breast cancer at the age of 28. Looking for mutual aid, she attended a cancer-support group, but found herself to be the youngest person in the room by 20 years. Ms. Schimmel founded Vital Options to provide a forum for young survivors whose concerns (education, career choices, dating, fertility, etc.) are often different from those of older survivors. In the beginning, Vital Options met in a social hall donated by a Los Angeles–area synagogue. By December 1985, Vital Options had raised enough money to establish its own office. Four years later, the organization offered a number of weekly peer-support groups, each facilitated by a trained therapist. These groups are tailored for cancer survivors between the ages of 17 and 40.

Y-ME is an example of a peer-support organization that offers national services and has established chapters in several states. In 1978, Y-ME was founded by Mimi Kaplan and Ann Marcou in an effort to meet with other women who had undergone breast-cancer treatment, as they had. Twelve women met at the YWCA in Park Forest, Illinois, as Y-ME's first support group. The following year, Y-ME established a 24-hour hotline, at first offering local help and then expanding to a national service in 1987. By 1989, Y-ME had chapters in Illinois, Connecticut, Florida, and the District of Columbia, which help breast-cancer survivors cope with their illness and address the concerns of their care givers, families, and friends. Although Y-ME does not directly organize breast-cancer support groups, it does provide support and technical assistance to those who want to start such groups. In July 1989, Y-ME published a manual containing guidelines for establishing cancer-support programs that is appropriate for breast cancer and other health-oriented peer support groups. In addition, Y-ME offers public-education programs, an annual conference on breast cancer, and a national newsletter.

Some self-help organizations operate primarily as telephone hotlines, providing two services: information and emotional support. Depending on the resources of the hotline, callers who seek information have their questions answered over the telephone, are sent publications, and are referred to other agencies. A caller who seeks emotional support and practical suggestions drawn from personal experience is matched with another cancer survivor, usually a "veteran" with a diagnosis similar to that of the caller. Typically, hotlines are staffed by trained volunteers who are cancer survivors or family members. Most provide services on a local rather than a national basis.

How Peer Support Differs from Professional Counseling

Peer support is a process of sharing emotional support and practical information learned through personal experience. Peer support and professional counseling are often complementary, and many cancer survivors benefit from both. Professional counseling and peer support differ, however, in a number of important ways.

Peer-support groups are member-owned and -operated. They develop their structure exclusively to address their own needs. Mutual-aid groups offer emotional support, education, skills development, advocacy, social opportunities, crisis intervention, and role modeling. They enhance self-esteem through common experience.

The goal of professional psychotherapy and counseling is to help patients who feel severely disturbed by their disease. Therapeutic efforts are directed to the interaction between an individual or group "client" and a professional listener. Effective professional therapy for cancer survivors provides comfort, support, and skills to cope with the impact of cancer outside of the therapeutic relationship. Psychotherapy is a "fee for service" from a trained professional.

Although there are traditional distinctions between peer support and professional therapy, there is a growing number of groups facilitated by professionals that encourage and nurture peer support.

> "I needed to find someone immediately who knew my terror; someone I could talk with on a personal—rather than clinical—level; someone who had 'been there.' I needed to find a survivor."
>
> —Janet Morrison, lymphatic-cancer survivor, *Washington Post*, March 9, 1983

Finding Peer Support

For some people, reaching out to others who have faced similar experiences is a natural response to a physical and emotional challenge. For others, self-reliance is the most comfortable response. Peer-support resources can benefit both types of survivors by providing individually tailored services.

There is no single right or wrong way to respond to the impact of cancer. Outreach of any kind, however, helps to demystify cancer and fight its isolating effects. The survivorship movement has developed a diversity of peer-support resources that offer a variety of approaches to dealing with cancer.

Taking the First Steps

If you want to explore the possible benefits of mutual aid but are dealing with your own reluctance to reach out, you may want to start by gathering information. The telephone can be a nonthreatening and effective way to reach out in privacy. You may begin by calling cancer hotlines, community support organizations, and public agencies for answers to your questions. This telephone contact can help you practice talking to others about cancer and its effect on your life.

At some point, you may want to meet face to face either with another survivor or with a group. Some survivors look for peer support shortly after they are diagnosed. More commonly, survivors reach out during or shortly after cancer treatment. Other survivors may wait weeks, months, or even years after treatment to share their experiences. The emotional impact of cancer may be felt for the rest of your life, and support can be sought as the need arises, not according to a fixed timetable.

Reaching out for peer support is a personal decision. No one else can decide when or if you should do so. Some people believe that peer-support groups provide no benefits because they think that cancer survivors are "not knowledgeable enough," "too emotional," or "not responsible enough" to manage without professional leadership. But the history of the survivorship movement, the growth of cancer-support groups, and the current endorsements of peer support by health professionals confirm that mutual aid can enhance the quality of life for most survivors.

How to Learn What Exists in Your Community

The next step in deciding whether peer support is right for you is to learn what is available in your community. Appendix A lists national organizations that can help you in your search, including their telephone numbers. Survivors may also try the following:

- Call the social-work department of your hospital.

- Call the national resource centers such as the National Cancer Institute, American Cancer Society, and National Coalition for Cancer Survivorship.
- Call the self-help clearinghouse in your area.
- If you are seeing a professional counselor, ask him or her for referral to a mutual-aid group.
- Look in the telephone directory, in the Yellow Pages under "Social Service Organizations" and in the white pages under "Cancer."
- Look in the community section of your local newspaper. Many now publish a weekly list of community support groups.
- Call or write to any organizations that may lead you to other resources. (Because many nonprofit networks have limited funds, including a stamped self-addressed envelope with your letter is helpful and speeds replies.)

Once you gather this information, you may change your mind and decide not to contact a support group. Such reluctance is quite common. If you are not ready to share your experience, keep the information you have collected for possible future use. At some later time, perhaps when you are no longer in treatment or your family no longer provides sufficient support, you may want to look into these resources for yourself or a loved one.

How to Assess What Is Right for You

Before you become a part of any survivorship community, ask yourself how you feel about discussing your cancer with others and how much energy you want to invest. If you feel you are ready for a survivor group, the following guidelines may help you evaluate whether a particular group is right for you.

- Be sure you feel comfortable with the people leading and participating in the group. After a few meetings, you should feel like a member of the group and not an outsider.
- Decide whether you want a group that is facilitated by a professional counselor or by other survivors. If you want to have the input of a professional, consider whether the professional serves as a passive adviser or an active leader. The role of a professional determines whether the focus of the group is peer support or professional counseling.
- Ask if the organization is advocating a particular philosophy concerning cancer survivorship. For example, some organizations put most of their energies into self-care techniques such as imagery or special diets. Others encourage survivors to adapt to certain perspectives, such as becoming an "exceptional" cancer patient. If you are comfortable with the philosophy, then try the group. If not, look elsewhere. If you are offered special cures or encouraged to discontinue established treatment, be suspicious and check with other veterans and oncology professionals. Cancer patients are often targets for quackery.
- See if the group is supportive of survivors with a diversity of perspectives and beliefs, without pushing one approach as right or wrong. The most useful groups understand that different people need different levels of privacy, sharing, and support.
- Assess how group discussions are focused. Does the group dwell on problems or seek out constructive solutions? Do they meet your need to share, give, and/or take? Are you asked to participate when the group etiquette demands it or when you feel like it? Does the group ask that a family member or a friend participate?
- If you are fortunate enough to live in a community that has a variety of mutual-aid organizations, shop around. Meet with the group a few times before you make a judgment about them. The nature and quality of a group varies from meeting to meeting, depending upon what members

bring to it at the time. You may visit a group on a night when the group is "down," perhaps because a member recently died. Give a group the opportunity to warm up to you, and you to them.
- Trust your own instincts. What works for your friends may not work for you. You have managed your life before cancer, and you are the best judge of your own needs. If your first experience leaves you anxious, depressed, overwhelmed, or confused, look elsewhere, or wait awhile and try the same group again.

Cancer is not a discriminating disease. It affects people of every age, race, gender, and life-style. Finding an exact match in the survivorship network may not be possible. But the search itself will put you in touch with interesting people and projects and perhaps result in long-term friendships.

Organizing Peer Support

In your search for a peer-support organization, you may discover that none exists in your community, or that existing ones do not meet your needs. As a result, you may consider creating your own program.

Look Before You Leap

Before creating a new organization, your first task is to look at what already exists. Creating a survivorship program can be both energizing and frustrating. Beginning and sustaining an organization demands personal energy as well as financial resources. These are limited commodities in the cancer community, and they need to be conserved. So consider working within an existing network rather than creating a new one. Sometimes it is easier to rebuild an old organization than to start a new one from scratch. However, if no organization provides a satisfactory fit, at the very least make sure your new program is complementary and not duplicative.

To evaluate existing programs, make a thorough search of the peer-support resources in your community. Then determine what issues, if any, they do not address, and what services, if any, they do not provide. Does your community need a telephone hotline, a support group, a newsletter, a hospital visitation program, or some other service? Are only certain populations within the cancer community served by existing programs? If you are a 65-year-old man with prostate cancer, support groups that cater to young adults or women with breast cancer may be of little value. You must honestly assess whether a new resource is needed. Other organizations can serve as models, but as the creator you will have to determine what will work for you and your particular community.

The requirements for a program in a large city, where people live closely together, have access to transportation, and may have a defensive mistrust of strangers, may be very different from the requirements for a new organization in a rural area, where transportation problems are balanced by a stronger sense of community and trust.

Before you begin the difficult task of founding a new organization, clearly define the concerns your group will address and be sure that there are others who share those concerns. In addition, your group must be accessible to prospective members. Find the best way to link people to your resource. Many cancer survivors who want to participate in your group may be too busy or too ill to do so. Traditional programs like group meetings can be adapted and expanded to accommodate survivors who are homebound, are physically handicapped, are isolated in rural communities, or have limited financial means to participate.

Creating even a modest organization or a one-time-only workshop can be a great deal of work, no matter how well planned in the creative stage. Careful evaluation of your time, energy, and financial resources is es-

> "Even in our first meeting we were like old acquaintances at a reunion, although we had not met before."
>
> —Founder of a cancer peer-support group in Pennsylvania

sential. If you do not have the resources to create a group on your own, then you must look to other survivors, and perhaps supportive professionals, to work with you as a team toward a mutual goal.

Developing a Peer-Support Group

There are many successful models for new peer-support groups. The development and maintenance of your group will depend as much on the skill and dedication of the planners as it does on the chosen model or the plan. Although the following suggestions have worked for a variety of peer-support groups, they are general guidelines and must be adapted to fit the individual circumstances of your community.

1. *Getting started*. Before you consider starting a cancer support organization, examine the history of peer-support organizations. The bibliography in the back suggests some books that help explain the unique role of peer support.

Even more important than library research, however, is field research. If possible, visit other programs, especially those that serve cancer survivors. Note what you like and dislike, how the group members interact, and how the structure of the group addresses (or fails to address) its goals. For example, you need to decide whether you will meet in a medical environment (hospital or doctor's office) or community environment (public building, church or synagogue, or member's home).

If you are interested in becoming a chapter or an affiliate of an existing organization, first make sure that a similar group does not already have a chapter serving your community. Contact the organization to learn whether it has specific guidelines you must follow to begin a new chapter. If you want to form an independent group, you may still wish to model your organization on a structure that has proved successful for other peer-support organizations.

2. *Identify a core group of people who are interested in working with you*. The most effective and lasting groups have a core group willing and able to do the necessary work.

Find other committed individuals, either skilled survivors, oncology professionals, or experienced community organizers, who complement your strengths and can assist in everything from designing the organization to addressing envelopes. Although some cancer-support groups are facilitated by professionals (social workers, nurses, psychologists, psychiatrists, or clergy), many are effectively led by cancer survivors or their family members. A growing number of groups are led by professionals who have a personal cancer experience.

3. *The first meeting*. The first meeting of your group will set the tone for the future. Before you determine the structure of the first meeting, you must decide what services you want your group to provide.

A group whose purpose is to offer emotional and social support to a limited group of participants may start with an informal gathering in a member's home. If your goal

> "I see myself more comfortable with the 'role of patient,' and see it in perspective next to my professional roles. My requirement is to shift between these two roles.... Now that treatment is over, I will explore 'recovery issues in myself,' taking my clues from you."
>
> —Pat Fobair, oncology social worker and breast-cancer survivor, speaking to other survivors in *Surviving!*, October/November 1988

is to provide education about surviving cancer, you may wish to begin with a meeting to plan a community-wide program, such as a conference on a current survivorship topic. If you wish to create a hotline program, your first meeting may need to be limited to a core group committed to performing the necessary development work.

Tasks in planning a meeting may include arranging the meeting space, preparing a presentation, and advertising the meeting to your target audience. You can attract participants by advertising in a local newspaper, placing fliers in community, health, and religious institutions, speaking with survivors in other cancer programs, and encouraging local health professionals to tell their patients about your plans.

4. *Planning for the future of your group*. At the close of the first meeting, there should be a general consensus on the need for the group to continue and, if so, where and when. Future meetings must strike a balance between focusing on the purpose of the group (for example, emotional support) and tending to the business of developing the organization. Group members should be invited to contribute time or resources to the group.

In planning the future of your group, you should resolve a number of questions to ensure that the purpose of the group is defined and the means exist to work toward that purpose.

- Are the group's goals clearly expressed? Are the goals useful, or should they be changed?
- Who may be a member of your group? Anyone? Only cancer survivors and their families? Only survivors of a specific type of cancer?
- When, where, and how often will you meet?
- How will you advertise?
- Will group discussions be facilitated by a professional, a lay leader, or both?
- What will be the focus of your first activities? Support-group meetings? Newsletter? Public-education program? An editorial in the local newspaper?
- How will you handle the business aspects of your group? Will you charge a membership fee? Will you elect officers? Will you write bylaws? Will you seek federal tax-exempt status so that donors can deduct their financial contributions from their income taxes and group purchases will not be subject to sales tax? How will you finance the group?

5. *Future troubleshooting*. Expect the group to experience a natural flux in attendance and enthusiasm. New problems and issues will arise. What do you do if members of the group disagree on its purpose? How do you handle a member who dominates the discussion? How do you attract more members? Where do you go if you lose your meeting space? What do you do if your fund-raiser is a flop? Be prepared to respond to these and other problems in a way that supports the goals and unity of the group.

Periodically evaluate the effectiveness of your group. Have you accomplished your initial goals? Have your goals changed? Are your services still needed? Does the group need mid-course redirection? Are the members of the core group working together, or is all the work falling on the shoulders of one or two people? Give your new group sufficient time to develop, grow, and become known in your community.

Resources to Help You Build and Sustain

You are not alone in your effort to create a survivorship organization. The first place to turn for help is in your own backyard. Medical centers, churches or synagogues, community centers, and private businesses may provide both space and advisers. Ask your oncologist, social worker, or nurse for support in starting a group. In addition to providing meeting space, your community may be a source of enough donated materials and personal assistance to get you started. An instant-print company may donate fliers that advertise your meetings, or a business-supply company may give you office equipment. A psychotherapist or an accountant may offer advice for free or at a discount.

In addition to local resources, there are several regional and national sources of assistance. The National Coalition for Cancer Survivorship offers technical assistance to individuals who want to start a local cancer-support organization. NCCS draws from its experience as a bridge between mutual-aid leaders and health professionals to provide a balanced list of suggestions to new organizations.

NCCS helps new groups in four ways. First, it helps leaders of new groups explore successful models represented by other cancer organizations. Second, it links new and established groups with other local, regional, or national groups that have similar survivorship programs. Third, NCCS sponsors conferences where leaders of community groups can discuss their programs and learn from people with years of experience in cancer support. Fourth, NCCS collects and disseminates the best available publications on group development.

Other important resources include the self-help clearinghouses—nonprofit organizations that help callers locate mutual-aid organizations and provide support services (training workshops, conferences, newsletters, speakers bureaus, consultation in developing and maintaining groups, development of resource materials, assistance with coalition building, and outreach efforts with professionals and the media). Make sure your group is listed with your regional self-help clearinghouse so they can refer survivors to your programs (see Appendix A).

One of the most difficult tasks of creating a new organization is managing the business aspects of the enterprise. Should you obtain tax-exempt status? How should you raise funds? Should you rent an office or work out of your home? When should you risk replacing that old typewriter with a personal computer and a facsimile machine? Should you have an all-volunteer or a paid staff? The Support Centers of America can help you answer these questions.

The Support Centers of America is a nonprofit organization founded in 1972 to increase the effectiveness of charitable organizations. Regional offices are located in San Diego, San Francisco, and Palo Alto, California; Chicago; Boston; Newark, New Jersey; New York; Oklahoma City and Tulsa, Oklahoma; Providence, Rhode Island; Houston; and Washington, D.C. These offices:

- sponsor workshops throughout the United States
- provide direct assistance to leaders of nonprofit organizations to help resolve specific problems

> "Can you fight for your life? That's a strange question to ask survivors. If the question is 'Can you fight for your life?,' then the answer is 'Hell, yes, what's to discuss?'"
>
> —Sally Henderson, survivor of breast cancer, colon cancer, lung cancer, and melanoma of the eye, coordinator of CanCare, a peer-support group in Charlotte, North Carolina.

- offer telephone service to answer questions about managing a nonprofit organization
- sponsor a business volunteer program that provides volunteer professionals, such as accountants, to small nonprofit groups
- refer callers to other resources in their communities that can provide technical assistance.

For information about the Support Center closest to your community, contact:

The Support Centers of America
1410 Q Street, N.W.
Washington, D.C. 20009
(202) 232-1234

Role Models—Examples of Four Mutual-Aid Groups

The cancer survivorship movement represents the diverse experiences of hundreds of mutual-aid organizations. Older, more established groups serve as role models for the development of newer groups. Anyone considering starting a mutual-aid organization can benefit from the successes and failures of the pioneers in cancer peer support.

The following are examples of four different types of cancer support organizations: telephone hotline, large community organization, small community organization, and peer-support group associated with a treatment center.

Telephone Hotline

The Cancer Guidance Institute in Pittsburgh, Pennsylvania, is a nonprofit agency that operates a 24-hour telephone service linking callers with trained volunteers who have experienced cancer themselves. The institute was founded in 1982 by Lynn Gray, a Pittsburgh schoolteacher, ten years after she was diagnosed with breast cancer. Ms. Gray felt that her experience developing peer-support programs for children in public schools could be channeled toward community support for cancer survivors. By the end of 1982, two staff members and one volunteer kept the hotline open 24 hours a day. After Ms. Gray died from breast cancer in 1983, the staff and volunteers of the Cancer Hotline of the Cancer Guidance Institute continued to develop and expand the hotline program.

By 1989, the hotline received approximately 40 calls per month from cancer survivors and their families in the Pittsburgh area. Callers speak with a volunteer and ask for information, or emotional or physical support (such as assistance with locating financial aid or medical equipment). Cancer survivors who want to speak with other survivors who have had similar experiences are matched with a veteran survivor by gender, type of cancer, and type of treatment. Volunteer survivors will contact only those callers who seek support for themselves. For example, a woman who calls the hotline and insists that "my husband needs to speak with another man who has been treated for prostate cancer" will be given information; however, a veteran volunteer will not call her husband unless he asks for a match himself. In addition to providing veteran matches, the hotline will mail educational materials to callers.

Western Pennsylvanians learn about the hotline from the local telephone directory, referrals from their oncologists, brochures in radiation-therapy and chemotherapy waiting rooms in hospitals, reference books on cancer, and local public-education programs. The Cancer Guidance Institute operates the Cancer Hotline and other programs, including a speakers bureau, community education programs, a newsletter, and a referral service for other cancer-support organizations. The institute is funded by membership subscriptions to its newsletter and charitable donations.

For more information contact:

Estelle Weissburg, Executive Director
Cancer Hotline of the Cancer Guidance Institute
1323 Forbes Avenue
Pittsburgh, Pennsylvania 15219
(412) 261-2211

Large Community Organization

The Living Through Cancer Survivorship Center (LTC) in Albuquerque, New Mexico, is a peer-support organization. It is a community of people with personal or family histories of cancer that provides support and educational services to survivors and their families. LTC was established in 1983 to show how "attitude, life-style, education, and appropriate support can combine to augment medical treatment and enhance the quality of life."

The first program sponsored under the Living Through Cancer name was a one-day conference on August 4, 1983. This conference, attended by 135 people, was designed for individuals in treatment for cancer, helping them live with the day-to-day realities of the disease and its treatment.

In direct response to recommendations from conference participants, five survivors, two of whom were still in treatment, founded LTC to create ongoing services. The organization began as a genuine grass-roots group with no paid staff or facility and no source of income. Educational programs, support groups, and organizational meetings were conducted in local churches and in members' homes. LTC began publishing a journal from the home of the president of its board.

Although the mission of LTC has remained unchanged since its formation, both the structure and the programs of the organization have matured through the years. By 1990, a larger board of directors with an active committee structure governed the organization. Membership grew to more than 400 individuals, and thousands of additional survivors, their families, and healthcare professionals participated in LTC programs. Services now include peer-support groups, counseling groups, one-on-one peer support, family potluck dinners, educational conferences and workshops, a lending library, and a bimonthly journal. LTC served as the lead agency in gathering together the core group of experts in cancer survivorship who formed the National Coalition for Cancer Survivorship.

More than 60 percent of LTC's funding comes from small private donations and memberships. LTC also has received grants of $500 to $7,000 from foundations and corporations. In addition to a variety of fund-raising activities, they also organize Viva!, an art show by New Mexican cancer survivors and their friends and families.

For more information, contact:

Barbara Waxer, Executive Director
Living Through Cancer Survivorship Center
323 Eighth Street, S.W.
Albuquerque, New Mexico 87102
(505) 242-3263

Small Community Organizations

The name of the Wildcat Ladies Breast Cancer Support Group in Washington, D.C., has many meanings and a special cachet. The Wildcat Ladies are a group of breast-cancer survivors who have operated successfully without the formal approval of any other established group.

The group first began as one of the American Cancer Society's "Post-Mastectomy Support Groups," which met for eight sessions and offered coping skills and support to women who had recently had surgery for breast cancer. The American Cancer Society provided a meeting place, informative literature, publicity, and oncology social workers as trained professional group leaders. Although the social workers offered guidance, literature, and support from their own perspectives, the true value of the groups lay in what the members offered one another.

The acknowledged "dean" of the groups was an 80-year-old woman who had been treated for breast cancer with a lumpectomy and radiation at age 30. She had her second breast cancer at age 80 and was coping with losses from the mastectomy and the annoyance of a troublesome breast prosthesis that never stayed in place. She offered and received help. Younger women, planning families, took advantage of her wisdom and hopefulness. Resourceful women showed her their ways to anchor a prosthesis.

The groups identified Mary Pollard, a young surgical nurse who was taking chemotherapy and radiation treatments, as their "medical consultant." She always came to meetings dressed in bright colors, with skillful makeup and a beautifully draped scarf to cover her bald head.

Women from a variety of social, financial, and educational backgrounds participated in the groups. In the beginning there were tears, but humor was always the most potent resource. Their jokes were very private, and were humorous only to other women struggling with similar issues.

In 1981, the American Cancer Society had a policy stipulating that these groups should disband after eight sessions, because some people thought that open-ended groups promoted dependency. At the eighth meeting, while others were exchanging platitudes and sharing refreshments, Mary Pollard stood up and announced that she was not ready to go. Partially masked by overt self-confidence and expertise was a very ill young woman who was now calling upon the group to give her strength and support.

In the true tradition of mutual aid, fueled by concern for a needy member and by some anger at a system that did not acknowledge their continued needs, some of the women came out of the closet marked "Post-Mastectomy" and began a wildcat, member-owned and -operated group. Approximately one-half of the women wanted to put their cancer experiences behind them and stopped attending the group after eight weeks. The other half began their own group, chose leaders, set goals, defined responsibilities, and planned programs to meet their needs. Their social-worker consultant helped the group find a convenient meeting place with free parking, recruit members, and gain credibility as a community resource.

Eventually Mary Pollard became physically weaker; however, her attitude seemed to grow stronger and more positive. Her refusal to let go had been the catalyst for getting the group started. As her illness progressed, group members did not become more fearful and disband. Instead, these women became closer, stronger, and more supportive of one another and of Mary through her last days. The first funds that they collected paid for flowers for Mary's funeral. After her death, the group retained its wildcat character, but changed its name to the Mary Pollard Support Group.

The group met regularly for five years. After 1986, they met on an as-needed basis, often organizing on an hour's notice to help a member or a stranger in crisis. They produced several community-education programs that each attracted over 50 women on an evening or a Saturday morning. Members provide support over the telephone and visit women in the community who ask for help. They serve as consumer advocates, raise money to help financially strapped survivors, and give parties for one another. Several volunteer in the American Cancer Society program Reach to Recovery.

The group never adopted a formal constitution or charged regular dues. No more than 15 women were active in the group at a time. Members enhanced one another's lives and, when necessary, dealt with dying. Through happy and sad times, they continued to provide one another with support, courage, humor, and strength.

For more information, contact:

Annette Jolles, A.C.S.W., L.C.S.W.
Department of Social Work 5W45
Washington Hospital Center
110 Irving Street, N.W.
Washington, D.C. 20010
(202) 877-6286

Peer-Support Group Associated with a Treatment Center

Stanford University Hospital in Stanford, California, operates Surviving, a program that consists of two peer-support groups, educational programs, and a nationally acclaimed newsletter. The program is dedicated to the problems of treatment and long-term survival in an effort to help patients regain a sense of control.

Stanford was one of the first treatment centers to sponsor peer-support programs for its patients. In 1980, two groups were formed, one for younger patients and one for older patients. The groups merged the following year and now meet weekly for 90-minute sessions facilitated by Pat Fobair, a clinical oncology social worker. Discussions focus on treatment issues for Hodgkin's disease (for which the majority of Stanford patients are treated) as well as other types of cancer.

In 1983, at the request of long-term survivors who sought peer support, Ms. Fobair began a support group for follow-up patients. This group meets for three hours once a month to discuss problems of long-term survival. Both groups serve cancer survivors throughout the Bay Area, as well as Stanford patients. In addition to the two support groups, Stanford provides individual social-work counseling to its patients.

Stanford's Surviving program also has two educational components. A coping-skills class teaches cognitive and behavioral therapy, including skills such as relaxation techniques, assertiveness training, and how to plan positive activities. The Surviving program is best known for its newsletter, *Surviving!*, written and created by cancer survivors for the benefit of survivors and their friends and families. First published in 1984, it now is distributed nationally to subscribers six or more times each year. *Surviving!* is dedicted to Dr. Henry S. Kaplan, former chairman of Stanford's Department of Radiology, who pioneered the treatment of Hodgkin's disease.

For more information contact:

Pat Fobair, L.C.S.W., M.P.H., Clinical Social Worker and Director of Rehabilitation Services
Stanford University Hospital
Patient Resource Center, Room H0103
Division of Radiation Oncology
300 Pasteur Drive
Stanford, California 94305
(415) 723-7881

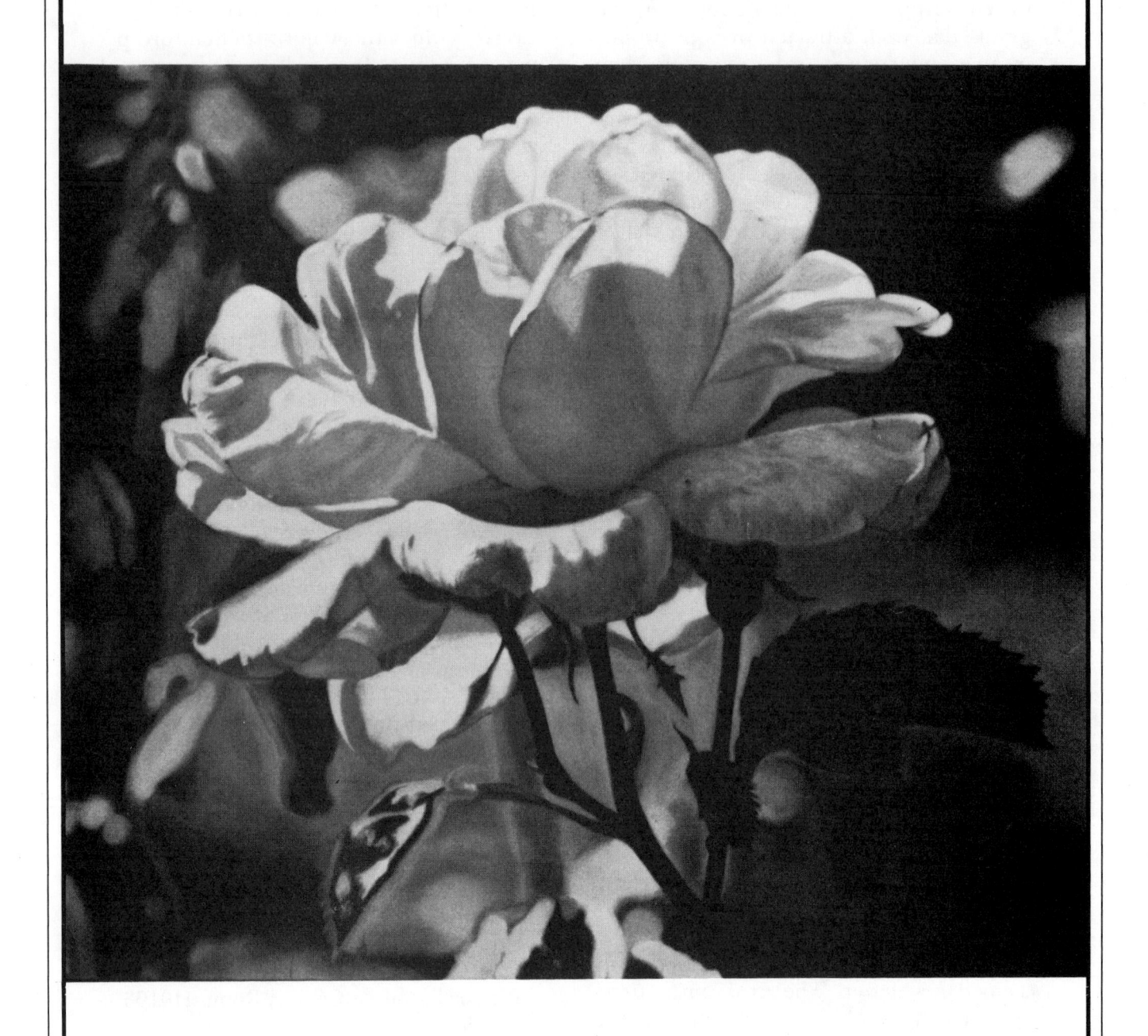

Alice Ferch
Yellow Rose #2
Oil on canvas
40″ x 26″

6

Taking Care of Business: Employment, Insurance, and Money Matters

Barbara Hoffman, J.D.

Most people think of cancer as primarily a medical experience, and secondarily an emotional experience. Such a perception, however, fails to appreciate the entire picture. Cancer is a *life* experience. As such, it affects survivors' access to employment, insurance, and financial support. Cancer survivors must advocate not only for appropriate medical care, but for their legal rights as well. Most cancer experiences involve legal issues:

- freedom from job discrimination
- protection from unprofessional medical treatment
- access to affordable health and life insurance
- right to refuse life-prolonging treatment
- availability of financial assistance

Your Job and the Law

Work is, in fact, financial and emotional medicine to millions of adults. It is not just a source of financial security and adequate health insurance, but provides self-esteem and identity.

A person who works 40 hours a week, 50 weeks a year, for 44 years will have spent 88,000 hours at his or her job. Most Americans do not have the option of not working. Employment is a substantial, necessary, and integral part of life. Despite this need, more than 1,000,000 Americans with a history of cancer face cancer-related hurdles in their quests for employment.

Employment Problems

Studies by health professionals and large companies report that about one in four cancer survivors faces job barriers because of a cancer history. Problems most frequently reported by cancer survivors are dismissal, failure to hire, demotion, denial of promotion, undesirable transfer, denial of benefits, and hostility in the workplace.

> Work on,
> My Medicine, work!
>
> —William Shakespeare, *Othello*

Although some actions, such as a blanket hiring ban against all individuals with cancer histories without consideration of their qualifications, can be arbitrary and blatant, cancer-based discrimination is more often subtle and directed against an individual.

Job discrimination affects all cancer survivors, young and old, rich and poor. Nevertheless, some groups of survivors experience higher rates of discrimination than others. Blue-collar workers tend to encounter more problems obtaining and keeping a job than white-collar workers. This difference may be attributed to a number of factors:

- Because blue-collar duties require more physical activity than white-collar duties, blue-collar employers are more likely to assume that a cancer survivor is unable to perform the physical demands of a job.
- Because blue-collar workers are more easily replaced than white-collar workers, blue-collar employers are less concerned with keeping a stable work force.
- Because the general educational level of a blue-collar worker tends to be lower than that of white-collar workers, blue-collar employers and employees are less knowledgeable about the prevention, treatment, and prognosis of cancer, and therefore more likely to believe the cancer myths at the root of discrimination.

In 1990, it is estimated that one out of every 1,000 20-year-olds is a survivor of childhood cancer. Childhood-cancer survivors confront additional hurdles not faced by older workers. For example, young survivors face particular difficulties in obtaining their first job because of their lack of experience. Some employers, especially police and fire departments, deny employment to young applicants with cancer histories seeking to gain that first step on the career ladder. As a result, younger cancer patients tend to be more concerned than older patients about revealing their cancer history when searching for work.

Adult cancer survivors who are denied job opportunities commonly experience stress and anxiety over economic insecurity, loss of independence, and reduced self-esteem. Many survivors who fear discrimination encounter "job lock." They hesitate to leave an undesirable job in the belief that by changing jobs they would risk losing hospital and medical insurance, pension rights, and other benefits.

Reasons for Employment Discrimination

Most employers base personnel decisions on economic, not charitable considerations. Many employers worry about the psychological impact of an applicant's cancer history on other employees. Although some employers, in evaluating the job qualifications of a survivor, consider the actual effect of that individual's cancer history on his or her personal abilities, many employers permit vague stereotypes about cancer to color their decisions.

The cancer myths discussed in chapter 1 have a particular impact on the employment opportunities of survivors. Belief in the death-sentence myth makes employers hesitant to invest in an individual they believe will die imminently. Co-workers are uncom-

> "About three o'clock or so I woke up in a total fright. I had been dreaming that I was wandering along the Beltway outside Washington trying to find the Raytheon plant that was located somewhere in those rolling hills. I was applying for a job after being turned down everywhere else. I had to find the plant to submit my résumé, but I was hopelessly lost. My cancer had rendered me unemployable, and my family was going to be destitute."
>
> —Former U.S. Senator Paul Tsongas, *Heading Home*

fortable working next to someone they believe will die soon. Insurance companies increase rates or refuse to issue policies, banks deny loans, and society disallows long-term planning on the assumption of a short-term life.

Belief in the contagious myth often results in physical and emotional isolation of those with cancer in the workplace. Employers often succumb to co-workers' demands to fire or transfer cancer survivors. In California, one survivor who applied for a job with a medical emergency-services company reported that he was asked by his interviewer, "Cancer, how did you catch that?" One recent study quoted a survivor who "was transferred from his job in a hotel kitchen for fear that he might 'contaminate' the food."

Belief in the myth of the decreased productivity of cancer survivors may lead to job termination or demotion. A senior executive in a large corporation who had demonstrated to his employer that he could perform his job while undergoing radiation therapy for Hodgkin's disease reported that he was nonetheless forced to resign because his superior feared he would no longer be a productive executive. The 45-year-old executive was unnecessarily forced to abandon his career.

As a result of the unproductive-worker myth, the unemployed are faced with few job opportunities and the underemployed are drained of their self-esteem. Yet studies by Metropolitan Life Insurance and Bell Telephone of their own employees found that, when these employees were compared with others of the same age, the turnover, absence, and work performance of cancer survivors were satisfactory. Of employees in the studies who left work for treatment, the majority were capable of returning to their jobs.

When Cancer-Based Discrimination Is Illegal

Federal law. Before 1970, few laws protected people from employment discrimination because of their medical histories. In 1973, a new law, the Federal Rehabilitation Act, sparked a movement to protect the rights of people with handicaps or a history of a serious illness.

Section 504 of the Federal Rehabilitation Act bans employment discrimination based on handicap by employers that receive federal financial assistance in the form of money or equipment. The Rehabilitation Act applies to federal, state, and local governments (police departments, fire departments, public agencies, United States Postal Service, etc.), most schools and universities, institutions that receive federal grants for research and development (hospitals, laboratories, technical institutes, defense con-

> "I lost my breast, not my brain."
>
> —Mastectomy survivor in response to being fired from her job as a paralegal

tractors, etc.), physicians who receive Medicare Part B funds, and health agencies that receive Medicaid payments.

The Rehabilitation Act defines "handicapped individual" as

> any person who (1) has a physical or mental impairment which substantially limits one or more of such person's major life activities, (2) has a record of such impairment, or (3) is regarded as having such an impairment.

Most cancer survivors are covered by at least one of these definitions. A survivor whose cancer affects his or her ability to do everyday activities, such as driving to work, has a "physical impairment which substantially limits one or more . . . major life activities." A survivor whose cancer at one time affected his or her ability to do everyday activities has a "record of such impairment." A survivor whose cancer did not affect his or her ability to do everyday activities, *but whose employer mistakenly believes his cancer is a handicap*, is "regarded as having such an impairment."

Department of Labor regulations explain that someone who has a history of a medical impairment is covered by the law because

> the attitude of employers, supervisors and co-workers toward that previous impairment may result in an individual experiencing difficulty in securing, retaining or advancing in employment. The mentally restored, those who have had heart attacks or cancer, often experience such difficulty.

In 1988, a federal court agreed that the Rehabilitation Act protected healthy cancer survivors from employment discrimination. The City of Houston Fire Department had a policy against hiring anyone with a history of lymphoma, regardless of whether the survivor was ill or in complete remission. Walter Ritchie, who had been successfully treated for lymphoma in 1981, applied in 1985 for a position as a fire cadet. Although Mr. Ritchie passed all of the required tests, the city refused to hire him, solely because of his cancer history. A federal court found that the city violated Mr. Ritchie's rights under the Rehabilitation Act by assuming that his cancer history made him unfit for the job. The court required the city to hire Mr. Ritchie and to consider applicants based on their individual abilities, not an irrelevant medical history.

The Rehabilitation Act protects only a "qualified" worker—that is, someone with the skills and background needed to perform the basic duties of the job. An employer may not deny a "qualified" cancer survivor salary, benefits, promotion opportunities, or working conditions equal to those offered to other workers. However, an employer is not required to hire someone who is "unqualified," a worker who cannot perform the basic duties of the job.

The Rehabilitation Act also requires employers to make a "reasonable accommodation" of an applicant or worker. Whether an accommodation is reasonable depends on the facts of the individual situation. An accommodation is not reasonable if it causes an undue hardship on the employer.

If you file a lawsuit, you have the initial burden of "stating a claim under the law." This means that you must allege facts that, if true, would entitle you to win your lawsuit unless your employer had a legitimate de-

AVERAGE NUMBER OF WEEKS MISSED FROM WORK DUE TO DISABILITY

Source: Mutual of Omaha Companies Group Operation, 1988 Annual Report, "Current Trends in Health Care Costs and Utilization." Based on survey of paid claims of approximately 25,000 group-policy beneficiaries.

	1986	*1987*	*1988*	*Average*
Cancer	8.9	9.0	13.4	10.4
Heart disease	7.6	8.7	10.0	8.8
Other circulatory	8.9	7.6	9.7	8.7
Musculoskeletal (arthritis)	8.2	8.0	9.1	8.4
Nervous system disorder	5.7	7.6	8.8	7.4
Accidents	7.1	6.0	7.0	6.7
Maternity	6.5	6.9	6.5	6.6

AVERAGE NUMBER OF WEEKS MISSED FROM WORK DUE TO TREATMENT

Source: "What Employers Need to Know About Cancer" (American Cancer Society, Illinois Division, 1987)

Colorectal cancer—9 weeks
Breast cancer—2 to 9 weeks
Uterine cancer—6 to 14 weeks
Skin cancer—1 day to 3 weeks

fense. "Stating a claim under the law" does not mean you automatically win; it does mean, however, that you have alleged sufficient facts to have your day in court. To state a claim that your employer has violated the law, you must state facts that show each of the following:

1. You have a cancer history (or your employer mistakenly thought you had cancer).
2. You were qualified for the job.
3. You were denied the position, fired, or treated differently despite your qualifications.
4. The employer sought to fill or filled the position with someone who was not handicapped or perceived as being handicapped.

The following facts would state a claim under the Rehabilitation Act: You have 20 years' experience as a public-school teacher (public schools are subject to the Act). You always received good performance evaluations (you are qualified to teach). You took two weeks off for breast-cancer surgery and can receive follow-up treatments without affecting your work schedule (you are able to perform the duties of your job). Yet the school board fired you the day you returned to work because it did not want the risk of having to hire a substitute teacher should you become unable to work in the future (discrimination because of speculative fear of future handicap).

The following scenario would not state a claim under the Rehabilitation Act: You work as a telephone operator for a small company that does not receive federal funds (employer not subject to the law). You have a laryngectomy and learn esophageal speech. Your employer transfers you to a lower-paying job after receiving customer complaints that they cannot understand you on the telephone (you are unable to perform reasonably the duties of a telephone operator).

Once you have stated a claim, the burden then shifts to the employer to raise a legitimate defense. The most common defenses are:

> "By amending the definition of 'handicapped individual' to include not only those who are actually impaired, but also those who are regarded as impaired and who, as a result, are substantially limited in major life activity, Congress acknowledged that society's accumulated myths and fears about disability and disease are as handicapping as are the physical limitations that flow from actual impairment. Few aspects of a handicap give rise to the same level of public fear and misapprehension as contagiousness. Even those who suffer or have recovered from such noninfectious diseases as epilepsy or cancer have faced discrimination based on the irrational fear that they might be contagious."
>
> —Supreme Court Justice William Brennan, *Arline* v. *School Board of Nassau County* [Fla.], 1987

1. You were not qualified for the job.
2. We are reorganizing and dismissed everyone in your department.

If the employer raises a defense, the burden shifts back to you to show that his defense is a pretext to hide the truth.

Most lawsuits, like federal-agency investigations, are either settled or dismissed. If you do go to trial and win your lawsuit, a federal judge may order your employer to compensate you for your harm, including back pay, reinstatement, and your attorney's fees.

A dramatic new civil rights law, the employment provisions of which take effect on July 13, 1992, will provide cancer survivors with greater federal remedies for employment discrimination. The Americans with Disabilities Act (ADA), signed into law on July 13, 1990, will prohibit employment discrimination by private employers against people with disabilities. Like the Rehabilitation Act, the ADA will prohibit discrimination against a qualified employee because he or she is disabled, has a history of a disability, or is regarded as being disabled. Although the ADA will not specifically protect cancer survivors, federal courts and agencies are expected to apply the law to cancer survivors just as they apply the Rehabilitation Act to prohibit cancer-based discrimination.

One of the purposes of the ADA is to protect workers not covered by the Rehabilitation Act. The ADA will not be limited to employers that receive federal funding. Like other civil rights laws, it will cover private employers (from mid-1992 to mid-1994, employers with 25 or more employees will be subject to the law; after mid-1994, employers with 15 or more employees must also comply with the law).

Like the Rehabilitation Act, the ADA will prohibit employers from requiring pre-employment examinations designed to screen out individuals with a disability, including a cancer history. An employer will be allowed to ask you medical questions only after you are offered the job and only if the questions are specifically related to the job.

The ADA will be enforced by the Equal Employment Opportunities Commission. If you believe you were treated differently, because of your cancer history by an employer covered by the ADA, you must file a com-

How to Enforce Your Rights Under Federal Law

Section 504 of the Rehabilitation Act can be enforced against employers that receive federal funds in two ways: by you through a private lawsuit, or by a federal agency.

The federal agency that provides the employer with federal funds may investigate an employer accused of discriminating against the handicapped. In most instances, the federal agency will either negotiate a settlement or decide that the employer did not violate the law. In the rare cases that are not dismissed or settled, the agency may refer the case to the United States Department of Justice for filing in federal court.

If you believe that your rights under the Rehabilitation Act were violated, you may ask the federal government to investigate. You should write directly to the agency that provides federal funds to your employer. For example, if your employer is a nursing home that receives Medicaid funds from the Department of Health and Human Services, you may contact the local office of the Department of Health and Human Services. If you do not know the name of the agency that provides federal funds to your employer, contact the Civil Rights Division of the Justice Department:

> Coordination and Review Section
> Civil Rights Division
> United States Department of Justice
> Washington, D.C. 20530
> (202) 724-2235
> (202) 724-7678 (for the hearing-impaired)

In addition to, or instead of, filing a complaint with a federal agency, you may choose to file a lawsuit in federal court. If you have also asked a federal agency to investigate, the judge who is assigned to your lawsuit may refuse to hear the case until the federal agency has completed its investigation. Although you are not required to have an attorney, your chances of success are greater if you are represented by an attorney with experience in employment-discrimination cases.

---

plaint with the EEOC to enforce your rights. The EEOC will attempt to settle the dispute. If no settlement is reached, the EEOC may appoint an investigator to evaluate your claim. If the EEOC determines that your rights may have been violated, it may sue on your behalf or may grant you the right to file your own lawsuit in federal court.

Your complaint should be filed with the closest of 50 regional EEOC offices. For more information about how to enforce your rights under the ADA and to obtain the location of your regional EEOC office, call the EEOC Public Information System at (800) USA-EEOC (872-3362).

If you prove that you were qualified for a job but treated differently because of your cancer history, you may be entitled to back pay, injunctive relief such as reinstatement, and attorneys' fees. The ADA will not, however, permit an award for compensatory or punitive damages.

State laws. Cancer survivors who face discrimination but are not covered by the Rehabilitation Act or the Americans with Disabilities Act must turn to state laws for

> ## How to Find an Attorney with Experience in Employment-Discrimination Cases
>
> Most communities offer a lawyer referral service through either the county or the state bar association. Typically, these services will provide you with the name or names of attorneys with expertise in a particular field, such as employment discrimination. The attorney you choose will meet with you at no charge, or at a discounted rate, to help you decide whether you should file a lawsuit. Most, however, will charge you their regular fee if, after the initial interview, you decide to retain them as your lawyer. Look in the telephone directory under state and county listings, as well as under "Lawyer Referral Services," "Legal Services," "Attorneys," and "Lawyers."
>
> In addition, some community cancer organizations keep a list of attorneys who possess the skill and express an interest in representing cancer survivors in employment-discrimination cases. For example, Candlelighters Childhood Cancer Foundation, 1312 18th Street, N.W., 2nd Floor, Washington, D.C. 20036, (800) 366-2223, retains a list of lawyers in the Washington, D.C., area. A few American Cancer Society units and divisions also retain such a list for their communities.
>
> If you meet maximum-income-level standards, you may qualify for free legal assistance by public legal-services organizations. Look in the telephone directory under "Legal Services" or under county offices for the organization in your area.

relief. Every state has a law that regulates, to some extent, employment discrimination against people with disabilities; however, the application of these laws to cancer-based discrimination varies widely.

Most state laws protect people who are "handicapped" or "disabled." In states that do not protect individuals who have a history of a handicap or who are regarded by others as having a handicap, you must actually be disabled from your cancer to be protected by the law. Other state laws borrow language from the Federal Rehabilitation Act to protect not only those who have a disability, but also those who are perceived to be disabled. Only California, the District of Columbia, Florida, Vermont, and West Virginia expressly prohibit discrimination against cancer survivors.

Although state discrimination laws differ substantially, they all have one thing in common with the federal law: only "qualified" workers are entitled to relief. For example, a Florida court ruled that Thomas Rateau, a cancer survivor who was denied a school-teaching position, was not qualified for the job he sought. After back surgery to remove a malignant tumor from his spine, Rateau applied for a job teaching high school. The school board refused to hire him because the job required frequent bending and lifting. The court held that, because Rateau's back pain would be aggravated by the daily duties of the job, he was not qualified for that teaching position, and therefore had no claim under the Florida Human Rights Act. The Rateau case illustrates that most antidiscrimination laws appropriately balance the employee's right to equal job opportunities with the employer's right to consider only qualified applicants.

Some states require all employers, public and private, large and small, to obey the antidiscrimination law. Other states limit the type of employer who must obey the law. For example, many states exempt from compliance employers who have fewer than 15 workers.

SUMMARY OF STATE HANDICAP DISCRIMINATION LAWS

Laws are subject to change by courts and legislatures. This chart represents the status of state laws as of September 1989. You or your attorney should learn whether any changes have been made in your state law since then.

Each state law defines who is protected by the law (the "protected class"). Most states protect a person with a "handicap" or a "disability." Some state laws expressly include within the protected class a person with a history of a handicap ("H") or a person who is regarded or perceived to be handicapped ("P"). (Refer to page 104 for a discussion of these terms.) Additionally, in some states that do not expressly include within the protected class someone who has a history of a handicap or is perceived as being handicapped, the enforcing agency or state court is likely to interpret the law as protecting those individuals ("h," "p"), as well as protecting persons who are currently actually handicapped.

State	Employer Covered	Protected Class	Enforced By
Alabama	public only	handicap	State Personnel Bd.
Alaska	public & private (min. 1 employee)	disability (H, P)	Commission for Human Rights
Arizona	public & private (min. 15 employees)	handicap (h, p)	Civil Rights Division
Arkansas	public & private employers that received public funds	handicap (h, p)	Grievance Review Committee
California	public & private (min. 5 employees)	handicap (people who are not cured or rehabilitated) medical condition (cured or rehabilitated cancer survivors)	Fair Employment and Housing Dept.
Colorado	public & private (min. 1 employee)	handicap (H, P)	Civil Rights Division
Connecticut	public & private (min. 3 employees)	disability (H)	Commission on Human Rights and Opportunities
Delaware	public & private (min. 20 employees)	handicap (H, P)	Human Relations Commission (private employees) Office of State Personnel (public employees)
District of Columbia	public & private (min. 1 employee)	handicap (H, P) (specifically includes cancer)	Commission on Human Rights
Florida	public & private (min. 15 employees)	handicap (h, p) (specifically includes cancer)	Commission on Human Relations
Georgia	public & private (min. 15 employees)	handicap (H, p)	Fair Employment Practice Board (public employees) state court (private employees)
Hawaii	public & private (min. 1 employee)	handicap (H, P)	Dept. of Labor and Industrial Relations
Idaho	public & private (min. 10 employees)	handicap (H, P)	state court
Illinois	public & private (min. 1 employee)	handicap (H, P)	Dept. of Human Rights
Indiana	public & private (min. 6 employees)	handicap (h, p)	Civil Rights Commission
Iowa	public & private (min. 4 employees)	disability (H, P)	Civil Rights Commission

State	Employer Covered	Protected Class	Enforced By
Kansas	public & private (min. 4 employees)	handicap	Commission on Civil Rights
Kentucky	public & private (min. 8 employees)	handicap	Dept. of Workplace Standard
Louisiana	public & private (min. 15 employees)	handicap (H, P)	state court
Maine	public & private (min. 15 employees)	handicap (H, P)	Human Rights Commission
Maryland	public & private (min. 15 employees)	handicap (H, P)	Commission on Human Rights Relations
Massachusetts	public & private (min. 6 employees)	handicap (H, P)	Commission Against Discrimination
Michigan	public & private (min. 4 employees)	handicap (H, p)	Dept. of Civil Rights
Minnesota	public & private (min. 1 employee)	handicap (H, P)	Dept. of Human Rights
Mississippi	public & private employers that received public funds	disability and handicap	State Personnel Commission
Missouri	public & private (min. 6 employees)	handicap (H, P)	Commission on Human Rights
Montana	public & private (min. 1 employee)	handicap (H, P)	Human Rights Commission
Nebraska	public & private (min. 15 employees)	disability	Equal Opportunity Commission
Nevada	public & private (min. 15 employees)	handicap	Equal Rights Commission
New Hampshire	public & private (min. 6 employees)	handicap (H, P)	Commission for Human Rights
New Jersey	public & private (min. 1 employee)	handicap (H, P)	Division on Civil Rights
New Mexico	public & private (min. 4 employees)	handicap (H, P)	Human Rights Commission
New York	public & private (min. 4 employees)	disability (H, P)	Division of Human Rights
North Carolina	public & private (min. 15 employees)	handicap (H, P)	Human Relations Council
North Dakota	public & private (min. 10 employees)	disability and handicap (h, p)	State Personnel Commission (public employees) state court (private employees)
Ohio	public & private (min. 4 employees)	handicap (H, P)	Civil Rights Commission
Oklahoma	public & private (min. 15 employees)	handicap (H, P)	Human Rights Commission
Oregon	public & private (min. 6 employees)	handicap (H, P)	Bureau of Labor and Industries, Civil Rights Division
Pennsylvania	public & private (min. 4 employees)	disability and handicap (H, P)	Human Relations Commission
Rhode Island	public & private (min. 4 employees)	handicap (H, P)	Commission for Human Rights
South Carolina	public & private (min. 15 employees)	handicap	Human Affairs Commission
South Dakota	public & private (min. 1 employee)	disability (H)	Human Rights Commission
Tennessee	public & private (min. 8 employees)	handicap (H, P)	Human Rights Commission

State	Employer Covered	Protected Class	Enforced By
Texas	public & private (min. 15 employees)	disability (H, p)	Commission on Human Rights
Utah	public & private (min. 15 employees)	handicap (h, p)	Industrial Commission, Anti-Discrimination Division
Vermont	public & private (min. 1 employee)	handicap (H, P) (specifically includes cancer	Civil Rights Division
Virginia	public & private (min. 1 employee)	disability (H)	Dept. for Rights of the Disabled and Council on Human Rights
Washington	public & private (min. 8 employees)	handicap (H, P)	Human Rights Commission
West Virginia	public & private (min. 12 employees)	handicap (H, P) (specifically includes cancer)	Human Rights Commission
Wisconsin	public & private (min. 1 employee)	handicap (H, P)	Dept. of Industry, Labor and Human Relations, Equal Rights Division
Wyoming	public & private (min. 2 employees)	handicap (H, P)	Fair Employment Commission

Specific prohibitions. Most state laws prohibit discrimination in "terms and conditions of employment"—that is, salary, benefits, duties, promotional opportunities, etc. Some state laws require employers to accommodate an employee's handicap, if it can be done so reasonably. The most protective laws prohibit employers from asking about your medical history until after they offer you a job.

Remedies. The type of remedy to which you may be entitled if you are a victim of discrimination depends not only on the state where you work but also on where your complaint is resolved (state agency or state court). Most states offer some or all of the following remedies:

- an order requiring the employer to "cease and desist" discriminatory activity
- an offer for a position for which you were denied
- reinstatement if you were fired or demoted
- back pay
- lost benefits (such as insurance and seniority)
- money to compensate you for your injury
- the costs of filing the complaint (court and attorney fees)

How to enforce your rights under state law. Most state antidiscrimination laws are enforced by state agencies. Every state except Idaho and Louisiana has a state agency that will consider an employment-discrimination complaint. The address and telephone number of each state agency are listed in Appendix A. Look in the state government section of your telephone directory for their local number.

Although each state has different procedures, most state agencies will handle a complaint in the following way:

1. An investigator will accept a complaint signed by you if you believe an employer has violated your rights under the state antidiscrimination law.

2. The investigator will ask the employer to present his or her side of the story.

3. If the investigator decides that you did not state a claim under the law, he or she will dismiss your case. If the investigator decides that you may have a legitimate claim against the employer, he or she will try to get you and the employer to reach a fair settlement.

4. If you and the employer cannot come to an agreement, the investigator may recommend that your case be heard by a judge.

Most states allow you to appeal a decision against you, either to a court or to a higher level in the state agency. The New York State Division of Human Rights, for example, ruled that a medical institute violated cancer survivor Dr. Lisa Goldsmith's rights under the New York Human Rights Law, which prohibits discrimination based on disability. Dr. Goldsmith had applied for admission in 1976 to the New York Psychoanalytic Institute, and three committees had to approve her admission. Two of the committees found that she was highly qualified and gave her excellent evaluations. The third committee rejected her application because of her cancer history. (Dr. Goldsmith had been treated for Hodgkin's disease, but had been in remission since April 1974.) The institute allowed reapplications, but turned Dr. Goldsmith down again in 1978.

She then filed a complaint with the New York Human Rights Division, which found that the institute's actions were unlawful because they were based solely on Dr. Goldsmith's cancer history. The institute appealed the decision to state court. There the Appellate Division of the New York Supreme Court affirmed the Human Rights Division's decision, reasoning that the institute denied a qualified applicant like Dr. Goldsmith the opportunity to enjoy a full and productive life after her cancer experience.

Idaho, Louisiana, and a number of states that have an enforcement agency allow you to enforce the law yourself by filing a lawsuit in state court. Because each state has different rules regarding when you may file a lawsuit in state court, and because choosing a forum (state agency or court) involves a number of factors (for example, which forum is likely to provide the swiftest solution, whether you can maintain an agency complaint and a lawsuit simultaneously), it is wise to consult with both a private attorney and a state representative before making a choice. Although you are not required to be represented by an attorney in state court, your chances of success are greater if you are so represented.

You may have additional legal rights if you are a union member. Some union contracts explicitly protect employees from discrimination based on handicap. In certain cases, unions may provide free legal assistance. Check with your union representative about the terms of your contract.

How to Avoid Becoming a Victim of Discrimination

State and federal antidiscrimination laws help cancer survivors in two ways: they discourage discrimination, and they offer remedies when discrimination does occur. Legal rights, however, are not the only answer. Enforcing your legal rights comes with a cost. Once you have sued your employer, he or she is not likely to welcome you back even if a judge orders that you be reinstated. Lawsuits cost time and money, as well as increase tension. Finally, after months or years of litigation you may lose your case.

Civil rights laws should be used as a last resort in the battle against cancer-based employment discrimination. The first step is to protect yourself from discrimination. If that fails, the next step is to attempt a reasonable settlement with your employer. If that fails, however, turning to a civil rights lawsuit may be the most effective next step.

The most constructive efforts against cancer-based discrimination eliminate opportunities for discrimination in the first place. Although each employment situation is unique, here are some steps you can take to lessen the chances that you will be denied a job.

1. If you are not asked directly whether you have ever had cancer, do not volunteer that you are a survivor unless it is directly relevant to the position (for example, as a counselor in an oncology center). In most situations, your cancer history will be irrelevant. There are very few jobs, for example, that require that a woman have two breasts. Unless it directly affects your ability to do that job, you have no obligation to disclose your medical history any more than any other personal, confidential information.

2. Stress your specific qualifications for the job. Do not apply for jobs for which you are not qualified. It is not illegal for an employer to reject you for a job for which you are not qualified, regardless of your medical history. No one has to hire you *because* you have a cancer history.

3. Try to lessen the impact of a gap in your work history by organizing your résumé topically (job skills and experience), instead of chronologically. If you have to explain a long period of unemployment during your cancer treatment, explain it if possible in a way that conveys that your illness is past, and that you are in and expect to remain in good health. For example,

> I had a cancerous eye removed two years ago, but I am now cancer-free, in excellent health, and at no greater risk for cancer than anyone else. Having only one eye in no way affects my abilities to do [the duties of the job].

Many employers may presume that no one can fully recover from cancer. Assume that the employer believes myths about cancer in explaining your absence from work or school. Be prepared to educate your interviewer about your type of cancer and why cancer does not equal death.

4. Do not lie on an employment application. If you are hired and the lie is eventually discovered, your dishonesty may be grounds for termination. Some state laws prohibit employers from asking you if you have ever had cancer unless it directly relates to your qualifications for the job (which it rarely does). Other states do not limit what an employer may ask. If an employment questionnaire asks, "Have you ever had cancer?" or "Have you had surgery in the past five years, and if so for what?," you should not simply say "yes" and assume that the employer realizes that you are in remission. One alternative is to answer the question asking for history and then explain your current health and prognosis. Some suggestions are:

- "I am presently fit to perform the duties of the job for which I am applying."
- "I currently have no medical condition that would interfere with my ability to perform the duties of the job for which I am applying."
- "I have not had cancer for X years and have a normal life expectancy."

Your answer should be an honest description of your health at the time of the application.

5. Seek the assistance of a job counselor. He or she can help you with your résumé and job interviewing skills. You should practice your answers to expected questions, like "Why did you miss a year of work?" or "Why did you leave your last job?" Answers to these questions must be honest, but should emphasize your current qualifications for the position and not past limitations, if any, resulting from your cancer experience.

6. If possible, seek out employers that are prohibited by federal law to discriminate based on disability. For example, federal departments, agencies, and institutions are required by the Federal Rehabilitation Act to have affirmative-action policies and are less likely to discriminate than are private employers.

7. Do not discriminate against yourself by assuming you are handicapped. Although cancer treatment leaves some survivors with actual disabilities, many survivors are capable of performing the same skills and activities as they had prior to diagnosis. You should make a realistic assessment of your abilities and the mental and physical challenges of the job you want.

> "I tried to return to work, but my employer said my old job wasn't there. (It's being filled by two part-time people.) I knew things like this happen but I didn't think it could happen in a small town. Of course, you probably know the rest of the story—no job, no health insurance. We shouldn't sit back and let things like this happen; we have to keep fighting."
>
> —James D. Moll, Hodgkin's disease survivor

Fighting Back Against Discrimination

If you suspect you are being treated differently at work because of your cancer history, think about negotiations before you leap into a lawsuit. It is best to try to assert your rights without appearing like an abrasive troublemaker. Most employers prefer qualified workers who contribute to a friendly atmosphere.

Here are some suggestions on how to be your own advocate and solve a small employment problem before it becomes a big one.

1. If you are encountering problems at work because of your cancer history, let your employer know that you are aware of your legal rights and would rather work out an informal agreement than resort to a legal solution. Be careful during settlement discussions that you do not say anything that could be used to hurt your claim should discussions ultimately fail and you end up in court.

For example, your doctor has agreed to give you Friday-afternoon appointments for your chemotherapy, but when you inform your boss, he says, "I'm sorry, but I'll have to let you go, because your job demands at least 40 hours per week." Be sure to let him know you will make up the time. You might say: "The state antidiscrimination law says that you cannot fire me if I am able to continue to perform my job despite my illness. My doctor and I believe I am able to continue working. Because I can stay at work until 1:00 P.M. on Fridays, I would be pleased to work an extra hour or two Monday through Thursday to make up the missed time. My doctor anticipates that I will need chemotherapy only for X weeks, so I should be back to my regular schedule by ———."

2. Be aware of the filing deadlines ("statutes of limitations") so that you do not lose your option to file a complaint. Many state antidiscrimination laws require you to file a complaint within 180 days of your employer's action. Once a deadline passes, it is very difficult to file a complaint. If you do file a complaint, however, and later change your mind, you may withdraw the complaint at any time.

3. If you need some kind of accommodation (for example, flextime or a reduction in duties), suggest several alternatives from which your employer could choose. If your employer offers accommodations, do not turn them down lightly. Such an offer may work in his or her favor should you end up in court.

4. If your employer seems to believe that people cannot survive cancer and remain productive. workers, educate him or her. Ask your doctor to write a letter explaining the type of cancer you had or have, and why you are able to work. For example, if your fellow workers are putting pressure on your boss to fire you because they are afraid you are contagious, send your boss a letter from your doctor or a journal article that explains that cancer is not contagious. Understandably, an employer is more likely to believe a doctor or a medical journal than you.

5. Ask oncology nurses and social workers to write or call your employer. They may be able to suggest employment alternatives, educate employers and fellow employees about cancer, and serve as a negotiator between you and your employer (see chapter 4).

6. Seek the support of your fellow workers. They have an interest in protecting themselves from future discrimination.

7. Keep careful written records of all job actions both that support your position and weaken your employer's position. Some employment actions, such as good performance evaluations, may be used in your favor to show that you were qualified for the job. Other actions, such as being moved from a job working with the public to a job that includes little interaction with the public after your hair falls out from chemotherapy, may be used against your employer to show illegal motives.

8. Reach out to community resources that may help you by serving as an advocate. Members of support groups may have valuable lessons to share from their employment experiences. Most state divisions of the American Cancer Society have a staff person who is familiar with state and federal discrimination laws.

9. Carefully evaluate your goals and plans. Be prepared to face the positive and negative aspects of enforcing your legal rights. Potential positive aspects include employment, monetary damages, and a vindication of your rights. Potential negative aspects include long court battles with no guarantee of victory (some cases drag on for five years or more), legal fees and expenses, stress, and an adversarial relationship between you and the people you sue. Articulate your desires and intentions clearly and strongly. Do not be afraid to enforce your rights. The more successful lawsuits that are filed by cancer survivors, the less likely it is that other employers will discriminate in the future.

Vocational Rehabilitation

Some cancer survivors, especially those who were physically disabled by their treatment, may benefit from vocational-rehabilitation services offered by public and private agencies. These services help people whose disabilities make it hard to find or keep a job. Depending on the agency, services may include financial assistance, job training and counseling, and the provision of special equipment.

One important way in which rehabilitation services help cancer survivors is to suggest job accommodations, or changes in the job or workplace, that fairly balance the worker's abilities with the employer's needs.

Cancer survivors can benefit from many types of job accommodations, including:

- offering flexible work hours to accommodate medical treatments
- "borrowing" sick days from future years
- changing job duties (such as reducing lifting)
- redesigning the equipment used to perform a job
- retraining a worker for a new skill

For example, an accommodation for a survivor whose larynx has been removed may include speech therapy and electronic speech aids. The Michigan Rehabilitation Services, Michigan's vocational-rehabilitation agency, fitted a field engineer with a special bullhorn that did not distort his newly trained voice.

Vocational rehabilitation may be appropriate for survivors at different stages of work, including those who are:

VOCATIONAL REHABILITATION RESOURCES

State

Every state has a vocational rehabilitation agency that provides direct services to individuals. You are covered by the agency in the state where you live, not where you work.

The Federal Rehabilitation Act requires state rehabilitation agencies to provide the following minimum services:
- evaluation of your rehabilitation potential
- counseling and guidance
- placement services
- rehabilitation-engineering services if you need physical accommodations, such as a special piece of equipment (the agency is not required to provide you with the equipment, but must help determine what type of equipment would assist you)

In addition to these minimum services, many states offer additional services, such as transportation and special equipment.

You can find your state rehabilitation agency in the telephone directory under one of the following state departments: Labor, Human Resources, Public Welfare, Human Services, or Education. In addition, some states have independent rehabilitation commissions, which would be listed under "Vocational Rehabilitation Services" or "Rehabilitation Services."

Federal

Although the federal Rehabilitation Services Administration does not provide direct services, it is responsible for ensuring that each state agency complies with federal law. If you believe your state agency is unreasonably denying you rehabilitation services, you may file a complaint with:

United States Department of Education
Rehabilitation Services Administration
Office of the Commissioner
Office of Special Education and Rehabilitation Services
330 C Street, S.W.
Washington, D.C. 20202
(202) 732-1282

For help in creating an accommodation for you, your employer may contact:
Job Accommodation Network
President's Committee on Employment of the Handicapped
P.O. Box 468
Morgantown, West Virginia 26505
(800) JAN-PECH (526-7234)

- entering the job market for the first time
- entering the job market after retraining
- unable to perform the duties of the previous job

Resources are available to help your employer create an appropriate accommodation. The Job Accommodation Network, a free service of the President's Committee on Employment of the Handicapped, was established in 1984 to provide information on practical job accommodations. The network has a toll-free number to reach a consultant who can suggest appropriate accommodations for a particular situation. Any company, regardless of size, may call the network whenever it has a disabled employee it wants to promote, help return to work after injury or illness, help perform a present job more easily, or hire for a vacant job.

Medical Malpractice

While cancer survivors are often victims of employment discrimination, many suffer from medical malpractice as well. The 1970s brought a dramatic rise in the number of malpractice cases. Although there is no evidence that actual malpractice increased during this time, and the majority of cases are still dismissed without payment to the patient, there are several reasons why patients are more willing to sue their doctors:

- Patients' expectations have risen as medical care becomes more sophisticated.
- Patients no longer view their doctors as infallible.
- Damage awards per case have increased manyfold.
- A growing number of attorneys advertise their willingness to handle malpractice cases.
- Courts have recognized greater patient rights.

Cancer survivors are at the center of the malpractice boom. They sue members of their treatment team for mistakes during surgery, chemotherapy, and radiation treatments. One of the most common medical-malpractice claims is the "failure to diagnose." The most common of these failures is the cancer diagnosis.

For example, in April 1976, Donald VanVleet complained of headaches and coughing up blood. His doctor referred him to a nose-and-throat specialist to treat the bleeding. In June, Mr. VanVleet returned to his doctor for another examination. Mr. VanVleet's doctor put a note in the chart that he should have a bronchoscopy; however, the doctor told neither Mr. VanVleet nor another doctor about this recommendation, so no bronchoscopy was scheduled. In April 1977, Mr. VanVleet again returned to his doctor, with similar symptoms. His doctor then took X rays and performed a bronchoscopy, which revealed advanced lung cancer. Mr. VanVleet died the following month. A North Dakota court awarded Mrs. VanVleet damages against the doctor because it found that he deviated from accepted medical practice when he failed to schedule a bronchoscopy in 1976.

A New Jersey woman won damages against her doctor for his failure to diagnose her breast cancer. Merle Evers found a tiny lump in her breast in March 1977. Her doctor examined her and told her that he found nothing suspicious and that she should not worry. By October 1977, the lump was four times larger. When her doctor's partner recommended no immediate treatment, she obtained a second opinion, which revealed cancer. Ms. Evers had a mastectomy in October 1977. She remained cancer-free from 1977 until 1983, when the cancer recurred in her lungs. A New Jersey court found that the delay in her diagnosis in 1977 significantly increased her risk of recurrence and awarded Ms. Evers damages for the suffering caused by the delay.

Similarly, in 1972, Cornelius O'Keefe complained of pain in his hip and leg. A

Veterans Administration hospital took X rays and sent Mr. O'Keefe home without a diagnosis. In 1976, Mr. O'Keefe had X rays taken at another hospital. A comparison of the 1972 and 1976 X rays showed that Mr. O'Keefe had cancer in his leg and hip bone that was localized in 1972 but had spread by 1976. To save his life, surgeons amputated his leg and hip. Mr. O'Keefe won damages for lost wages, pain, and suffering against the Veterans Administration because the Oklahoma court found that, had he been told of his cancer in 1972, he could have been treated with surgery less radical than amputation.

Delay in diagnosis can be reasonable, however, and therefore *not* grounds for malpractice. On March 28, 1978, Margherita Henning's doctor examined her for a lump in her breast. He took a mammogram, and found no visible difference from the mammogram he had taken in 1976. He told Ms. Henning to observe the lump and return immediately if she noticed any changes, otherwise to return in a month. Ms. Henning found no changes, and returned to her doctor's office on May 8, 1978. At that time, her doctor suspected a change in the lump and scheduled a biopsy. When the biopsy revealed early breast cancer, her doctor referred her to two oncologists. Ms. Henning's treatment was unsuccessful, and she died. A New Mexico court held that her doctor had met the duty of skill, knowledge, and care that he owed Ms. Henning under the circumstances, that he diagnosed her breast cancer at the earliest possible stage, and that the one-month delay had had no effect on her outcome.

Responsibility of Care

Anyone who provides your medical care has some responsibility for the quality of that care. Hospitals are responsible for their employees and, under some circumstances, for physicians who have admitting privileges. Physicians are responsible for their own work, as well as that of their employees.

All doctors and other care givers have a duty to give their patients reasonable professional medical care. This means that your doctor must act with the minimum level of skill and learning common to other doctors in his or her community and field of expertise. A specialist in one field is measured against other specialists in that same field.

What is "reasonable" depends on professional standards determined by state laws, accrediting agencies, professional societies, hospital rules, expert opinions, and common medical practice. Examples of unreasonable care are:

- Your doctor negligently delays diagnosing your cancer, a delay that significantly changes your prognosis and/or treatment.
- Your surgeon fails to remove all malignant tumors that could reasonably be expected to be removed by a surgeon.
- You are harmed by inappropriate radiation therapy or chemotherapy that was given at a frequency, dose, or time considered not medically professional.
- Your doctor fails to perform an important test that most other, similar doctors would consider essential (for example, your mother and grandmother had breast cancer, you discover a suspicious lump in your breast, and your doctor decides to wait a few months without performing any diagnostic tests).
- Your doctor was grossly negligent in treating you (for example, stating that he or she was an expert in treating your type of cancer, when in fact you were his or her first cancer patient).
- Your doctor erroneously and negligently diagnoses a malignancy when in fact none exists, and consequently you are subjected to needless worry and/or treatment.

Your doctor does not have a duty to guarantee a particular result or to provide you with the most up-to-date form of treatment.

Although many patients are unhappy with the outcome of their treatment, very few have a legitimate malpractice claim against their doctor.

Bringing a Malpractice Case

Every state sets a statute of limitations, a deadline by which you may file a lawsuit. Kentucky, Louisiana, Ohio, and Tennessee have short statutes of limitations, only one year. Maryland (five years) and Nevada (four years) have relatively long statutes of limitations. In every other state, you must file a lawsuit within two or three years from when you were actually injured or when you learned of your injury.

You cannot sue your doctor simply because he or she makes an error in judgment. To bring a malpractice claim against your doctor, you must show three things:

1. Your doctor treated you for a medical condition.

2. You were harmed by your doctor's treatment.

3. Your doctor did not exercise reasonable professional care.

Your doctor's treatment must actually have caused your injury. It need not have been the only cause of your injury, but it must have been a "substantial factor." In determining the cause of your injury, a court will consider if you contributed to your own injury—for example, by smoking or failing to follow your doctor's instructions.

If you win a malpractice case, you may be entitled to an award that restores you, at least financially, to the condition you would be in if your doctor had not made a mistake. For example, you may win lost wages, reimbursement for medical expenses, and an award for "pain and suffering."

Confidentiality of Medical Records

Until the 1960s, few people other than your health-care provider saw your medical records. Because of changes in the way medical care is purchased, and because of consumer advocacy by patients, many people, including yourself, are now likely to have access to your medical records.

The main reason for this change is that patients no longer directly pay for the majority of their medical expenses. Insurance companies, employers, and government agencies currently pay approximately 70 percent of all medical bills, and thus have an interest in seeing your medical records to verify the legitimacy of the bill. When you buy health insurance, for example, you are probably asked to sign a form giving the insurance company permission to look at your medical records at any time to review a charge.

Additionally, one of the results of the consumer movement and cancer-survivorship movement is an increasing effort by survivors to obtain copies of their medical records. Cancer survivors and other patients may want to see their medical records for a number of reasons:

1. So they can be more informed about their own health care, which will allow them to play a more active role. (You cannot be an effective member of your health team if you are not privy to the game plan.)

2. To make it easier to seek a second opinion or change primary-care providers.

3. To help them protect their privacy by ensuring that the information about them in their records is accurate.

4. To provide a base of information that may be helpful in dealing with potential long-term consequences of cancer, such as recurrence, secondary tumors, and latent physical effects of treatment.

> "As recently as 1979, the American Medical Association opposed giving patients access to their own records, citing the need to protect patients from being misled by the information in the record or from trying to treat themselves.... Perhaps because of the continued demand for release of medical records by patients and the debunking of many of the myths about the 'harm' to patients caused by access, the AMA has moderated its position. In 1984, the AMA finally came to the view that doctors should 'on request of the patient...provide a copy or a summary of the record to the patient.'"
>
> —Sidney M. Wolfe, M.D., *Medical Records: Getting Yours*, Public Citizen Health Research Group, 1986

In general, there are two types of medical records: your doctor's records and your hospital's records. Doctors are just becoming comfortable with allowing patients access to their medical records.

Doctors' records are usually shorter than hospital records. If you are receiving chemotherapy or radiation on an outpatient basis, however, your doctor's records may be more lengthy than your hospital records.

Hospital records are usually organized into different sections. When you request your hospital records, clearly state whether you want your entire record or only a specific section. The most common sections are:

- face sheet: a cover page with general information about you and your insurance
- admission record: your status at the time you were admitted to the hospital
- progress notes: results of tests, treatment, and your daily care while in the hospital
- surgery report: record of any inpatient surgery
- pathology: results from studies of biopsies or other tissue samples
- laboratory reports: results of lab tests such as blood and urine tests
- X-ray report: results of X rays
- vital-sign sheets: graph of temperature, blood pressure, pulse, and respiration
- doctor's order sheets: doctor's directions to nurses and other hospital personnel
- discharge summary: your diagnosis and condition at time of discharge

Laws that regulate your right to your medical records. Your right to obtain your medical records depends on state law (unless you are seeking records from a federally owned hospital, as discussed below). Thirty-three states have laws that regulate patients' access to medical records. (Most states have laws that regulate access to mental-health medical records; these laws are not discussed here.) Twenty-one states have no law guaranteeing your right to see your hospital or physician's records. Twenty-three states give you the right to see both types of records.

State laws that regulate your right to see your medical records vary in several ways:

1. what types of records are covered
- hospital records (public and/or private)
- doctor's records

2. whether any exclusions apply (for example, some states allow a doctor to refuse to release your medical records if he or she believes that reading them will "harm" you)
3. who may see your records
- you or your family
- your lawyer
- another doctor

4. what type of access you have
- to read your record (all or part)
- to photocopy your record (all or part)

5. when you have access
- at your request
- only by court order
- only for a lawsuit
- only when the hospital or doctor agrees

For more information about the law in your state governing access to hospital records, contact the medical-records department of your hospital, your state's office of the American Medical Records Association, or your state's hospital association. For more information about the law in your state governing access to physicians' records, contact the state agency that licenses physicians. This may be called the State Licensure Board or the State Board of Medical Examiners.

Federal, not state, laws govern your right to your medical records if you were treated in a federal hospital (Department of Veterans Affairs, military hospital run by the Department of Defense, or Public Health Service program). The federal Privacy Act gives you the right to inspect and copy your medical records that are maintained by a federal agency. Each federal agency determines how it will permit access.

How to obtain your medical records. If you were treated in a state, local, or private hospital or doctor's office, state law will govern your right to see your medical records and the steps you must take to obtain them. If the state where you were treated does not have a law, the doctor or hospital can decide whether to give you access to your records.

Your first step is to contact the medical-records department of the hospital or your physician's office. Ask them what steps you must follow to obtain a copy of your records. If state law does not establish guidelines and procedures, your hospital or doctor may do so. If you make a written request, keep a copy of your letters. If your request is denied, ask the hospital or doctor to state in writing why they will not let you see your records and how you can appeal the decision.

One way to obtain your records if your request is denied is to find a friendly doctor who will ask the provider to send them to him or her, and will then share them with you. American Medical Association rules require your treating physician to transfer your records to your new physician at your request. If you cannot locate another doctor, you may wish to have a lawyer obtain your medical records (either by bringing a lawsuit or by threatening to do so).

If you are seeking medical records kept by a federal agency, you can ask for them in writing, in person, or by telephone (although some agencies require that your request be written). The medical-records department of the hospital in which you were treated can tell you what steps you must take to see your records. When you ask for your records, find out what procedures you should follow if your request to see them is denied.

If you make a written request, always keep a copy for yourself. Your letter should include the following:

1. "I am seeking my medical records under both the Freedom of Information Act (5 U.S.C. Section 552) and the Privacy Act (5 U.S.C. Section 552a)."

2. Put on the letter and the envelope "Attention: FOIA/Privacy Act request." Filing a request under these laws gives you certain rights.

3. State the type of record you want (for example, your entire medical record or just your laboratory reports).

4. State when and where you were treated.

5. State your full name, current address, and name and address at the time you were treated.

6. State that you expect a response within ten business days.

Under the Privacy Act, the hospital must let you know within ten business days whether it will give you access to your records. If it will, it must do so within 30 business days. The hospital is allowed to charge you its actual cost to photocopy your record. If the hospital denies you access to your records, the Freedom of Information Act gives you the right to appeal to the head of the federal agency that holds your records. You have the right to have them corrected should you find a mistake.

Public Citizen, a consumer-rights group founded by Ralph Nader, may be able to help you if you are unsuccessful in obtaining your records from a federal agency. For information and possible help in appealing a denial of access, write to: The Freedom of Information Clearinghouse, Public Citizen, 2000 P Street, N.W., Washington, D.C. 20036.

Insurance Issues

No law guarantees that all cancer survivors can buy adequate, affordable health and life insurance. Nevertheless, there are a number of laws, resources, and helpful suggestions that can make your search for insurance more productive.

The most common nonmedical concerns that cancer survivors express center on questions about health and life insurance. In general, insurance is a commodity for sale to individuals whom private companies determine to be a sufficiently low economic risk, and most companies consider cancer survivors to be a high risk. Obstacles in obtaining, collecting, and keeping insurance hinder cancer survivors' efforts to receive needed medical care without declaring bankruptcy. Because few people can pay for the costs of oncology care solely from their own pockets, most survivors depend on health insurance to weather the enormous financial impact of cancer.

Securing Health Insurance

More than 37 million Americans under the age of 65 have no health insurance. An estimated 50 million more have minimum coverage that is insufficient to meet medical expenses for a serious illness. Although most Americans obtain health insurance through their jobs, more than two-thirds of the uninsured are employed or are the dependents of employed individuals. Cancer survivors represent a disproportionate number of these uninsured and underinsured Americans.

Because most adults in the United States obtain health insurance through their employment, the loss of employment often results in lost or decreased health insurance. Survivors who are not covered by group policies, which spread the risk among a large applicant pool, are the most vulnerable to insurance problems.

Roughly one in four cancer survivors is unable to obtain adequate health insurance. It is not uncommon for an insurance company to double premiums once it learns that a subscriber has a cancer history. Insurance companies construct barriers to health insurance by rejecting new applications, canceling policies, reducing benefits, increasing premiums, requiring long waiting periods before pre-existing conditions are covered by the insurance, and excluding coverage for certain pre-existing conditions.

Cancer survivors who have health insurance may find some of their claims rejected because the insurance policy does not cover "experimental treatment." Unfortunately, what your doctor considers current, standard, aggressive cancer treatment may be considered "experimental" by your insurance company. For example, many oncologists use chemotherapy drugs to treat their patients for diseases other than the specific types of cancer indicated on the "package insert" (description of the drug and its uses and side effects) required by the Food and Drug Administration. Although the Food and Drug Administration permits doctors to prescribe drugs for any use if there is competent medical evidence to support that use, insurance companies and Medicare often refuse to pay for chemotherapy that is used in a way not listed on the package insert.

If your policy explicitly excludes coverage of "experimental treatment," your insurance company will probably reject claims for treatments that the FDA has approved only for investigational, and not general, use. If you participate in an experimental trial to test a cancer drug, find out if the pharmaceutical manufacturer will pay for the treatment.

Should your insurance company refuse to pay for a claim for treatment approved by the FDA for general use, appeal the company's decision. Ask your physician to write a letter explaining why that treatment choice was justified in your case. Your physician should attach copies of medical articles, if any, that support the treatment. Although every appeal is not successful, each appeal further encourages your insurance company to pay for the most current and promising treatment as determined by your physician.

Your Legal Right to Health Insurance

As long as it otherwise complies with state and federal law, an insurance company can decide what type of insurance it will sell and to whom. The company can decide what type of risk it will insure as long as it applies the same standards to all similar risks. When you apply for an individual or small group policy, the company will probably "medically underwrite" you. This means that the company considers your medical history in deciding whether, and at what cost, to insure you.

In general, you do not have a "legal right" to adequate health insurance. Whether termination from a plan, denial of benefits under a plan, or refusal to issue insurance violates a law is determined by two factors: the terms of the policy and the applicable law (federal and state).

Contractual rights. An insurance policy is a contract between you (the insured) and your insurance company (the insurer). Your obligations under the contract are to pay your premiums on time and to provide your insurance company with the information it requests to process your claim. Your insurance company's obligations are to pay you benefits and provide other services as spelled out in the policy. If you meet your obligations, but your insurance company refuses to pay benefits (or perform another duty, such as renew your policy) in accordance with the terms of the policy, you may be able to sue your company for breach of contract.

Federal laws. No federal law guarantees a right to adequate health insurance. Two laws (COBRA and ERISA), however, provide cancer survivors with opportunities to keep the health insurance they have obtained at work even after they are no longer employed.

COBRA. The Comprehensive Omnibus Budget Reconciliation Act requires employers to offer group medical coverage to employees and their dependents who otherwise would have lost their group coverage due to individual circumstances. Public and private employers with more than 20 employees are required to make continued insurance coverage available to employees who quit, are terminated, or work reduced hours. Coverage must extend to surviving, divorced, or separated spouses, and to dependent children.

By allowing you to keep your group insurance coverage for a limited time, COBRA gives you valuable time to shop for long-term coverage. Although you, and not your former employer, must pay for the continued coverage, the rate you pay may not exceed by more than 2 percent the rate set for your former co-workers. Continuation of coverage must be offered regardless of any conditions, such as cancer.

Eligibility for the employee, spouse, and dependent child varies under COBRA. The employee becomes eligible if he or she loses group health coverage because of a reduction in hours or termination due to reasons other than gross employee misconduct. The spouse of an employee becomes eligible for any of four reasons:

1. death of spouse
2. termination of spouse's employment (for reasons other than gross misconduct) or reduction in spouse's hours of employment
3. divorce or legal separation from spouse
4. spouse's eligibility for Medicare

The dependent child of an employee becomes eligible for any of five reasons:

1. death of parent
2. termination of parent's employment or reduction in parent's hours
3. parent's divorce or legal separation
4. parent's eligibility for Medicare
5. dependent's ceasing to be a "dependent child" under specific group plan

The continued coverage under COBRA must be identical to that offered to the families of your former co-workers. If your employment is terminated, you and your dependents can continue coverage for up to 18 months. Your dependents can continue coverage for up to 36 months if their previous coverage will end because of any of the above reasons. Your group plan may give you the right to convert to an individual plan. Some states require insurance companies to permit you to convert from a group plan to an individual policy. If you do, expect your premiums to increase.

Continued coverage may be cut short if:

1. your employer no longer provides group health insurance to any of its employees
2. your continuation-coverage premium is not paid
3. you become covered under another group health plan (if the plan limits coverage for pre-existing conditions, you can continue COBRA coverage for 18 months)
4. you become eligible for Medicare

The employee or family member has the duty to inform the group-health-plan administrator of a change in family status. The employer is responsible for notifying the group health plan of an employee's death, termination of employment, or reduction in hours. Employees and beneficiaries are given 60 days from the date they would lose coverage to make a decision about continued coverage.

COBRA was amended in 1989 to provide additional help for disabled employees who leave their jobs. They can continue coverage for up to 29 months, when they become eligible for Medicare. Disabled employees can be charged 150 percent of the premium between 18 and 29 months.

COBRA is enforced by the Pension and Welfare Benefits Administration of the United States Department of Labor. The first step to resolving a COBRA complaint is to try to work out a settlement with your employer. If no adequate solution can be reached, you should write the Department of Labor at:

Pension and Welfare Benefits Administration
U.S. Department of Labor, Room N-5658
200 Constitution Avenue, N.W.
Washington, D.C. 20210

STATES THAT REQUIRE THE RIGHT TO CONVERT A GROUP HEALTH POLICY TO AN INDIVIDUAL POLICY

(June 1990)
Reprinted with permission,
National Association of Insurance Commissioners

Arizona	Kansas	New Mexico	Tennessee
Arkansas	Kentucky	New York	Texas
California	Maine	North Carolina	Utah
Colorado	Maryland	Ohio	Vermont
Connecticut	Minnesota	Oklahoma	Virginia
Florida	Missouri	Oregon	Washington
Georgia	Montana	Pennsylvania	West Virginia
Illinois	Nevada	Rhode Island	Wisconsin
Iowa	New Hampshire	South Dakota	Wyoming

ERISA. The Employee Retirement and Income Security Act may provide a remedy to an employee who has been denied full participation in an employee-benefit plan because of a cancer history. ERISA prohibits an employer from discriminating against an employee for the purpose of preventing him or her from collecting benefits under an employee-benefit plan. All employers who offer benefit packages to their employees are subject to ERISA.

Some employers fear that participation of cancer survivors in group medical plans will drain benefit funds or increase the employers' insurance premiums. A violation of ERISA may occur when an employer, upon learning of a worker's cancer history, dismisses that worker for the purpose of excluding him or her from a group health plan.

If the employer fires the employee for the purpose of cutting off that employee's benefits, regardless of whether the employee is considered handicapped under the statute, then the employer may be liable for a violation of ERISA. Employee-benefit plans are defined widely, and include any plan with the purpose of providing "medical, surgical, or hospital care benefits, or benefits in the event of sickness, accident, disability, death or unemployment." An employer may also violate ERISA by encouraging a person with a cancer history to retire as a "disabled" employee. Most benefit plans define disability narrowly to include only the most debilitating conditions. Individuals with a cancer history often do not fit under such a definition and should not be compelled to so label themselves.

Under certain circumstances, ERISA may provide grounds for a lawsuit to workers with a cancer history. ERISA covers both participants (employees) and beneficiaries (spouses and children). Thus, if the employee is fired because his or her child has cancer, the employee may be entitled to file a claim. ERISA, however, is inapplicable to many victims of employment discrimination, including individuals who are denied a new job because of their medical status, employees who are subjected to differential treatment that does not affect their benefits, and employees whose compensation does not include benefits.

ERISA is enforced by the Pension and Welfare Benefits Administration of the United States Department of Labor. The first step to secure your benefits is to file for all those you are entitled to under the plan. Your plan administrator must furnish you with a summary of the plan that tells you how the plan works, what benefits it provides, how they may be obtained or lost, and how you can enforce your rights under ERISA.

You must be notified within 90 days whether your claim is accepted or rejected. If you are not paid benefits to which you are entitled within 90 days, you may request a review of the denial, unless the plan administrator requests additional time to respond to your claim. You have at least 60 days from the date of denial to decide whether you will appeal the decision. If you do appeal and your claim is denied upon review, you must be told the reason for the denial and the plan rules upon which the decision was based.

If you are still dissatisfied with the decision, you may file a complaint in federal court. You do not have to have an attorney to file a complaint in federal court, but the assistance of an attorney at this stage is usually beneficial. The federal government does not have an informal administrative procedure to handle appeals from denial of benefits. Information about how to enforce your rights under ERISA may be obtained by writing the Department of Labor at:

Pension and Welfare Benefits Administration
U.S. Department of Labor, Room N-5658
200 Constitution Avenue, N.W.
Washington, D.C. 20210
(202) 523-8521

In certain cases, the Department of Labor may try to negotiate a solution before your case is filed in federal court.

State laws. Every state has an insurance commission or department that enforces state regulation of insurance companies. The commission determines what types of policies must be offered and when rates may be raised. States regulate insurance sold by insurance companies; they do not regulate self-insured policies (policies that companies fund and administer for their own employees). State regulations cover all aspects of health insurance, including rates, policy conditions, termination or reinstatement of coverage, and the scope of coverage and benefits.

Some states have laws that establish "high-risk pools" for those who are unable to obtain health insurance because of their medical histories. Risk-sharing pools are designed to ensure that all individuals have the opportunity to purchase health insurance regardless of pre-existing conditions such as cancer.

State laws that create high-risk pools require major insurers to participate in the plan and share the risks. Risk pools usually provide a package of benefits with a choice of deductibles. Although the premiums are higher than those for individual insurance, most states impose a cap on the amount that can be charged. Many states have a waiting period for individuals with a pre-existing condition before the new policy will pay benefits. A waiting period of six months for pre-existing conditions like cancer is common. For example, if you are receiving cancer treatments in January and you join a high-risk pool with a six-month waiting period, some or all of your medical bills will not be covered by the plan until the following July. Some states, however, will waive the waiting period if you pay a specified premium surcharge. All aspects of these pools vary from state to state.

If you live in a state with a high-risk pool, contact your state insurance department for information about how to participate in the pool. Even if your state does not offer such insurance now, you should ask whether it plans to do so. Many states are considering creating high-risk pools.

Some Blue Cross and Blue Shield associations offer individual policies to individuals regardless of their medical histories. As of December 1989, Blue Cross and Blue Shield in Maryland, Michigan, New Hampshire, New Jersey, New York, North Carolina, Pennsylvania, Rhode Island, Vermont,

STATES THAT MANDATE INSURANCE COVERAGE FOR MAMMOGRAPHY

(Compiled with the assistance of the
National Alliance of Breast Cancer Organizations)

As of June 1990, the following states required insurance coverage for mammography. The provisions in these laws vary from state to state according to age, cost, and frequency of testing. The most comprehensive state laws mandate that insurance cover a baseline mammogram for women ages 35 to 39, a mammogram every two years for women ages 40 to 49, and a mammogram every year for women age 50 and over.

Because many states are considering passing such laws, and many others are revising their laws, you should check with your insurance carrier, state insurance commissioner, or community cancer organization for current information in your state.

Arizona (law passed in 1988)
Arkansas (1989)
California (1988)
Colorado (1989)
Connecticut (1988)
Florida (1988)
Georgia (1990)
Illinois (1989)
Iowa (1989)
Kansas (1988)
Kentucky (1990)
Maine (1990)
Maryland (1986)
Massachusetts (1987)
Michigan (1989)
Minnesota (1988)
Nevada (1989)
New Hampshire (1988)
New Mexico (1990)
New York (1988)
North Dakota (1989)
Oklahoma (1988)
Pennsylvania (1989)
Rhode Island (1988)
South Dakota (1990)
Tennessee (1989)
Texas (1987)
Virginia (1989)
Washington (1989)
West Virginia (1989)
Wisconsin (1990)

Virginia, and the District of Columbia guaranteed acceptance (open enrollment) into individual plans. Some of these plans are offered continuously, whereas others are offered only for a brief period each year. These plans generally have a waiting period for cancer (and any other pre-existing condition) coverage from three months to one year. Contact your local Blue Cross and Blue Shield offices to learn what is available in your state.

Types of Health-Insurance Coverage

You may purchase a private health-insurance policy as an individual or through a group. An individual policy is issued to you and covers only you and/or your dependents. A group policy is issued to a policyholder, such as an employer or an organization, and insures those who are affiliated with the policyholder (for example,

> ### STATE-MANDATED HIGH-RISK POOLS
>
> In August 1989, 25 states had laws establishing high-risk health insurance pools:
>
> | | |
> |---|---|
> | California | Nebraska |
> | Colorado | New Mexico |
> | Connecticut | North Dakota |
> | Florida | Oregon |
> | Georgia | Rhode Island |
> | Illinois | South Carolina |
> | Indiana | Tennessee |
> | Iowa | Texas |
> | Louisiana | Utah |
> | Maine | Washington |
> | Minnesota | Wisconsin |
> | Missouri | Wyoming |
> | Montana | |

employees or members of the organization). There are two main types of private health-insurance plans: fee-for-service and managed health plans.

Fee-for-service plans are traditional health-insurance policies. You pay premiums to an insurance company, which then pays for health-care services as covered by the policy. You may choose to be treated by any physician or medical facility. Your insurance company pays part or all of the cost of each service. You are responsible for paying all bills not covered by your policy.

In a managed health-care plan, you pay a membership fee or premium to an organization that provides health services directly from doctors and other providers affiliated with the plan. Because most services are prepaid, you usually do not have to fill out claim forms. Health Maintenance Organizations (HMOs) are the most common form of managed health-care plan today. Because you will be covered only for services provided by doctors and hospitals affiliated with the plan, make sure oncologists and hospitals you trust are members of any HMO you consider joining.

There are five general levels of protection that are provided by fee-for-service health-insurance policies:

Basic protection. Basic protection pays for daily room and board and regular nursing services while you are in the hospital, and for certain hospital services and supplies (such as X rays, laboratory tests, medication, and inpatient and outpatient surgery) and some related expenses. Blue Cross and Blue Shield are the major providers of basic insurance.

Hospital indemnity. A hospital-indemnity policy pays benefits only for your care in a hospital. These policies are a source of extra cash during an illness, because benefits are paid directly to you in cash for you to use as you see fit. Hospital-indemnity policies are relatively inexpensive and simple; you need only submit your hospital bill to collect. A fixed amount is paid for each day you are in the hospital, regardless of the actual charges. Some may not pay for the first few days you are in the hospital. However, the benefits are limited (only cover a portion of your bill), and usually do not keep up with inflation. If you have a good, comprehensive health-care policy, you probably don't need hospital insurance.

Major medical. Major medical covers most medical costs associated with serious illness. These plans usually have a large deductible, the amount you or another insurance plan (such as a basic policy) must pay before you receive reimbursements. The deductible in major medical plans is usually $1,000 to $5,000. Although plans vary, in general, the higher your deductible, the lower your premiums will be. Major-medical plans usually require you to make co-payments. Typically, the policy will pay 75 to 85 percent of the bill, and you pay the remainder. Most major-medical policies have a stop-loss feature; this is the point at which out-of-pocket expenses cease and the major-medical policy pays 100 percent of your claims for the remainder of the calendar year. Major-medical plans do limit how much you may collect during your lifetime, and sometimes limit how much you may collect per illness. A "comprehensive policy" includes both basic coverage and major medical.

Catastrophic. Catastrophic policies are like major medical in that they cover the costs of serious illness. They are helpful if you have a major-medical plan with low lifetime maximum benefits. Catastrophic policies are relatively inexpensive and usually have a very high deductible (usually $10,000 to $50,000). Once you reach the deductible, even if those expenses are paid by your major-medical policy, the catastrophic policy will pay 100 percent of your expenses. If you are considering buying a catastrophic policy, make sure it will apply to its deductible any expenses paid by your other health-insurance plans. You want as many of your medical bills applied to the deductible as possible because the sooner your expenses reach the deductible, the sooner the catastrophic policy will pay all of your expenses. Avoid a catastrophic policy that applies only your out-of-pocket expenses to the deductible.

Disability income. You may also buy insurance to pay you a percentage of your regular income should you become unable to work. You should make sure that the benefits will begin within a few months of your disability and will provide you sufficient income while you are not working. Most policies require that you be totally disabled to receive benefits. Others provide some income if you are able to work only part-time. Each company may have a different definition of "disabled." Make sure that the policy will replace significant income lost due to any disability, whether partial or total.

Public Health Insurance

Medicare. Medicare is health insurance for the elderly and disabled funded by Social Security taxes. It is the primary health insurance for 30 million Americans.

Medicare has two parts. Part A is the hospital program, which covers the hospital, a skilled nursing facility, home health care, and hospice care. Part B is the supplemental medical-insurance program, which covers physicians' fees, outpatient laboratory tests, outpatient radiation and chemotherapy, medical equipment, prosthetic devices, and other expenses.

Although the United States Department of Health and Human Services is responsible for the administration of Medicare, the day-to-day operation of the program is handled by private insurance companies that have contracted with the government as either Part A intermediaries for hospitals or Part B carriers. In each state, the federal government contracts with a private company, such as Travelers, Aetna, or Blue Cross, to handle your medical claims. You may not choose which company will handle your Medicare claims.

There are five ways to be eligible for Medicare:

1. You are 65 years old or older, and are entitled to either Social Security, widow's, or Railroad Retirement benefits.
2. You are disabled and you have received Social Security, widow's, or Railroad disability benefits for at least 24 months.
3. You have end-stage renal disease and require dialysis for a kidney transplant.
4. You are over the age of 65 and are not eligible for either Social Security or Railroad Retirement, and you pay a monthly premium for Medicare coverage.
5. You are legally blind.

You are automatically enrolled in Medicare if you are 65 years old or older and are entitled to either Social Security, widow's, or Railroad Retirement benefits. Otherwise,

> ## Cancer Insurance
>
> Some insurance companies market "cancer policies," policies that pay benefits only for cancer treatment. Such policies are generally available only to people who have never had cancer. Because of the many disadvantages of cancer policies, many states have banned or severely restricted their sale. Most insurance experts recommend buying good basic and major-medical plans instead of disease-specific policies, for five reasons:
>
> **1.** Because major-medical plans usually cover the costs of cancer treatment, additional "cancer policies" usually duplicate other policies and are an unnecessary expense.
>
> **2.** Premiums are very high for limited benefits.
>
> **3.** Cancer policies often exclude coverage of complications from cancer treatment.
>
> **4.** Some policy salesmen try to mislead consumers and prey on their fears about cancer.
>
> **5.** Sales and administrative expenses for cancer policies tend to be much higher than other policies.

you must fill out an application for enrollment. If you are denied benefits under either Part A or Part B, you may appeal the decision.

Because Congress has considered several changes in Medicare recently, especially for catastrophic illness, your coverage may have changed. For more information about Medicare, you can obtain consumer pamphlets by contacting your local Social Security office or by writing to:

United States Department of Health
and Human Services
Health Care Financing Administration
(HCFA)
Baltimore, Maryland 21207

or by calling the HCFA hotline at (800) 888-1998.

Medicaid. Medicaid is a jointly financed federal-state insurance program for low-income families. The federal government administers Medicaid through the Health Care Financing Administration (HCFA) of the Department of Health and Human Services. Each state has a single agency (usually the Department of Social Services or the Department of Public Welfare) that administers Medicaid in that state.

The federal government requires certain basic benefits; each state then determines what additional benefits it will provide and who is eligible. Because states have some role in determining who is eligible for Medicaid and what benefits are paid, Medicaid coverage varies widely from state to state. All states, however, must give you a fair hearing before the state agency if your Medicaid claim is denied. The types of expenses covered by Medicaid may include hospitals, physicians, prescription drugs, and home aids. For more information about Medicaid, contact your state public-welfare department.

Maximizing Health-Insurance Coverage

Group plans. In general, the best option for cancer survivors is to be enrolled in a group health-insurance plan. Because group-plan premiums are based on the illness risk of the group and not that of an individual, group policies are usually far less expensive than are individual policies for similar coverage, and often provide better benefits.

Most group plans cover you and your immediate family. Group plans do vary, however, depending upon the carrier. For example, although a majority have pre-existing condition clauses, some states, like New York, require large employers to offer group health insurance to their employees with no waiting period for pre-existing conditions. Most group plans offer either hospital benefits or major-medical coverage.

If you are looking for a job, consider whether you will be covered by the group health plan. If you have a job, check with your personnel department or union to learn if you are eligible for a group plan through work.

If you are unable to join a group health-insurance policy through your job or your spouse's job, join an association or organization that offers group health insurance to members. Many national and regional organizations sell group health coverage to their members. Hundreds of fraternal, political, and professional organizations offer such plans. There are a number of ways to find such organizations.

1. Choose the type of organization that meets your personal interests. Fraternal organizations include social-service clubs, volunteer organizations, and religious groups. Professional organizations represent the interests of lawyers, health-care workers, accountants, union members, and other workers. Some colleges and universities offer group plans to members of their alumni associations. Group policies are also available from some political organizations, such as the National Organization for Women and the American Association of Retired Persons, as well as the National Association for the Self-Employed.

2. Use your public library to locate the names and addresses of organizations. Ask the reference librarian for books, such as the *Encyclopedia of Associations,* that list the names and addresses of associations by topic.

3. Look in your local telephone book and the AT&T Toll-Free Directory under headings such as "Associations," "Clubs," "Organizations," "Religious Organizations."

4. If you own a bank credit card, ask your bank if it offers a group health-insurance plan to its credit-card members.

If you were covered by a group plan at work and lose your job, there are several steps you can take to try to remain covered by the plan.

1. Learn how long your insurance will continue after your last day of work.

2. Ask if you can convert your group coverage to an individual policy (see following section).

3. Ask whether you are eligible for extension under COBRA (see p. 119).

4. If your spouse is covered by a group plan, find out whether it will cover you.

5. Consider a short-term policy that covers medical expenses other than cancer to protect you until you find a new job that offers health insurance.

Individual plans. Few health-insurance plans cover 100 percent of your medical expenses. Before you consider buying any health-care plan, especially one to supplement your current insurance, carefully review all of the benefits of each plan to make sure you obtain the maximum amount of coverage for your premiums. For example, if you are eligible for Medicaid, you probably do not need additional insurance, because Medicaid pays almost all medical costs. The following chart may help you compare insurance policies.

When you look for private health insurance, keep the following suggestions in mind:

POLICY/PLAN COMPARISON WORKSHEET
MAJOR MEDICAL INSURANCE

Insurance company												
Policy/plan name												
Premium	$			$			$			$		
Deductible if any	$			$			$			$		
Co-payment percent: Company ___ You ___	___%	___%		___%	___%		___%	___%		___%	___%	
Maximum benefits payable	$			$			$			$		
Is the policy renewable?	Yes ☐	No ☐		Yes ☐	No ☐		Yes ☐	No ☐		Yes ☐	No ☐	
The following services should be covered by any policy you consider:	**Self**	**Spouse**	**Depndt**	**Self**	**Spouse**	**Depndt**	**Self**	**Spouse**	**Depndt**	**Self**	**Spouse**	**Depndt**
Blood and blood components (transfusions)												
Cosmetic surgery (as a result of accident/injury)												
Dental treatment (as a result of accident/injury)												
Diagnostic tests (examples: X rays, laboratory)												
Durable medical equipment (rental of hospital bed, wheelchair, etc.)												
Outpatient mental-health service												
Outpatient treatment services (examples: chemotherapy, radiation therapy)												
Obstetric services												
Oxygen/oxygen supplies												
Physician/surgeon services												
Physical therapy												
Prescription drugs												
Professional nursing services												
Prosthetic appliances (limbs, eyes, orthopedic braces)												
Radiation therapy												
Rehabilitation services												
Respiratory therapy												
Room and board (semiprivate)												
Surgery and supplies												
Transportation (ambulance)												
List additional services covered.												
EXCLUSIONS: List services *not* covered.												

1. Before you apply for insurance, you may wish to check your status with the Medical Information Bureau, Inc., a company that keeps data about you on file for insurance companies. When you apply for health, disability, or life insurance, you are usually asked to sign a form giving the company permission to provide the Medical Information Bureau with information about your medical history. Although their files are very current, a computer automatically erases reports that are more than seven years old. Under the Fair Credit Reporting Act of 1970, you have a right to verify the information in your file to ensure its accuracy. Contact:

Medical Information Bureau, Inc.
P.O. Box 105
Essex Station
Boston, Massachusetts 02112
(617) 426-3660

Ask for a form requesting disclosure of any information in your file. Medical information may be sent only to the "licensed medical professional" of your choice, but MIB will send nonmedical information directly to you. You may request a correction form from MIB to submit along with documentation to clear up errors in your file.

2. If you have health insurance, no matter how inadequate, do not give it up until you have obtained other insurance and all waiting periods for benefits have passed.

3. Compare the costs and protection offered by several private companies before deciding which policy to buy. An efficient way to do this is to have an independent broker (one who does not work for a particular company) shop among the companies in your area to obtain the best possible plan for your needs. You may get a list of all licensed insurance brokers in your area from the state insurance department or find them listed in the Yellow Pages. With or without an agent's assistance, you should carefully compare the conditions and limits of each policy. A policy may cover most expenses but only up to a maximum amount that could easily be reached with a serious illness. Some hospital-indemnity policies may not pay for the first few days you are in the hospital, whereas others will.

4. Do not buy duplicate coverage. For example, "cancer insurance" usually duplicates a basic or major-medical plan. One comprehensive policy is better than several policies with overlapping or duplicate coverage.

5. Look for policies that will cover care related to a pre-existing condition with the shortest possible waiting period. Many policies will not cover you for cancer-related care if you were diagnosed before you bought the policy.

6. Look for policies that guarantee you the right to renew the policy. These are called "noncancelable" and "guaranteed-renewable" policies. Your state insurance commissioner may have a list of companies that issue guaranteed-renewable policies in your state.

7. If you pay your own premiums directly, you will save money by paying quarterly or annually rather than monthly.

8. Buy a policy only from a licensed insurance agent. Agents must be licensed by your state and carry proof of their license. Ask to see proof that their company is licensed (a business card is not proof). The government does not sell Medicare Supplements. If someone tells you that he or she is from the government and then tries to sell you a health-insurance policy, report that person to your state insurance department.

9. If you can, plan ahead. Do not wait to buy health insurance until you or a family member is ill.

10. If you do not have adequate coverage for chemotherapy, ask your doctor to try to obtain free chemotherapy drugs from a pharmaceutical company. Many have limited free programs for indigent patients (see Appendix A).

Once you have chosen a policy to buy, consider the following:

1. Complete the application carefully and accurately. If the insurance company learns that you omitted important information, the company may refuse coverage for a related illness or cancel your policy. Keep a copy of the application for your files.

2. Pay for your policy by check, money order, or bank draft. Make the check payable to the insurance company, not to the agent. Do not pay cash.

3. Carefully read your policy to make sure it is what you intended to buy. Some companies will give you at least ten days to review the policy and will cancel it for a full refund if you decide not to keep it. Some states require insurance companies to give you this right to review and cancel.

4. The company should deliver the policy to you within 30 days. If you contact the company, and more than 60 days pass without a response, contact your state insurance department.

Getting the Most from Your Health Insurance

Cancer treatment often involves numerous bills from a variety of parties: hospital, physicians (surgeon, anesthesiologist, oncologist, radiologist, etc.), support services (nurse, social worker, nutritionist, therapist, etc.), radiology group, pharmacy (drugs and medical supplies), and consumer businesses (wigs, breast inserts, special clothing, etc.). Your insurance company will pay some of these parties directly, in part or in whole. You must pay other bills, and submit copies to your company for reimbursement. If you have more than one policy, you must submit the right bill to the right company in the right order.

Keeping track of dozens of expenses, often amounting to tens of thousands of dollars, can be confusing and exhausting. The key to collecting the maximum benefits to which you are entitled under your insurance policy is to keep accurate records of your medical expenses.

Here are some suggestions to help you keep track of your claims:

1. Make photocopies of everything you send to your company, including letters, claim forms, and bills.

2. Keep all correspondence you receive from your insurance company.

3. Even if you are unsure whether a particular expense is covered by your policy, submit a bill. The worst that can happen is that your expenses will not be reimbursed.

4. Keep accurate records of your expenses, claim submissions, and payment vouchers. One way to do this is by using a record-keeping chart. You may wish to use the following chart, developed with the assistance of Helen Johnson, a consultant to the Post Treatment Resource Program of Memorial Sloan-Kettering Cancer Center in New York City.

You have a right to appeal to your public or private insurer any decision it makes about your claim. Claims are frequently delayed or rejected in part or in full because of errors in filling out the claim forms. Before you challenge the insurance company's rejection of your claim, make sure that you have accurately provided all of the information requested. If the insurance company asks you for more information to complete your claim, be certain that you send them all of the information they request.

If you are having trouble collecting on your claim:

1. Contact your insurance company in writing and insist that they reply in writing. Send copies of all documents and keep the originals for your files.

2. Keep a record of your contacts with the insurance company (copies of all letters you send and notes from every telephone call). Write down everything you do, the names of people you talk to, dates, and other facts.

TAKING CARE OF BUSINESS

Page No. _____

MEDICAL INSURANCE RECORD FOR _____

						Primary Policy					Second Policy				
DATE OF SERVICE	PROVIDER	SERVICE	AMOUNT OF BILL	DATE BILL RECEIVED	CHECK NO.	DATE TO COMPANY	DATE FROM COMPANY	AMOUNT RECV'D	BALANCE I OWE	AMOUNT TOWARD DEDUCTIBLE	DATE TO COMPANY	DATE FROM COMPANY	AMOUNT RECV'D	BALANCE I OWE	AMOUNT TOWARD DEDUCTIBLE

3. Contact the state or federal agency that regulates your insurance provider if you do not receive a satisfactory and timely answer from your insurer (see p. 132). Every state has an insurance department or commission that helps consumers with complaints. Look in the state-government listings in the telephone directory.

4. Contact cancer-support organizations in your community. Some, such as the Candlelighters Childhood Cancer Foundation, offer ombudsman programs to help survivors and their families maximize insurance reimbursement.

5. If your claim is still not settled, consider filing a complaint in small-claims court or hiring a lawyer to sue your company.

If you are unable to manage your own insurance claims, there are private companies in some communities that will organize your bills and submit them to your insurance company for you. Most of these companies take a percentage of the benefits they obtain for you as their fee. Look in the Yellow Pages of the telephone directory under "Insurance Claims Processing Services" for such companies. Avoid companies that charge an hourly rate. Review your claims before they are filed with the insurance company to make sure the claims accurately represent your care and have not been altered to increase the chance of reimbursement. When choosing a claims processing company, be sure to inquire about its reputation. Find out how long it has been in business. Ask about the qualifications of the owner and staff. Your local Better Business Bureau or state Department of Consumer Affairs may be able to tell you if they have received complaints about a particular company.

WHO REGULATES YOUR INSURANCE POLICY

If Your Insurer Is...	It Is Regulated By...
Private company (e.g., nonprofit like Blue Cross and Blue Shield; for-profit company like Prudential)	State insurance department
HMO	Several state and federal agencies. Start with your state insurance department
Private employer or union self-insurance or self-financed plan	U.S. Dept. of Labor (Office of Pension & Welfare Benefits)
Medicaid (called "MediCal" in California)	State Dept. of Social Services
Medicare Supplemental Security Income Social Security Benefits	U.S. Social Security Administration
Veterans Benefits CHAMPUS	Dept. of Veterans Affairs

Life Insurance

Life insurance provides two types of benefits: replacement of wages if a wage earner dies, and replacement of retirement income if a retired family member dies. Although most people agree that life insurance is practical protection in the event of unforeseen tragedy, many are confused about who needs life insurance and why. Insurance experts recommend buying life insurance when:

1. You have young children (all adult wage earners in the family should be covered).

2. You have a family without young children where one spouse would suffer financial hardship if the other spouse died suddenly.

3. You are supporting an aged parent who depends on you for income.

When you apply for life insurance, your medical history becomes of vital interest to the insurance company. Companies will not issue life insurance to an individual they believe to be terminally ill. Although the questions asked on applications vary, common questions that affect the chance of cancer survivors for securing life insurance are:

- Have you been treated for cancer in the past twelve months?
- Has another insurance company ever rejected you, and if so, why?

You must answer these questions honestly. If you do not, and the company discovers the truth, they may cancel your policy or deny some or all of the benefits. If the company is suspicious about your medical history, it may check your file at the Medical Information Bureau (see p. 129).

The company may ask you to submit to a medical exam, paid for by the company, so it can further evaluate your health. It may also conduct an investigation of your daily habits and medical history.

Once the company has collected the information it requires, it determines whether it will issue you life insurance and if so what rate you will be charged. Different companies have different systems for determining what your rate will be.

Some companies market policies for people with serious health problems. Before buying such a policy, read it carefully. The

> "There have certainly been times when I have felt greater uncertainty about my long-term survival than I have at other times. In each of the last three autumns, I have wondered whether to plant the tulip and daffodil bulbs for the spring bloom or not to bother. Now again this past spring, a glory of living color rewarded me, and once again I have planted for next spring's blooming."
>
> —Robert M. Mack, M.D., "Lessons from Living with Cancer," *New England Journal of Medicine*

benefits are often limited (you may have no coverage for the first two policy years) and can be relatively expensive.

The following suggestions may increase cancer survivors' abilities to obtain adequate life insurance.

1. Try large companies that carefully grade type and stage of cancer.

2. Obtain estimates from several companies. An efficient way to do this is to have an independent agent (one who does not work for a particular company) shop among the companies in your area to obtain the best possible plan for your needs. You may get a list of all licensed insurance brokers in your area from the state insurance department.

3. If you are unable to obtain a life-insurance policy with full death benefits, consider a graded policy. If you die from cancer within the first few years of the policy (usually three years), a graded policy returns only your premium plus part of the face value of the policy to your beneficiaries. If you die after the waiting period has passed, the company will pay the full face of the policy.

4. Try to obtain life insurance through a group plan (see p. 126). Many employers and organizations that offer group health insurance also offer group life insurance.

The insurance company does not make an individual evaluation of the health of each plan member of a large group; however, your health may be considered if you participate in a plan with a small number of members (for example, if you are one of 30 workers). If your health is considered, you may be excluded from the plan, denied full benefits, or required to pay an extra premium.

Whether you will be able to buy life insurance and what rate you will pay depend upon the type of cancer you have, when you were diagnosed, and your prognosis. When you apply for life insurance, you are rated and assigned a risk factor. If you are rated within a short time of being diagnosed with a malignancy, the company may decline to issue you a policy at all. If your prognosis improves, you may be issued a policy, but you may be charged an extra premium. The amount of this premium varies depending upon your individual medical history.

How do companies determine these figures? Large companies and reinsurers publish risk selection guides based on reports by their medical staffs. Underwriters then use these guides to evaluate your medical files and determine what policy, if any, they will issue you. Some companies, however, do not differentiate substantially between different types and stages of cancer.

> "When I had to give up my Empress Club card with Canada Airlines International, I felt like a spectator watching life from the outside. The loss of the Club card, a symbol of my success as a salesman, symbolized my loss of full participation in life."
> —Chris Castle, multiple-myeloma survivor

Money Matters

The Expenses of Cancer Treatment

Cancer can have a devastating financial impact on survivors and their families. There are two main types of expenses associated with cancer care: direct medical costs and nonmedical expenses.

Direct medical costs are those resulting from cancer treatment (physicians' fees, hospital expenses, pharmacy bills, etc.). Most of these expenses are covered by basic health-insurance plans. The extent of direct medical costs to the survivor depends on the type of cancer (treatment can cost hundreds of thousands of dollars), the scope of insurance coverage, and the community in which the survivor is treated.

Everyone recognizes that medical care for a serious illness can be quite expensive. Few people, however, are prepared to meet the nonmedical costs of illness until they are faced with mounting bills. Most nonmedical costs related to cancer care are not covered by health insurance. Depending on the scope of your insurance policy, you may have to pay for transportation to and from treatment, child care, a nurse's aide, a housekeeper, a counselor (see chapter 4), treatment-related consumer products, wigs, etc. In addition, many survivors find that their insurance premiums are increased, sometimes manyfold, after their diagnoses.

Cancer can have an especially harmful financial impact on survivors who are not employed, do not have adequate health insurance, or do not have savings or other financial resources. The cost of cancer care is particularly high for those who require expensive long-term care, including long stays in a hospital or nursing home.

To make matters worse, while survivors' costs are increasing, their income is often decreasing. Survivors who face employment discrimination may experience a loss of income and insurance benefits. As a result, many cancer survivors must dip into their savings or borrow money to pay for cancer care.

If the costs of cancer care far exceed your resources, you may want to contact a financial counselor to help you plan a budget. Look in the telephone directory under "Consumer Credit Counseling Services" for a *nonprofit* service that can help you manage your bills. A nonprofit service is likely to provide free or inexpensive assistance; a for-profit company will charge you a fee for their service.

If you cannot locate a nonprofit service in your community, contact:

National Foundation for Consumer Credit, Inc.
8701 Georgia Avenue
Silver Spring, Maryland 20901
(301) 589-5600

This office will supply you with the name of a credit counseling service in your area (if you write, send them a stamped, self-addressed envelope). NFCC is a nonprofit umbrella membership organization of more than 400 nonprofit consumer credit counseling services. NFCC provides confidential financial counseling for people having trouble managing their bills. No one is turned away because of inability to pay.

Financial Support

Financial support services. A number of organizations provide financial support for the costs of direct medical care and related expenses. For example, some organizations have programs that provide free transportation to and from treatment when a volunteer is available. Others offer "lending libraries" of wigs, hospital beds, wheelchairs, and other products. Some organizations offer stipends to families who cannot pay their bills.

The type and amount of financial assistance available varies from community to community. Many of these services are not advertised, but are available for the asking. Resources to contact for financial assistance include:

- social-service department of your hospital
- cancer organizations (see Appendix A)
- labor unions
- community-service organizations
- religious organizations
- social and fraternal organizations
- pharmaceutical companies that offer free drugs to indigent patients (see Appendix A)
- local congressional representative's office
- local public-assistance office

Worker's compensation and unemployment insurance. Two sources of state financial assistance to survivors whose jobs are affected by their health or who otherwise lose their jobs are worker's compensation and unemployment insurance.

Worker's-compensation laws. Worker's-compensation laws provide for fixed awards to employees or their dependents in case of *employment-related accidents and illness*. The purpose of worker's-compensation laws is to compensate workers who are injured on the job without the complexities of litigation. In short, worker's compensation provides no-fault health benefits.

Worker's-compensation laws are commonly applied to cases where an employee is hurt in an accident at work. Workers who contract occupational cancers (for example, miners, shipyard workers, nuclear-power-plant employees) may be entitled to worker's compensation. In some cases, workers have recovered benefits where an injury at work aggravated a pre-existing cancerous condition.

Workers benefit from these laws because, in order to collect compensation, they do not have to prove that their employer negligently harmed them; employers are strictly liable to their workers who are hurt on the job. Employers benefit because they agree to pay a fixed benefit to an injured employee in return for protection from being sued; worker's compensation is the only remedy the worker is entitled to receive. A worker who accepts worker's-compensation benefits for an injury may not then sue his employer for causing that injury.

Worker's-compensation laws are state laws. State laws vary as to the amount of compensation, the types of employment covered, duration of benefits, etc. Federal employees are covered by a separate law, the Federal Employees Compensation Act. For information about the law in your state, contact your state Department of Labor or Worker's Compensation Division.

Unemployment-disability laws. Some states provide for unemployment-disability benefits for people who are unable to work because of illness or injury *unrelated to their jobs*. Typically, to receive disability benefits, the worker and his or her physician must fill out a form provided by the employer. Benefits

> "A year after I had my lung removed, my doctor asked me what I cared about most.... I told him that what was most important to me was garden peas. Not the peas themselves, of course, though they were particularly good that year. What was extraordinary to me after that year was that I could again think that peas were important, that I could concentrate on the details of when to plant them and how much mulch they would need instead of thinking about platelets and white cells. I cherished the privilege of thinking about trivia."
>
> —Alice Stewart Trillin, lung-cancer survivor, "Of Dragons and Garden Peas: A Cancer Patient Talks to Doctors," *New England Journal of Medicine*

(some percentage of the weekly wage) are paid until the disability ends or a fixed period of time has passed. State laws do not guarantee the worker's job back. An employer may replace the worker for any legitimate business reason. For information about the law in your state, contact the state Department of Labor or Unemployment Division.

Social Security benefits. One source of federal financial assistance is social security. The Social Security Act creates several programs for providing financial assistance to qualified individuals, including disability insurance benefits, unemployment compensation, and supplemental security income for the disabled.

1. Retirement benefits. To be eligible for retirement benefits, you need not be disabled or poor. All that is required is that you be of a certain age and have paid into the Social Security system. You can retire at age 62 with partial benefits or at age 65 with full benefits. Under certain circumstances, children of retirees may receive additional benefits.

2. Spouses', survivors', and dependents' benefits. A widow, widower, surviving divorced spouse, child, or parent of a person who was entitled to Social Security benefits may directly receive those benefits if certain conditions are met.

3. Supplemental Security Income (SSI) benefits. The SSI program is designed to provide funds to people with income below the federal minimum level who are 65 or older, or are blind or disabled. Eligibility is determined by need, not whether you have paid into Social Security when you worked. Although SSI payments can be quite small, in many states an individual receiving SSI benefits will automatically be eligible for Medicaid.

4. Disability-insurance benefits. Disability benefits are designed to provide income to people who are unable to work because of a disability. You are entitled to receive disability benefits *while* you are disabled before the age of 65 if:

a. you have enough Social Security earnings to be insured for disability

b. you apply for benefits

c. you are disabled or had a disability that ended within the 12-month period before you applied for benefits

d. you have been disabled for five consecutive months

In some cases, spouses of disabled claimants are also entitled to benefits. The Social Security Administration considers you disabled if you have a severe impairment that makes you unable to do your previous work or any other gainful work. Your disability must have lasted, or be expected to last, for at least 12 months.

The amount of benefits is based on a sliding-scale percentage of wages determined by elaborate, frequently changing formulas. An employed person may not collect benefits. Workers may not receive both worker's compensation and Social Security disability for the same illness.

The medical records of individuals who apply for Social Security disability are evaluated according to regulations issued by the Social Security Administration. Individuals who are denied benefits may appeal to an administrative-law judge.

To determine whether your cancer is a disability under the law, the Social Security Administration considers what type of cancer you have, the extent of metastasis, and how you are responding to treatment. Small localized tumors that respond to therapy usually do not constitute an impairment. For example, early-stage breast cancer that is successfully treated with surgery is not considered a severe impairment. Cancer that has spread beyond regional lymph nodes, however, is usually so considered. Otherwise, your diagnosis is evaluated on a case-by-case basis.

To apply for disability benefits, you must obtain a form from your local Social Security Administration office (look in the telephone directory under "United States Government, Department of Health and Human Services"). The SSA gives your application to the state disability agency to determine, according to a complex formula, whether you are disabled under the law. If you are denied benefits, you may appeal to a federal administrative-law judge, who will hold a hearing to consider all of the evidence. If you are found to be disabled (but not permanently disabled), your case will be reviewed at least once every three years. When your condition improves and you are able to return to work, benefits will be discontinued.

Veterans' benefits. The Department of Veterans Affairs offers a variety of benefits to veterans. Although most disability benefits apply to veterans whose disability is service-connected, which cancer seldom is, some benefits are available to cancer-survivor veterans.

Depending on when you served, your age, and your income, you may be eligible for a non-service-connected pension. An additional allowance may be paid if you are in a nursing home, need a home aide, or are housebound because of your illness.

Hospital care in VA facilities is provided to veterans who meet certain standards, such as those who are eligible for Medicaid, need care related to exposure to cancer-causing substances (such as dioxin, Agent Orange, or nuclear fallout), have a VA pension, or have a limited income. Outpatient care and medical equipment are also available under certain circumstances.

The Department of Veterans Affairs also offers a variety of other benefits to qualified veterans, including life insurance, burial benefits, death pension to your dependents if your death is non-service-connected, and civil-service preference certificates if you seek government employment.

For more information, look in the telephone directory under "United States Government, Department of Veterans Affairs" (formerly Veterans Administration) for the number to reach a VA representative. Toll-free telephone service is available in all 50 states. If you are a beneficiary or policyholder in the Government Life Insurance programs, call (800) 422-8079 for 24-hour information about your insurance coverage.

Deducting medical expenses from your taxes. Part of the money you spend on medical care for yourself, your spouse, and your dependents may be itemized deductions for federal income-tax purposes. Keep track of

> The Social Security Administration has a national toll-free hotline to answer your questions about available benefits: (800) 234-5772.

physician fees, prescription drugs, dental expenses, home-nursing fees, hospital bills, medical-insurance premiums that you (not your employer) paid, laboratory bills, and transportation and lodging if you sought medical care away from home.

At the end of the calendar year, add up all of your medical expenses. From this number, you must then subtract a percentage of your gross income (in 1990, you must first subtract 7.5 percent of your gross income). You may deduct the balance from your income subject to federal income tax.

For example, if your gross income was $20,000 and you had $10,000 in medical expenses, you could claim a tax deduction of $8,500 for your medical expenses.

Total Medical Expenses	10,000
7.5% of Gross Income	−1,500
	(7.5% of $20,000)
Medical Deduction	$8,500

The Internal Revenue Service has a number of free publications that describe potential deductions related to health care. An IRS counselor will also answer over the telephone your questions about the tax regulations.

Planning for the Future—Wills and Estates

Financial planning for the future is important to ensure that your desires for yourself and your property are carried out according to your intentions. Additionally, careful financial planning may provide a crucial source of income should cancer or another serious illness strike. Wills and trusts are important tools in providing for the future.

Living wills and your right to die. A living will is a statement that tells your family and your doctor that you do not want your life prolonged by medical procedures if your condition becomes hopeless and there is no chance you will recover. Similar to your right to refuse medical treatment (see p. 55), you have the right to state *in advance of being incapacitated* that you do not want to be kept alive by certain procedures.

Physicians can prolong life with a variety of modern medical techniques, including surgery, drugs, respirators, tube feeding, and kidney dialysis. You may list on your living will the types of procedures you do not want performed on you, or you may sign a form living will, which directs your doctor not to take steps to prolong your life. You may use the living will to tell your doctor that you want only care to keep you comfortable, such as pain medication.

Preparing a living will. If your state has a living-will law, the form you must sign is printed in the state law. You may obtain a copy at a law library or from an attorney. In addition, the Society for the Right to Die, a nonprofit organization, provides state forms and instructions. If your state does not have a living-will law, you may write your own living will or use the society's living will. You must sign and date any living will in the presence of two adult witnesses. Most forms allow you to name a person of your choice (your "proxy") to make decisions about your medical care once you are unable to make such decisions.

> "The anticipation of death has made it essential for me to give thought to emotional and practical preparations for my children, my mother, my helpmate and partner, and other important people in my life. I have a sense of great satisfaction in having arranged for such practical matters as wills, death benefits, trust funds, and a retirement plan. For the most part this activity has been associated not with a sense of impending doom or imminent death but with a sense that making these arrangements now frees me from future concern."
>
> —Robert M. Mack, M.D., "Lessons from Living with Cancer," *New England Journal of Medicine*

Society for the Right to Die
250 West 57th Street
New York, New York 10107
(212) 246-6973

Choose as a proxy someone you are confident will be willing and able to carry out your wishes. You may wish to appoint two proxies, the second to make decisions if the first is unable to do so. Critical medical decisions, such as withdrawing life-support equipment, are very difficult, and should be entrusted only to those family members or friends who would make the same decision you would about your treatment.

To keep your living will current, you should review it regularly, and write your initials and the date you reviewed it on the document. If you change your mind about an instruction, write in your new instruction, initial it, and date it. If you change your mind about having a living will, destroy all copies.

Make sure that the people who will be involved in your medical care have a copy of your living will. Give a copy to your doctor to be kept in his or her files. Keep another with your personal papers (not in a bank safety-deposit box) so that others can find it if necessary. You may wish to place a card in your wallet that states you have a living will and where it can be found.

Validity of a living will. By January 1990, 40 states and the District of Columbia had a living-will law. If your state does not yet have a living-will law, expressing your personal requests on paper will encourage your physician to treat you according to your wishes. A physician who ignores your desire to refuse treatment may be liable for damages. Making a living will is not considered evidence of suicide, so it will not affect your life insurance.

Traditional wills. A traditional will is a written document that states how you would like your property to be distributed after you die. Although contemplating writing a will may cause anxiety (few people are comfortable thinking about their own death), it is essential if you want to control how your property is distributed after your death.

A traditional will is a way for you to ensure that your decisions about your property and family are respected. Even the simplest will should perform three tasks:

STATE LIVING-WILL LAWS

Compiled with the assistance of the Society for the Right to Die

Alabama Natural Death Act (passed in 1981)
Alaska Rights of Terminally Ill Act (1986)
Arizona Medical Treatment Decision Act (1985)
Arkansas Rights of the Terminally Ill or Permanently Unconscious Act (1987)
California Natural Death Act (1976)
Colorado Medical Treatment Decision Act (1985)
Connecticut Removal of Life Support Systems Act (1985)
Delaware Death with Dignity Act (1982)
District of Columbia Natural Death Act (1982)
Florida Life-Prolonging Procedures Act (1984)
Georgia Living Wills Act (1984, 1986, 1987)
Hawaii Medical Treatment Decisions Act (1986)
Idaho Natural Death Act (1977, 1986)
Illinois Living Will Act (1984)
Indiana Living Will and Life-Prolonging Procedures Act (1985)
Iowa Life-Sustaining Procedures Act (1985, 1987)
Kansas Natural Death Act (1979)
Louisiana Life-Sustaining Procedures Act (1984, 1985)
Maine Living Wills Act (1985)
Maryland Life-Sustaining Procedures Act (1985, 1986)
Minnesota Adult Health Care Decisions Act (1989)
Mississippi Withdrawal of Life-Sustaining Procedures Act (1984)
Missouri Life Support Declarations Act (1985)
Montana Living Will Act (1985)
Nevada Withholding or Withdrawal of Life-Sustaining Procedures Act (1977)
New Hampshire Terminal Care Document Act (1985)
New Mexico Right to Die Act (1977, 1984)
North Carolina Right to Natural Death Act (1977, 1979, 1981, 1983)
North Dakota Act (1989)
Oklahoma Natural Death Act (1985)
Oregon Rights with Respect to Terminal Illness Act (1977, 1983)
South Carolina Death with Dignity Act (1986)
Tennessee Right to Natural Death Act (1985)
Texas Natural Death Act (1977, 1979, 1983, 1985)
Utah Personal Choice and Living Will Act (1985)
Vermont Terminal Care Document Act (1982)
Virginia Natural Death Act (1983)
Washington Natural Death Act (1979)
West Virginia Natural Death Act (1984)
Wisconsin Natural Death Act (1984, 1986)
Wyoming Act (1984)

1. Explain how your property should be distributed.

2. Appoint someone to take care of your minor and/or disabled children.

3. Appoint an executor (the person you choose to make sure the instructions in your will are followed).

If you die without a valid will, your state will distribute your property according to state probate laws. The result may or may not be the same result you intended. State probate laws are designed to promote fairness and predictability in estate management. They are not designed to protect your family's long-term financial needs after your death.

Before you prepare a will, complete the following steps to ensure that your will reflects your carefully considered intentions:

1. Discuss with your family their long-term financial needs.

2. Make a list of your property (major items such as house, car, insurance policies, heirlooms).

3. Decide whom ("beneficiaries") you want to receive what.

4. If you have minor and/or disabled children, decide whom you want to be responsible for their care and ask that person if he or she is willing to serve as your children's "testamentary guardian."

5. Select your will's executor and ask that person if he or she is willing to be responsible for distributing your assets.

You may write your own will (see bibliography). However, your will is more likely to withstand any legal challenge if it is prepared by an attorney. If your will is challenged and declared invalid, the state may disregard your intentions and distribute your property according to its probate laws. The money you save in writing your own will while you are alive may be lost several times over in court battles over your will after your death.

Each state has laws that establish formalities a will must meet to ensure that your wishes are enforced. For example, some states require that two adults witness your signing of the will, whereas other states require three witnesses. Some states recognize a handwritten will, but other states require that it be typed.

Every state requires, at a minimum, the following three elements to recognize a will as valid:

1. If you are preparing a will, you must be capable of making decisions about your property. You must understand what the purpose of the will is, know the nature of your property, know the beneficiaries you name, and be acting of your own free will.

2. Your will must be witnessed by "disinterested witnesses." These are adults who do not stand to gain by your death and who are not named in your will as beneficiary, executor, or trustee.

3. You must sign and date the will in the presence of the disinterested witnesses. You must also make it known to them that you intend the document to serve as your will and that you are signing it without coercion.

After you prepare a will, you must make certain it remains safe and reflects your current wishes:

1. Give a copy of your will to your attorney and keep a copy for yourself. Because your safety-deposit box may be sealed temporarily after your death, an attorney's office is the safest place to keep a will.

2. Review your will every few years to determine whether it reflects your current intentions and assets. If you decide to change your will, have an attorney make the changes or write a new will to ensure that your new instructions, and not the old ones, are followed.

Trusts and estates. A trust is a financial and legal relationship in which one party (the trustee) holds title to property for the benefit of another party (the beneficiary). There are several different types of trusts, which accomplish different purposes. For example, one way to avoid having to "spend down" your money (reduce your assets) to qualify for Medicaid is to give your money to a family member or friend in the form of a trust. Under the terms of such a trust, the family member or friend would be asked to spend the money on your care.

By establishing a trust, you may appoint a "trustee" to use his or her discretion in making all decisions about your assets, or you may restrict the types of decisions the trustee may make. Some trusts may take effect only once you become disabled, whereas others transfer decision-making powers to a trustee as soon as you sign the documents. You should choose as your trustee someone who is able to make competent financial decisions, such as operating your business, borrowing money, managing real estate, and filing your tax returns.

Trusts can be quite complex, must comply with state laws, and have a variety of tax consequences. You should contact an attorney to help you draw up such a trust to be certain that it will accomplish the purpose you intended. An attorney or a financial adviser could help you determine if you would benefit from a trust, or could gain the same results by granting a power of attorney. A power of attorney is less complicated and expensive than a trust; however, it is not as flexible as a trust can be.

Power of attorney. You may grant another person the right to make decisions for you by granting a "power of attorney." This is a simple and inexpensive procedure in which you nominate another person (your "agent") to act in your place and on your behalf.

When you give a power of attorney to your agent, you permit him or her to manage your assets, such as your bank accounts, stocks, and house. Many cancer survivors can relieve themselves of the burden of paying bills and making financial decisions by granting that authority to a responsible person.

A few states permit you to grant a power of attorney to make decisions about your medical care (see p. 140). If you grant a "durable power of attorney," your agent may continue to make decisions for you when you become unable to do so for yourself. You may grant a power of attorney to one or more adults, including a family member, friend, lawyer, or business associate. You may revoke the power of attorney at any time.

Because granting and revoking a power of attorney involve the power to manage your property and must comply with state laws to be valid, you should consult with an attorney for help in preparing the documents that will express your intentions and be accepted by banks and other institutions.

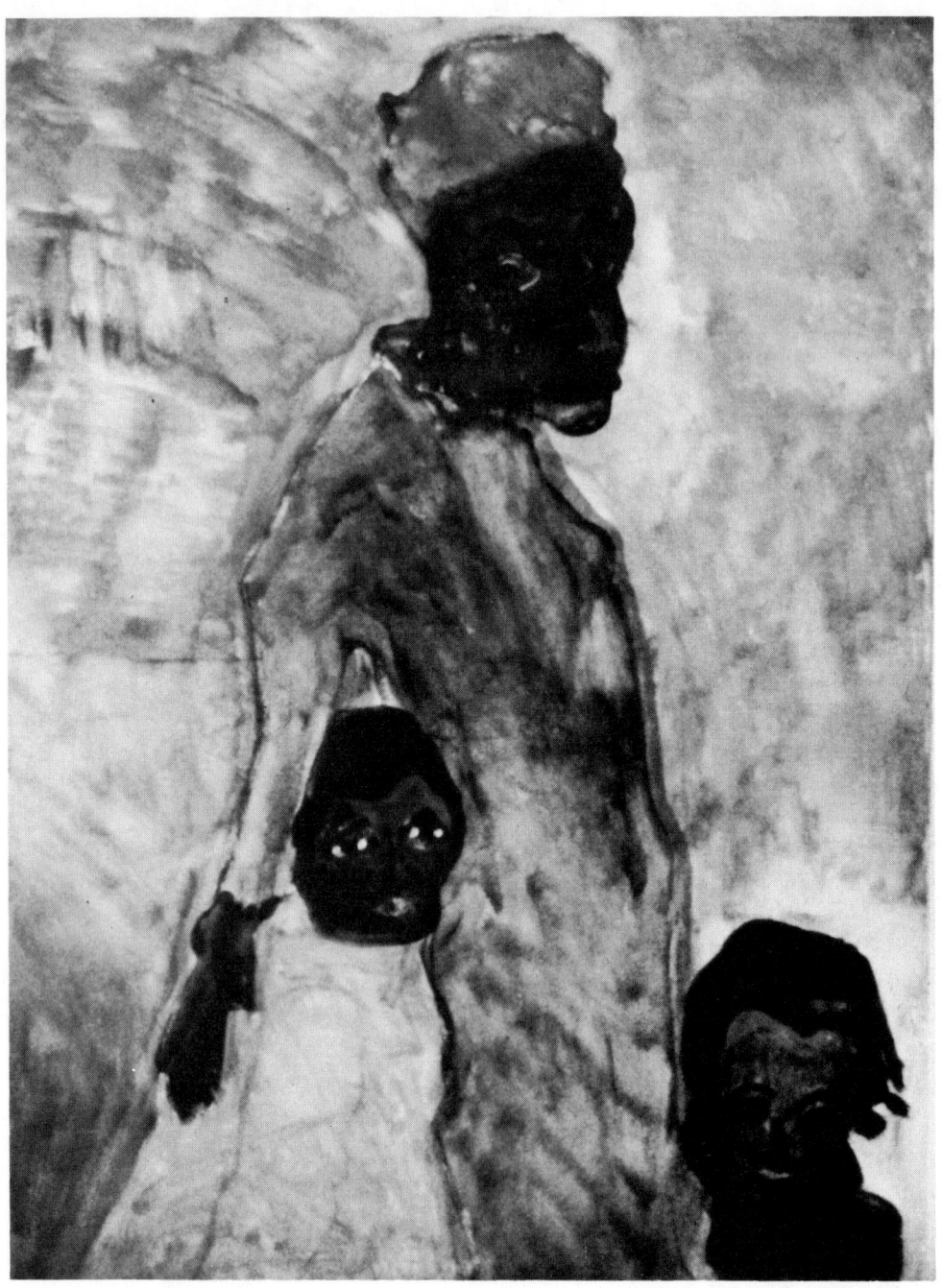

Gloria Maccabee
Mother & Children
Oil on canvas
40″ x 30″

7

Cancer and the Family

Katharine G. Baker, D.S.W., L.C.S.W.

Sue decided to go with her husband, Joe, when he went back to the doctor's office to get the results of the biopsy he had had on Tuesday. Even though it meant taking the morning off from work, she wanted to be with him in case he got bad news. When the doctor said the word "cancer," her mind went blank for a minute and she felt numb all over. As the doctor continued to talk calmly about treatment and prognosis, she forced herself to concentrate on what he was saying. She even reached automatically into her purse for a pad and began to take notes. Later all she could remember saying to Joe was "We're all in this together, dear."

Everyone in a family—husband, wife, lover, parent, child—responds with anguish to the serious illness of a loved one. How family members interact with one another and with the survivor, as well as whether they are able to offer support, care, respect, humor, perspective, and help in decision making, can affect the quality of the survivor's healing environment.

Families tend to cycle through periods of closeness or distance, depending on the stage of life they are in. Families with small children generally value togetherness and have a focus on child rearing and home activities, whereas families with adolescent and young-adult offspring generally have more emotionally distant relationships. Some family relationships are intensely close, almost smothering. Others are comfortably friendly and connected. Some are cool or distant, with infrequent formal contact, and others are completely cut off, with no contact at all. Whichever relationship pattern is most familiar to families of cancer survivors will probably be the one which continues as the family deals with cancer.

Serious illness seems to intensify the relationship styles and patterns that are already in place in a family, although no family and no period in the family cycle is ideally suited to tolerating cancer in any of its members. Close families often become closer and support one another through hard times, but they can also be suffocatingly overinvolved with each other. Distant family members may have difficulty pulling together and supporting one another, but

> "My life is a quilt, and cancer is just one patch in that quilt."
>
> —Barbara Lazarus, Ed.D.

they can also permit more independence and autonomy among their members when serious illness occurs.

For a family with young children that places a high value on togetherness, a diagnosis of cancer in one of the parents can strain the emotional resources of the family. The parent with cancer may initially need as much care as the children, or more, while having to give up many parenting tasks (at least temporarily). A family with adolescent and young-adult offspring may place less value on family togetherness, but often has more energy available to focus on the survivor.

Although serious illness may be a more expected part of the life cycle during old age, it is never welcome and always causes severe disruption in family relationships, finances, and routine living. If the family has had prior experience with illness—i.e., accidents, heart attacks, or long-term disabilities—the family as a whole may have developed some useful coping skills along the way. But no family is ever really ready to hear that a loved one has cancer.

When someone is diagnosed with cancer, the natural inclination of that person's closest relatives is to focus on the immediate demands of the cancer, to provide care, support, nurturance, and understanding. At the same time, family members must also recognize that they will need to take care of themselves during what may be a very long period of uncertainty and stress. In order to be truly helpful to the survivor and deal adequately with all the demands of family life, they must keep themselves healthy, strong, calm, and emotionally balanced. Individuals with years of experience in living closely with a cancer survivor have come to acknowledge that they have some specific rights and obligations to themselves.

Dealing with the Shock of Diagnosis

The diagnosis of cancer usually comes as a devastating blow to the whole family. Disbelief, denial, rage, confusion, anxiety, and a host of other tumultuous feelings race through your head when you hear that someone you love has cancer. If you are the "close one"—the husband, wife, or lover of the survivor—you may experience an intense fear of loss. In the initial state of shock you may not be able to sleep or eat. Some family members are unable to concentrate on even the simplest tasks. They cry or wander around in a daze. Some may find themselves going over and over the facts, preoccupied suddenly with how they will be able to take care of themselves and go on living without the other person. The wife of one survivor found herself mentally planning her husband's funeral and thinking about whom she would remarry so that she would not be alone.

The greatest fear and confusion may surface in the middle of the night, when you feel most vulnerable. One woman awoke screaming as she dreamed that her car's brakes had given way on a steep hill. A man reported dreaming that his wife had stepped out the front door of their house and into a deep hole on the doorstep. As he ran to rescue her, he found himself staring into a dark pit that yawned hundreds of feet

> ## Barriers to Communication with a Cancer Survivor's Family
>
> Serious illness often accentuates existing communication problems within a family. A cancer experience can result in three major barriers to communication.
>
> **1. *Conspiracy of silence*.** Some survivors and family members engage in a "conspiracy of silence" to avoid discussing cancer in a misguided attempt to protect each other from stress. Refusing to talk about problems does not make them go away. Invite conversation. A survivor might say to a family member, "My cancer has made us seem like strangers. Instead of going through our private hells separately, how can we best talk about it?" A family member might say to a survivor, "I know your cancer is hard for both us of to talk about, but if you ever want to talk, I'm always here to listen."
>
> **2. *Premature mourning*.** One harsh reality of cancer—that approximately half the individuals diagnosed in 1990 will eventually die from the disease—often leads family members to mourn prematurely the loss of a loved one. While family members may be mourning an anticipated death (in part because pessimism may be safer than the potential disappointment of hope), the survivor may be recovering from cancer, may live with it for years, or may want to enhance the quality of his or her life, even if it is nearing an end.
>
> Premature mourning, by both family members and the survivor, can be a very natural process of preparing for the threatened loss of a loved one. Even outliving the odds can be upsetting. When family and friends go through the pain of premature mourning at the time of diagnosis, they are hesitant to re-experience the pain of the actual loss at a later date. Thus even good news of increased survival time, or even cure, can feel like a double-edged sword to the premature mourner.
>
> **3. *Need to help*.** When someone close to you is seriously ill, it is only natural to feel a desire to help, frustration at your powerlessness and a loss of control over life. Family members should be careful not to let their own agenda for fighting cancer get in the way of the survivor's personal needs and priorities. You do not have to stamp out cancer or pain in order to help a survivor. Usually, the survivor needs more mundane things from you, such as your time and friendship, help with errands, and a comforting touch.
>
> —Neil Fiore, Ph.D., psychologist

down into the earth. His wife lay at the bottom of it, silently staring up at him. Another man dreamed that he was caught in the midst of a wild forest fire and could not read the instructions on the side of a small manual fire extinguisher.

These dreams are dramatically expressive of the helplessness felt when cancer strikes a family. Distracted thinking is common. You may find yourself dialing phone numbers and forgetting whom you have called, driving to the store and forgetting the grocery list, repeating yourself in conversations, missing appointments at work, or having a series of small accidents at home.

You may also find yourself lashing out angrily at those you love best (including the survivor). Some family members find themselves intermittently denying that the whole thing is happening, believing that they will wake up tomorrow morning and it will all have been a bad dream. They may become

Bill of Rights for Family Members of Cancer Survivors

As family members of cancer survivors, we have the following rights:

■ *The right and obligation to take care of our own needs.* Even though we may appear at times to be selfish, we must do what is necessary to keep our own peace of mind so we can be better able to help our loved ones.

■ *The right to ask for help from others in caring for our loved ones.* Although our loved ones may object to the involvement of others, we must assess our own limitations of strength and endurance, and determine when we need assistance in caring for them.

■ *The right to determine the limits of our ability to help our loved ones.* By avoiding undue sacrifice, exhaustion, and resentment, we will be more genuine in the assistance we offer.

■ *The right to balance our own needs with those of our loved ones.* An appropriate balance will help lessen family tension and encourage attention to the ongoing needs of all family members.

—Neil Fiore, Ph.D.

---

obsessed with magical mental bargains made with themselves or God: "If I am nice enough . . . quick enough . . . smart enough . . . careful enough, this will all go away. . . . God will make everything turn out right."

These thoughts, feelings, and behaviors are symptoms of extreme anxiety. Most cancer survivors themselves go through a similar roller coaster of fear, anger, denial, fantasy, nightmares, and unusual behaviors. But family members in a crisis often do not share their fears with people with whom they are closest. It does not seem fair to tell your husband or wife how frightened you are that he or she may die when he or she is fearing the same thing.

You know you are supposed to be calm and clearheaded and supportive, but you cannot help thinking of yourself at the same time. Your tears may be for the pain of your loved one, but they are also for yourself. Shame, embarrassment, and guilt may intensify the emotional turmoil for family members of a cancer survivor. A common result of this emotional upheaval is that even the close family members may become distant and angry with one another. The cancer survivor may become emotionally isolated from the family at a time when connection and support are vital to the beginning stages of survival.

What should families do to get through this initial period of shock and disorientation without damaging family relationships and mutual support? No single solution will work for every family, but here are some suggestions that may help your family deal with the acute state of adjustment to cancer in the family.

■ Maintain family routines.
■ Continue to eat, sleep, and exercise regularly.
■ Engage in lovemaking as the survivor's energy level permits. Cuddling and touching are important.
■ Go to work.
■ Continue to buy presents and new clothes for the survivor.
■ Go to movies, out to dinner, and on trips.
■ Try to keep a sense of humor about life.
■ Try to communicate openly with the cancer survivor about all aspects of daily living. Survivors need help in not feeling isolated, because it often seems that everyone is talking *about* them, but not *to* them.
■ Find a regular time of the day to talk with the survivor, allowing time to listen carefully

> "We went home dazed, but neither of us panicked. As always, Bogie's attitude was: what has to be done has to be done—no need for dramatics. I took my cue from him."
>
> —Lauren Bacall, *By Myself* (discussing Humphrey Bogart's battle with lung cancer)

as well as to express your own thoughts and feelings. Be prepared also for the fact that the survivor may occasionally not want to talk. Do not force communication.

■ Talk to a close friend or relative about your own thoughts and feelings as well as about your irrational fears, anger, and unusual behaviors. The survivor need not know every detail of such feelings.

■ If you are holding too much in or feeling overwhelmed by more anxiety than a friend or a relative can handle, find a counselor who can listen to your thoughts and feelings and can help you put the situation in perspective (see chapter 4).

A cancer diagnosis often demands immediate decisions about what doctors to work with, whether or not to get a second opinion, what treatments to choose, where to get treatment, and how to manage a myriad of responsibilities at home and work. If you are the closest family member, you will probably be involved in many of the survivor's decisions. The most important contribution you can make to decision making is insisting on an atmosphere of respect for the survivor. Ultimately survivors must make the key decisions about what happens to their bodies, and family members must acknowledge and support their autonomy. But family members can help survivors make those decisions. You can help the survivor keep a log of symptoms, side effects, and progress between doctors' visits. You can also encourage the survivor to keep a list of questions to ask doctors. Most important, you can help establish a tone of calm and dignity in these highly stressful interactions.

You can be most helpful on a practical level by providing a second set of ears during the medical consultation. It is difficult to recall large amounts of complex information when you are under stress. You can facilitate thoughtful preparation for meetings with doctors and recollection of new information by listening and taking notes for later discussion. One wife of a survivor asked all the doctors with whom she and her husband met if she could tape-record the consultations so that they would not miss any information. None of their doctors objected to this request.

In addition, family members should decide with the survivor whom to talk to about the illness. What, when, and how to communicate about cancer are complex questions that reflect precancer relationships. Will the people you talk to about the cancer be able to understand and be supportive, or will they become so frightened that their anxiety overwhelms your own? Will they be able to keep connected with the survivor on a personal level, or will they begin to write him or her off as "doomed" because of the diagnosis? Will a network of supportive friends and family move into helpful roles, or will the family gossip network take over, as relatives talk *about* the survivor, but not *to* him or her? Can family and friends make positive contributions to the treatment information-gathering process, or will they bombard the survivor with anecdotes about Great-aunt Julia's magical Mexican cure or Uncle Larry's long, painful death?

In most families, once a few key people have heard the news of a cancer diagnosis, within days everyone knows something (accurate or inaccurate) about it. It is therefore important to decide how the information will be shared, what to say, and how much to talk about prognosis and treatment choices. If the survivor wants family or friends to be actively involved, inform them early on. If the survivor wants to make crucial decisions about treatment alone, then you may want to delay sharing information.

Family members should decide for themselves whom they will talk to about their own fears, anxieties, and adjustments. Most family members need to find at least one close person who will provide support, understanding, and friendship during a loved one's illness. But they need to inform the survivor of what they are saying to whom and for what purpose. Respect for the survivor's autonomy is crucial in these communications and can help reduce their nonmedical stress, such as walking into a room full of talkative relatives at a family reunion and having the entire room suddenly fall silent.

Family Involvement in Treatment

As soon as the cancer survivor has chosen a doctor and a course of treatment, medical procedures usually begin fairly rapidly. Whether or not family members agree with the choices the survivor has made, their primary role is to support those choices in every way possible.

Family members must decide how much to be involved in treatment. This decision depends on a number of factors: how much family involvement the survivor wants, the physical condition of the survivor, and the actual availability of close family members to be involved in treatment. Moreover, if the income of the survivor is drastically curtailed during convalescence, the healthy relative may have to work long extra hours to meet the family's financial commitments and may have little time to help with treatment.

For a couple, the degree of involvement in treatment will also reflect the quality of the relationship before the cancer diagnosis. Some relationships place a strong value on togetherness. The survivor's partner may wish to be there for all therapies and may want to be involved with home treatments. Other relationships place a stronger value on autonomy and will promote independent self-care for the survivor to the extent that it is physically possible.

Varying degrees of family involvement are apparent at many oncology centers. At one clinic where survivors were being taught to give themselves daily injections, several spouses went into the classroom and even learned to give the injections themselves. Other spouses stayed in the waiting room, having accompanied the survivor to treatment, but not actually participating in its administration. Some survivors were there on their own, without family members. There is no right or wrong degree or kind of involvement in treatment.

Understanding, anticipating, and helping the survivor cope with the side effects of treatment are also important areas for family involvement. Survivors may experience extreme discomfort, pain, nausea, diarrhea, weakness, fatigue, sleep and appetite disturbance, hair loss, or physical disfigurement following treatment. Loving family members may feel a sense of helplessness in not being able to ease the survivor's discomfort. Love itself, however, can be comforting.

Physical and verbal expressions of affection from family members can be very important during treatment. Survivors need frequent hugs, kisses, touching, and holding. Within the limits of their physical energy, most appreciate lots of contact with their children. They also need opportunities for sexual expression. Many survivors want to remain involved in daily routines and mundane family matters. They need to hear

> ## Reminders for Family Members When Involved in Survivor Decisions
>
> - Try to remain calm and thoughtful.
> - Keep a hopeful attitude. You never know when a medical breakthrough, a new treatment, or a cure will come along.
> - Participate in meetings and information gathering to the extent that the survivor wants you to.
> - Be an extra set of ears, take notes, or tape-record meetings.
> - Remember that the survivor has the final say in what doctor and treatment are chosen, as well as who gets told about the cancer.
> - Let the survivor know if you seek personal support from a friend or relative.

the news of the day from family members, where people went, what they did, and how they enjoyed themselves.

Most families divide up their involvement with the survivor according to their interests, talents, and the nature of the relationship they had before the diagnosis. For example, one son of a businessman convalescing from cancer surgery focused his involvement on their common business and financial interests. He reviewed his father's will with him and made provisions for his father's business while he was recovering. One daughter who was an artist decorated her father's bedroom with cheerful paintings and worked with him on creative visualization of himself as a healthy person. Another son, in college, sent tape recordings of interesting lectures. A young daughter at home played chess with her father almost every afternoon and also went over her math homework with him in the evening. His wife took nutritional-cooking classes and improved the entire family's eating habits. She became the family's "central switchboard," receiving calls from concerned friends and relatives, passing the phone to her husband as he felt able to communicate, and sharing information with the family network to the extent that he wished her to. She also found a cancer-support group, which they attended as a couple. Even the family dog played a role, by lying near her husband's bed and being available for recuperative walks.

Family members can nevertheless become anxious, frustrated, and exhausted during the early stages of treatment. This is often a period of intense emotional and physical stress for the entire family. Fear of loss can be very close to the surface. Family members must learn to take turns being helpful and supportive. If you become a "martyr" to the cancer and try to handle all the care, you will burn out long before the crisis is past. No one person can do it all, and everyone needs a break from time to time. Going out with friends, attending church, playing games and planning a picnic or a weekend trip are important methods of relief for family members under stress. The survivor may not be able to go with you at this early stage of recovery. Some survivors will want to hear all about the family expedition afterward and will be glad that family life continues as normally as possible. Others may be sad, envious, or resentful that they cannot join in family activities. Asking a close friend to spend some time with the survivor while you are away may help ease the pain of not being able to participate.

Here are some suggestions for helping family members cope with the early stages of treatment:

> "Occasionally Bogie would make me go to dinner at a friend's house. Because he wasn't up to it, he said, was no reason why I should stay home all the time. Secretly he wanted me with him constantly, just to know that I was there, but realistically he felt I had to get out once in a while. So I did—once in a while, but not for long."
>
> —Lauren Bacall, *By Myself*

- Maintain family routines. Include the survivor in family chores. Allow the survivor to be responsible for doing something that is helpful to the family. Participating in chores gives survivors a feeling of being useful and expands their role beyond just being a patient. Family holidays and birthdays should not be postponed, but need to be celebrated as usual, with the survivor taking part as much as possible.
- Follow the survivor's preferences in your involvement with actual medical care. Even if you need to be actively involved in treatment procedures, avoid constantly reminding or nagging the survivor to take medication or see the doctor. Cancer survivors are not mentally incompetent and can remember these aspects of treatment themselves, unless they have some additional disability. If so, you may need to take a more active role in their medical care.
- Let your involvement be reflective of your own interests and talents and your precancer relationship with the survivor.
- Take a break from time to time, but tell the survivor what your plans are and who will be available if problems arise while you are away.
- Keep lines of communication open so that no family member is either left out or overburdened. Check in with one another on at least a weekly basis to ensure that family members are expressing what is on their minds.
- Familiarize yourself with professional resources in the community. Nurses, social workers, clergy, counselors, and community organizations can help family members as well as survivors.
- Let neighbors, friends, relatives, and cancer volunteers help with child care, transportation, shopping, cleaning, telephone calls and messages, cooking, errands, and visiting with the survivor while family members rest or work.

When Mommy or Daddy Has Cancer—The Special Needs of Young Children

When the parent of small children is diagnosed with cancer, the family must think not only of the immediate emotional and treatment needs of the survivor, but also of the needs of the children. A small child does not understand what a serious illness is and usually experiences cancer as a withdrawal of the parent's love. Both parents may be frightened by and preoccupied with treatment decisions. One parent will be away from the home, in the hospital or receiving treatment. The other parent may be working long hours and visiting the survivor parent frequently, but often will not be able to take young children along to the hospital or clinic. Routines are inevitably disrupted in ways that little children cannot understand.

Such family uncertainty and heightened

> When Maureen Tyler was diagnosed with breast cancer, her daughter, Becky, had just turned five and was about to enter kindergarten. Becky was too young to understand any threat to her mother's life, although she heard the fear in her parents' voices as they discussed the diagnosis. After Maureen had decided to have the mastectomy recommended by her doctor, she sat down with Becky and told her about the lump in her breast. Becky knew that she had been breast-fed as a baby, and it was hard for her to understand that this nurturing part of her mother had something wrong with it. Her mother let her feel the lump and explained that Grandma would come to take care of Becky while she was in the hospital to have the breast with the lump taken away.
>
> She also explained that she would be tired for a while after she came back from the hospital, but that she would still be the same loving mommy except for the change in one part of her body.
>
> That night, when Becky's father put her to bed, she asked him to tell her the whole story again, and they acted it out with her teddy bears. When her mother left for the hospital, Becky clung to her for a minute and then patted her mother's breast and said good-bye to it.
>
> Because she was so young, Becky was not allowed to visit her mother in the hospital, but she and her grandmother drove by it and looked up, trying to imagine which window was Mommy's. Her mother called her every evening on the telephone, and Becky drew lots of pictures expressing her childlike understanding of what had happened. When her mother came home she tired easily, and Becky had to learn to bring her mother a glass of water or the morning mail. She also had to learn to play alone more. She wanted to see where the surgery had been, and she touched the scar gently. She continued to re-enact the surgery from time to time with her teddy bears, but gradually she lost interest as Mommy seemed more like her old self.

anxiety often lead to regressive behaviors in young children. When their parents are less available, less calm, and less nurturing, children can become demanding, whiny, or withdrawn. Parents may have difficulty meeting the needs of young children when they are caught up with serious health concerns, but their children will experience fewer long-term negative consequences from the parental illness if the parents can make thoughtful plans for them.

The most important single aspect of planning for young children when a parent has cancer is child care. It is not always easy to find a responsible, consistent, and familiar adult to care for your child during the crisis of a parental cancer diagnosis. But a trusted grandparent, aunt, uncle, neighbor, or regular sitter can be very important in easing the impact of the experience for young children.

Knowing where a parent is and when he or she will be coming back, and maintaining regular telephone contact are reassuring to a young child. If a parent will be away for more than a few days, sending him or her cards and school artwork can help the child feel a sense of connection. Children need to be prepared for the fact that when the parent comes home he or she will not be as strong or active as before. It is hard for small children to understand that a parent cannot pick them up, carry them around, or play with them as before. Giving young children a particular caretaking task (such as carrying the newspaper or the mail to their parent) can help them feel that they have a part in the parent's recovery.

Children also need to have fairly specific explanations of any changes in their parents' appearance or abilities. This explanation must of course be given in very simple language, appropriate to their age level. Drawing pictures or explaining through doll play can also be helpful. Observing and touching changed body parts following surgery can be reassuring to a child, as long as the parents do not present the changes negatively. Hiding the changes and keeping them secret can be frightening to a young child, who often picks up on any secrecy in adult behavior, even though nothing is said out loud.

In spite of the best parental intentions and careful preparation, many young children will become very distressed when a parent receives a cancer diagnosis. Often children believe that somehow they have caused the cancer. If only they had been less naughty, Mommy or Daddy would not have become sick or had to go to the hospital. Such children may become very withdrawn and obsessively "good," hoping that good behavior will make the parent well.

Young children may, conversely, express family tensions through negative behaviors such as whining, crying, throwing temper tantrums, wetting the bed, sucking their thumbs, or refusing to go to school, to eat, or to go to bed. In school or in the neighborhood they may pick fights with their playmates or do poorly in their schoolwork.

When a parent is not well or is going to the hospital for surgery or other treatments, all significant adults in the child's life should be informed. Teachers, day-care staff, babysitters, Sunday-school teachers, sports-team coaches, neighbors, friends, and relatives need to know what is going on so that they can be alert to any changes in a child's behavior and can offer extra attention and support.

Both parents need to be involved in planning arrangements so that their children's routines will be minimally disrupted, but the healthy parent will clearly have to take on more responsibility for implementation. Friends, neighbors, and relatives are unusually eager to help a family in which a parent has cancer. Child care is a good direction for channeling their helpfulness.

Family Involvement over the Long Haul

After the survivor returns home from the hospital, after the radiation, the chemotherapy, and other treatments are past, after the hair has grown back, the nausea has subsided, the blood tests are normal, and the scar has begun to fade, most families must still deal with a continuing anxiety that the cancer might come back. They fear that an ache, a pain, a bruise, or a more subtle change in body awareness could signal me-

> "Home was humming with activity and expectation. The children, so excited about Daddy's coming home, were briefed by me about not jumping all over him. Harvey [the dog] would have to be kept at bay."
> —Lauren Bacall, *By Myself*

tastasis. Most survivors and their families live with the long-term uncertainty of remission rather than the clarity of cure.

For some cancer survivors and their families, the experience of cancer truly has no long-term impact. The diagnosis was made early in the course of the disease, and treatment was completely successful. These people return to former activities and relationships relatively untouched by cancer except as a brief episode of anxiety and discomfort.

For most, however, the experience of cancer will have lifelong effects. Denial of the seriousness of the illness, of its disruption of family relationships and routines, and of its potential for recurrence is a common emotional response to an experience of helplessness and fear. Many people, unable to understand or master a situation, would rather pretend it had not happened. The long-term emotional consequences of denial, however, may have disruptive effects on the family, resulting in relationship conflicts, emotional problems, or disturbing misconduct among the children.

It is in the best interests of the family to realize that cancer changes the perspectives of all the members. Each realizes, "If it could happen to him, it could happen to me." Having faced the real and immediate possibility of the loss of a loved one, each thinks more seriously of the possibility of his or her own death and begins then to re-examine the quality of present daily relationships. Cancer can offer the chance for personal growth to family members as well as to survivors.

After getting through the shock of diagnosis, the stress of making treatment decisions, and the acute phase of cancer care, survivors and their families have an opportunity for significant change in the way they relate to one another. Many families are able to become more direct in the way they express thoughts and feelings. Minor irritations, frustrations, and conflicts take on less significance, and differences of opinion are resolved more rapidly. The sense that "We only have one life to live, so let's do it right" can become an inspiring and guiding principle for families of survivors.

Despite these long-term changes in outlook and interaction, when the crisis has passed, cancer survivors and their families begin to shift the focus from cancer to normal living. They start socializing with old friends outside the survivor network again and are less interested in attending cancer-support groups. From a practical and psychological point of view, it is best to strike a balance between a focus on the outside world and preparation for future cancer-related problems.

Survivors and family members usually maintain an awareness of cancer as a part of their lives for many years to come. While they strive to live as normally as possible, many cancer survivors and their family members continue to follow developments in cancer research, identifying quietly with newly diagnosed cancer survivors and reflecting periodically on the length of time since their own diagnosis.

Sometimes, in spite of the best care, cancer will recur. The family will then move back through the stages described early in this chapter. There will be the disappointment and renewed shock at the diagnosis of recurrence, the need for decision making

> **TO MY DAUGHTER**
>
> You have the breasts now
> Your baby nipple buds
> will bloom one day
> a discovery of roses
> Cherish them
> as you would your very inmost self.
> Let them and you
> be free of these cells
> that can't stop growing,
> that are fed by female blood.
> May you grow beautiful babies
> and beautiful breasts.
> You will never remember
> how you kissed the scar,
> just like a scraped knee,
> to make it better,
> but I will.
> You will never remember
> how I looked with two breasts,
> you are only two years old.
> But I will.
>
> copyright © 1981 by Claire Henze

with regard to old or new treatments, and the period of acute care as the recurrence is dealt with medically. Anxiety and fear of loss may reappear with renewed intensity at this time.

But these stages are also different, because the survivor and the family have been there before. They are better prepared with successful coping mechanisms. Experienced survivors and their families know who are their most effective and supportive resources. They know how to swing into high gear as a family group, how to divide up the tasks and responsibilities, how to deal with the medical experts and how to promote attitudes of survival.

Nevertheless, anxiety can be more intense, because a recurrence of cancer is often viewed as an even more serious threat to life than a first-time diagnosis. Anger and resentment can boil to the surface, because the cancer has recurred in spite of all the careful precautions and changes that the family has made. Some family members experience guilt that "we didn't try hard enough or weren't careful enough," that "we are being punished" for not having dealt with the cancer effectively enough the first time. Family members may feel bad about not taking good enough care of the survivor, not protecting him or her enough, or not insisting on implementing all the good habits they had planned. They may also feel anger toward the medical experts for not curing their loved one.

Some survivors and their families live with a series of cancer recurrences or in chronic states of illness for many years. The most

> **TO MY SON**
>
> Perhaps because of me
> you will be a man to whom
> breasts are not just boobs, knockers,
> jugs, tits
> and calendar art.
> Perhaps you will know
> that any part of the body
> is as worthy as another,
> that there is beauty in
> asymmetry,
> that a breast only covers
> the heart underneath,
> that skin is the most erogenous organ,
> that women are strong,
> that men may weep
> and that only lizards
> grow new tails.
>
> copyright © 1981 by Claire Henze

important task for family members during recurrence is to maintain constructive attitudes, allowing themselves time to pursue their own interests, using the help of outsiders as necessary, but keeping open, affectionate communication with the survivor.

With recurrence of cancer, death may become inevitable. The survivor and the family must decide together how to respond to this development. Family members may now begin to distance themselves from the survivor and ally themselves increasingly with the medical professionals, as the pain of impending loss becomes more real. Though receiving and sharing accurate medical information is necessary and responsible at all times during treatment, it is especially important that the survivor not become isolated during this most stressful period. The family connections woven so carefully over a lifetime need to stay in place. The survivor's wishes and values for living should continue to be respected.

Many survivors and their families choose to enter a hospice program at this stage (see chapter 4). Even during the hospice stage, survivors and family members need to try to express their thoughts and feelings clearly and directly to one another, not only about cancer, but about the deepest values in living. At this time they can lay to rest any unresolved differences, as they review their lives together and say good-bye. Acceptance of the limitations of medical intervention and of human mortality does not diminish the survivor's potential for continuing emotional growth up to the very moment of death. A peaceful and respectful leave-taking can be the final affirmation of connection to a loving family.

When the survivor dies, family members will enter a period of grieving that reflects the quality of the relationship they had with their loved one, as well as that person's role in the family. Most people go through an initial stage of numbness, then attend to the

> Bob had just turned 51 when he was diagnosed with advanced pancreatic cancer. The diagnosis came as a terrible blow to him and his wife, Nancy. Their youngest son had just left for college, and they were looking forward to active years ahead.
>
> After a period of pain and weeping with Nancy, Bob decided that he would not subject himself to experimental treatments but, except for pain medication, would let the disease take its course. The doctors told him he had about six months to live. In fact, he survived for a year.
>
> Bob continued to go to work regularly until two weeks before he died. During that year, Bob taught Nancy how to get along on her own. Although she had always had a career, there were many aspects of family finances with which she was unfamiliar. They did estate planning with a good lawyer and accountant, and she joined a new firm that offered generous benefits.
>
> Nancy and Bob took two cruises to islands they had visited before and loved. The boys came home for visits regularly and called their father on the telephone several times a week. Christmas was particularly hard, because they all knew it would be the last one for Bob, but there was a lot of laughter and love and closeness during the holiday. Nancy and

practical demands of informing family and friends and planning the funeral. After the ceremonial aspects of death have passed, family members are faced with the task of reorganizing their lives without the person they have lost. For some this means living alone or managing finances or household responsibilities for the first time. For others it means learning how to be a single parent.

Resuming regular activity, exercising, returning to work, and socializing with old friends are recommended following bereavement. Talking about the person who has died with family members and friends who knew him or her is also suggested. Families are also encouraged to celebrate holidays and other special anniversaries throughout the first year of mourning with special acknowledgment of the one who has died. If intense feelings of despair continue for more than two or three months, however, you may wish to seek bereavement counseling. Hospice programs can provide counseling, as can many churches, synagogues, and mental-health clinics. Bereavement counseling will help you gradually come to accept your loss, to begin to reorganize your life to include new relationships, and to remember the person who has died as he or she was through all the fullness of life, in which cancer was but one experience.

A family experience with cancer opens new pathways to understanding both life and death. Those who can accept the ambiguities of this understanding have called cancer "an incredible journey."

Bob instinctively provided emotional balance for each other: when she was feeling low, he was strong for her, and when he got depressed, she could pull him out of it. They spent some time with Bob's elderly parents and with their closest friends.

Bob decided he wanted to be involved with a hospice program before he had medical needs. A hospice worker came once a week to take Bob's blood pressure, offer nutritional advice, and help with practical problems. Later she began to prepare them for the final period of Bob's illness.

The end came very quickly. Bob chose to die at home with his family around him. The hospice provided a hospital bed, a daily home-health-care worker, and professional nurses. Nancy slept on the sofa near his bed, and the boys came home to sit with him, hold his hand, and play music for him. He gradually weakened, and died at five in the morning, when the rest of the family was asleep.

The family held the simple funeral Bob and Nancy had planned. The hospice worker came to the service and continued to be available to Nancy throughout the year following Bob's death. Nancy grieved for her loss, but she had no regrets about her relationship with Bob and the final year they had spent together.

Postscript

Fitzhugh Mullan, M.D.

Great strides have been made in recent years in the prevention, diagnosis, and treatment of cancer. These advances provide not only better health for our population as a whole, but special benefit and hope to everyone whose life is touched by cancer. Nonetheless, the diagnosis of cancer is always an unwelcome and unexpected intruder in the life of an individual or a family. It remains a one-way ticket across a wide and swift river to a land on the far bank—the land of cancer survivorship, with its own biology, its own psychology, and its own community. It is a land where family and friends, doctors and nurses can visit but where the survivor becomes a permanent resident. It is a land that, until recently, received very little attention and had few maps and no constitution.

The land across the river is changing quickly, and for the better. This book is but one example of the consciousness and articulateness of survivors today, who are bringing a new sense of community and mutual support to the hills and dales of the land across the river. This land lacks neither population nor energetic, gifted, brave people. It has always had ample numbers of new recruits as well as seasoned veterans. What has been missing, though, is community recognition, identity, and pride. Too often cancer has been treated as an embarrassment and a cause for mortal fear, with families and individuals having little sense that help, information, role models, guidance, or succor might be available from others with cancer. The people living on the far bank have tended to live alone, paying little attention to the other denizens of the land and taking little strength or sustenance from one another. It has been an undercivilized existence.

The survivorship movement is changing that, mapping and civilizing that land. Survivors are talking publicly and writing about their experiences so that others can understand the land and its topography. They are meeting together and sharing their experiences, frustrations, and hopes, staffing telephone hotlines, and organizing support groups, potluck dinners, and fashion shows. They have given testimony on Capitol Hill, in statehouses, and before presidential commissions. "Sixty Minutes," *Newsweek,* and *The New York Times,* among others, have featured the growing activism of cancer survivors. These efforts will make the land on the other side of the river warmer, less solitary, and more habitable. All of the terrain, of course, is not beautiful, but a hard journey will surely be less onerous if the traveler is armed with good maps and the counsel of those who have gone before.

The authors of this book have recorded their counsel on the preceding pages in the spirit of mapping the land and building the community. Their anecdotes and their art, their advice, poems, charts, humor, sorrow, and wisdom are testimony that no one is alone in the battle against cancer, no matter how newly diagnosed, sick, or discouraged. Survivorship, in fact, has proved revitalizing to many, forging new intellectual, spiritual, and personal connections. Life for many, as the book records, is no longer measured in time but in quality.

Most of all, the book and the concepts behind it are to be shared. Survivors need to be encouraged to talk about their illnesses and their experiences, to read and write and participate in cancer-support programs. Survivors as well as their families, their doctors, and their nurses need to be recruited to the movement, and they in turn need to recruit others. Survivors can do a lot for one another—simple human acts that will benefit everyone involved.

Although a great deal has been done to begin the process of civilizing the land across the river, it remains primitive compared with what it might become. This book gives an exciting glimpse of the challenges that lie in front of us all.

Appendix A

Cancer Survivorship Resources

Medical Information

National Cancer Institute

National Cancer Institute
Cancer Information Service
Building 31, Room 10A18
Bethesda, MD 20892
(800) 4-CANCER (800-422-6237)
(800) 638-1234 (if you call from Alaska)

Provides answers to questions about cancer, as well as a wide variety of free consumer publications about cancer prevention, diagnosis, and treatment. Also operates Physician Data Query (PDQ), which provides information about treatment, including the most current results from investigational trials. Spanish-speaking staff members are available to callers from the following areas (daytime only): California, Florida, Georgia, Illinois, New Jersey (area code 201 only), New York, and Texas.

Comprehensive and Clinical Cancer Centers Supported by the National Cancer Institute

Comprehensive medical centers investigate new methods of diagnosis and treatment of cancer and provide new scientific knowledge to doctors who treat cancer. To be designated a comprehensive medical center by the National Cancer Institute, the hospital must meet ten specific criteria, which include basic and clinical research and patient care.

Clinical cancer centers receive support from the National Cancer Institute for cancer research for the investigation of promising new methods of cancer treatment.

In addition to the following medical centers designated by the National Cancer Institute to be comprehensive* or clinical† cancer centers, more than 1,000 medical centers throughout the United States provide cancer diagnosis and treatment. For information about medical centers in your area, call the National Cancer Institute, 1-800-4-CANCER.

Alabama
University of Alabama Comprehensive Cancer Center*
1918 University Boulevard
Basic Health Sciences Building, Room 108
Birmingham, AL 35294
(205) 934-6612

Arizona
University of Arizona Cancer Center†
1501 North Campbell Avenue
Tucson, AZ 85724
(602) 626-6372

California
The Kenneth Norris Jr. Comprehensive Cancer Center*
University of Southern California
1441 Eastlake Avenue
Los Angeles, CA 90033-0804
(213) 226-2370

Jonsson Comprehensive Cancer Center (UCLA)*
10-247 Factor Building
10833 Le Conte Avenue
Los Angeles, CA 90024-1781
(213) 825-8727

City of Hope National Medical Center†
Beckman Research Institute
1500 East Duarte Road
Duarte, CA 91010
(818) 359-8111, ext. 2292

University of California at San Diego Cancer Center†
225 Dickinson Street
San Diego, CA 92103
(619) 543-6178

Colorado
University of Colorado Cancer Center†
4200 East 9th Avenue, Box 8190
Denver, CO 80262
(303) 270-3019

Connecticut
Yale Comprehensive Cancer Center*
333 Cedar Street
New Haven, CT 06510
(203) 785-6338

District of Columbia
Howard University Cancer Research Center*
2041 Georgia Avenue, N.W.
Washington, DC 20060
(202) 636-7610 or 636-5665

Vincent T. Lombardi Cancer Research Center*
Georgetown University Medical Center
3800 Reservoir Road, N.W.
Washington, DC 20007
(202) 687-2110

Florida
Sylvester Comprehensive Cancer Center*
University of Miami Medical School
1475 Northwest 12th Avenue
Miami, FL 33136
(305) 548-4850

Illinois
Illinois Cancer Council* (includes institutions listed and several other organizations)

Illinois Cancer Council
36 South Wabash Avenue
Chicago, IL 60603
(312) 226-2371

University of Chicago Cancer Research Center
5841 South Maryland Avenue
Chicago, IL 60637
(312) 702-9200

Kentucky
Lucille Parker Markey Cancer Center†
University of Kentucky Medical Center
800 Rose Street
Lexington, KY 40536-0093
(606) 257-4447

Maryland
The Johns Hopkins Oncology Center*
600 North Wolfe Street
Baltimore, MD 21205
(301) 955-8638

Massachusetts
Dana-Farber Cancer Institute*
44 Binney Street
Boston, MA 02115
(617) 732-3214

Michigan
Meyer L. Prentis Comprehensive Cancer Center of Metropolitan Detroit*

110 East Warren Avenue
Detroit, MI 48201
(313) 745-4329

University of Michigan Cancer Center†
101 Simpson Drive
Ann Arbor, MI 48109-0752
(313) 936-2516

Minnesota
Mayo Comprehensive Cancer Center*
200 First Street Southwest
Rochester, MN 55095
(507) 284-3413

New Hampshire
Norris Cotton Cancer Center†
Dartmouth-Hitchcock Medical Center
2 Maynard Street
Hanover, NH 03756
(603) 646-5505

New York
Memorial Sloan-Kettering Cancer Center*
1275 York Avenue
New York, NY 10021
(800) 525-2225

Columbia University Cancer Center*
College of Physicians and Surgeons
630 West 168th Street
New York, NY 10032
(212) 305-6730

Roswell Park Memorial Institute*
Elm and Carlton Streets
Buffalo, NY 14263
(716) 845-4400

Mount Sinai School of Medicine†
One Gustave L. Levy Place
New York, NY 10029
(212) 241-8617

Albert Einstein College of Medicine†
1300 Morris Park Avenue
Bronx, NY 10461
(212) 920-4826

New York University Cancer Center†
462 First Avenue
New York, NY 10016-9103
(212) 340-6485

University of Rochester Cancer Center†
601 Elmwood Avenue, Box 704
Rochester, NY 14642
(716) 275-4911

North Carolina
Duke University Comprehensive Cancer Center*
P.O. Box 3843
Durham, NC 27710
(919) 286-5515

Lineberger Cancer Research Center†
University of North Carolina School of Medicine
Chapel Hill, NC 27599
(919) 966-4431

Bowman Gray School of Medicine†
Wake Forest University
300 South Hawthorne Road
Winston-Salem, NC 27103
(919) 748-4354

Ohio
Ohio State University Comprehensive Cancer Center*
410 West 12th Avenue
Columbus, OH 43210
(614) 293-8619

Case Western Reserve University†
University Hospitals of Cleveland
Ireland Cancer Center
2074 Abington Road
Cleveland, OH 44106
(216) 844-8453

Pennsylvania

Fox Chase Cancer Center*
7701 Burholme Avenue
Philadelphia, PA 19111
(215) 728-2570

University of Pennsylvania Cancer Center*
3400 Spruce Street
Philadelphia, PA 19104
(215) 662-6364

Pittsburgh Cancer Institute†
200 Meyran Avenue
Pittsburgh, PA 15213-2592
(800) 537-4063

Rhode Island

Roger Williams General Hospital†
825 Chalkstone Avenue
Providence, RI 02908
(401) 456-2070

Tennessee

Saint Jude Children's Research Hospital†
332 North Lauderdale Street
Memphis, TN 38101
(901) 522-0694

Texas

The University of Texas
M. D. Anderson Cancer Center*
1515 Holcombe Boulevard
Houston, TX 77030
(713) 792-3245

Utah

Utah Regional Cancer Center†
University of Utah Medical Center
50 North Medical Drive, Room 2C10
Salt Lake City, UT 84132
(801) 581-4048

Vermont

Vermont Regional Cancer Center†
University of Vermont
1 South Prospect Street
Burlington, VT 05401
(802) 656-4580

Virginia

Massey Cancer Center†
Medical College of Virginia
Virginia Commonwealth University
1200 East Broad Street
Richmond, VA 23298
(804) 786-9641

University of Virginia Medical Center†
Box 334
Primary Care Center, Room 4520
Lee Street
Charlottesville, VA 22908
(804) 924-2562

Washington

Fred Hutchinson Cancer Research Center*
1124 Columbia Street
Seattle, WA 98104
(206) 467-4675

Wisconsin

Wisconsin Clinical Cancer Center*
University of Wisconsin
600 Highland Avenue
Madison, WI 53792
(608) 263-6872

Professional Medical Societies

Cancer patients traditionally have attracted a broad spectrum of medical assistance, from highly skilled and qualified health professionals who practice state-of-the-art medicine to quacks who market worthless, even harmful, pseudo-panaceas. To ensure that you receive professional medical care only from a trained care giver and certified facility, you may learn more about your treatment team from several professional medical societies.

The American Board of Medical Specialties
One Rotary Center, Suite 805
Evanston, IL 60201
(708) 491-9091

The American Board of Medical Specialties is the umbrella organization for all specialty boards that certify physicians. It keeps a national list of physicians who have been certified in their specialties, and can tell you if your physician is board-certified in his or her specialty. Board certification does not guarantee a physician's expertise, but it does signify meeting rigorous standards established by his or her peers. The organization also publishes the *ABMS Compendium of Certified Medical Specialists*, the only biographic directory that is authorized by all specialty boards. The *Compendium*, which is available in public and medical libraries, is published every even-numbered year, with an annual supplement.

American College of Radiology
1891 Prespon White Drive
Reston, VA 22091
(703) 648-8900

The American College of Radiology provides a list of accredited mammography facilities. It conducts a voluntary peer review of mammography facilities to determine if they meet accreditation standards designed to ensure that mammographies are performed by qualified staff, and that equipment used is specially designed and properly maintained for mammography.

American College of Surgeons
Office of Public Information
55 East Erie Street
Chicago, IL 60611
(312) 664-4050

The American College of Surgeons provides a geographic list of Fellows of the American College of Surgeons (who are board-certified surgeons), including type of specialty. It prefers written requests.

College of American Pathologists
325 Waukegan Road
Northfield, IL 60093-2750
(708) 446-8800

The College of American Pathologists surveys hospital and nonhospital laboratories to determine if they meet CAP standards for accreditation. CAP standards are voluntary. Approximately 4,000 laboratories in the United States have asked CAP to survey their facilities and received accreditation. You can call CAP to find out if a particular lab is accredited (be prepared with the name and address of the lab).

Community Health Accreditation Program, Inc.
350 Hudson Street
New York, NY 10014
(800) 669-1656

The Community Health Accreditation Program accredits home-care organizations for minimum standards of safety and care. It will provide callers with a list of accredited and nonaccredited agencies in your community.

International Pain Foundation
909 N.E. 43rd Street, Suite 306
Seattle, WA 98105-6020
(206) 547-2157

The International Pain Foundation has publications about pain for the general public. Affiliated with the International Association for the Study of Pain, it is a professional organization that fosters and encourages research, promotes education and training, and facilitates dissemination of new information in the field of pain.

Joint Commission on Accreditation of Healthcare Organizations
Public Information Coordinator
Department of Corporate Relations
One Renaissance Boulevard
Oakbrook Terrace, IL 60181
(708) 916-5632

This joint commission of the American Hospital Association, the American Medical Association, the American College of Physicians, the American College of Surgeons, and the American Dental Association establishes standards for hospital care. The commission accredits hospitals that meet its standards. The Public Information Coordinator can tell you if a particular hospital is accredited.

Visiting Nurse Associations of America
3801 East Florida Avenue, Suite 806
Denver, CO 80210
(800) 426-2547

The Visiting Nurse Associations of America will provide a caller with names of visiting-nurse associations in his or her community. There are more than 500 non-profit visiting-nurse associations in the United States that provide community-based home care services, including skilled nurses, therapists, and home health-care aides.

Office of Disease Prevention and Health Promotion

The Office of Disease Prevention and Health Promotion is an office of the United States Department of Health and Human Services that operates two programs that are of particular service to cancer survivors.

National Health Information Center
P.O. Box 1133
Washington, DC 20013-1133
(800) 336-4797
(301) 565-4167 (Maryland only)

The National Health Information Center is a health-information referral organization. It provides callers with the names, addresses, and telephone numbers of organizations that can reply directly to their questions about cancer and other health issues. It produces publications on a variety of health issues, including nutrition, work-site health-promotion programs, and special concerns of the elderly and minorities. The center does not answer specific medical questions.

National Information Center for Orphan Drugs and Rare Diseases
P.O. Box 1133
Washington, DC 20013-1133
(800) 456-3505

The National Information Center for Orphan Drugs and Rare Diseases is a component of the National Health Information Center. It provides callers with the names, addresses, and telephone numbers of organizations that can reply directly to their questions about rare diseases (those affecting 200,000 or fewer persons in the United States) and orphan drugs (medicines not widely researched or available). It provides the names of drug companies that manufacture orphan drugs so that the caller can learn about the availability of the drugs. This organization also provides written information about certain rare conditions from their medical library.

Community Resources for Cancer Survivors and Consumers

National Professional and Mutual-Aid Organizations

American Cancer Society
Tower Place
3340 Peachtree Road N.E.
Atlanta, GA 30026
(404) 320-3333
(800) ACS-2345 (national and local information)

The American Cancer Society is an information-and-referral service providing general information on prevention, diagnosis, research, treatment, support, publications, and the organization itself.

American Red Cross
431 18th Street, N.W.
Washington, DC 20006
(202) 737-8300

A network of local chapters provides various community services, including nursing health programs and voluntary blood donations. Contact your local chapter first. If you cannot find a chapter listed in your telephone directory, the national office in Washington will help you locate the chapter nearest you.

Association of Brain Tumor Research
6232 North Pulaski Road, Suite 200
Chicago, IL 60646
(312) 286-5571

The Association of Brain Tumor Research raises funds for brain-tumor research and provides public education about brain tumors.

Better Together Club
P.O. Box 4277
Syosset, NY 11791-9706
(800) 422-8811

Free club organized by ConvaTec (a Squibb Company) that provides practical information about living with an ostomy and offers referrals to enterostomal therapists.

Candlelighters Childhood Cancer Foundation, Inc.
1312 18th Street, N.W., Second Floor
Washington, DC 20036
(800) 366-2223

Candlelighters is an international organization of parents whose children (through adolescence) have or have had cancer. It provides guidance and emotional support for families as well as identifying needs and serving as intermediary to other resources. Services include support groups, several newsletters, blood and wig banks, housing, transportation, baby-sitting, and limited financial assistance.

CanSurmount
Begun as a grassroots support program, CanSurmount is currently a program of the American Cancer Society that brings together survivors, family members, survivor volunteers, and health professionals to provide mutual support and education. Contact your local American Cancer Society unit for information about CanSurmount in your area.

Center for Medical Consumers
237 Thompson Street
New York, NY 10012
(212) 674-7105

A center for education and information, this organization provides referrals to national health organizations. It publishes a monthly consumer newsletter called *Health Facts,* which updates general medical and health news, including oncology. It has a medical consumer's public library, including books and clippings from medical journals.

Children's Oncology Camps of America
c/o Dr. Edward S. Baum
Children's Memorial Hospital
2300 Children's Plaza
Chicago, IL 60614
(312) 880-4564

Children's Oncology Camps of America publishes an annual national directory of children's oncology camps.

Consumer Health Information Research Institute
300 East Pink Hill Road
Independence, MO 64057
(800) 821-6671

This is a nonprofit organization that provides information about questionable medical practices, including unorthodox cancer treatment. The Consumer Health Information Research Institute categorizes health services into (1) folklore, (2) quackery, (3) unproven, (4) investigational, and (5) proven.

Corporate Angel Network
Westchester County Airport Building 1
White Plains, NY 10604
(914) 328-1313

The Corporate Angel Network alleviates costs of cancer patients receiving specialized treatment in NCI-approved treatment centers by arranging transportation aboard corporate aircraft on routine flights when seats are available.

DES Action U.S.A. (East Coast office)
Long Island Jewish Medical Center
New Hyde Park, NY 11040
(516) 775-3450

DES Action U.S.A. (West Coast office)
2845 24th Street
San Francisco, CA 94110
(415) 826-5060

DES Action is a national organization with over 30 chapters in the United States, and affiliates in Canada, Australia, The Netherlands, and France. Offers counseling, educational materials, and a newsletter about diethylstilbestrol (DES), a synthetic hormone that was once given to women during pregnancy to prevent miscarriages. DES increases the risk of certain types of cancer in those women and their daughters who were exposed to the drug in the womb.

Encore
YWCA of the United States
726 Broadway, 5th Floor
New York, NY 10003
(212) 614-2827

Encore provides postmastectomy group and rehabilitation programs, including support groups, and special water and floor exercises. Contact the YWCA in your area first to learn about a local Encore program. The national office of the YWCA trains staff, certifies each program, and can help you locate the nearest Encore program in your community.

I Can Cope
Begun as a grassroots support program, I Can Cope is currently a program of the American Cancer Society that addresses the educational and psychological needs of survivors and family members through a series of eight classes. Contact your local American Cancer Society unit for information about I Can Cope in your area.

International Association of Laryngectomees

This voluntary umbrella organization promotes and supports rehabilitation programs for laryngectomees. Contact your local American Cancer Society unit for information about services for laryngectomees in your area.

Let's Face It
Box 711
Concord, MA 01742
(508) 371-3186

Let's Face It is the United States branch of an international mutual-help network for the facially disfigured. It provides mutual support, educational services, and a newsletter.

Leukemia Society of America, Inc.
733 Third Avenue
New York, NY 10017
(212) 573-8484

Chapters offer patients with leukemia and other hematic cancers financial assistance, transportation, and consultation services for referrals to other means of local support.

Make Today Count
101½ South Union Street
Alexandria, VA 22314
(703) 548-9674

Make Today Count is a national organization of more than 200 chapters that provides emotional self-help to survivors and their families. Chapters' activities include formal programs, group discussions, chapter newsletters, social activities, workshops and seminars, and education activities.

National Alliance of Breast Cancer Organizations (NABCO)
1180 Avenue of the Americas,
2nd Floor
New York, NY 10036
(212) 719-0154

NABCO fosters unity among organizations and individuals in the fight against breast cancer and serves as a resource for persons who have concerns about breast cancer and other breast diseases. NABCO also seeks to affect public and private policy in the areas of insurance reimbursements, funding priorities, and health legislation dealing with breast cancer at the national, state, and local levels. NABCO prefers written inquiries.

National Brain Tumor Foundation
323 Geary Street, Suite 510
San Francisco, CA 94102
(415) 296-0404

This organization raises funds to support brain-tumor research and provides information and support services to patients and families. It publishes a resource guide for patients and their families.

National Cancer Care Foundation and Cancer Care, Inc.
1180 Avenue of the Americas,
2nd Floor
New York, NY 10036
(212) 221-3300

Cancer Care provides national information about and referrals to nonmedical resources for cancer survivors. It offers professional, community, and national education programs, oncology social-work services, support groups, and financial assistance to cancer survivors, primarily in New York, New Jersey, and Connecticut.

National Coalition for Cancer Survivorship
323 Eighth Street, S.W.
Albuquerque, NM 87102
(505) 764-9956

NCCS is a national coalition of individual cancer survivors, health professionals, institutions, and regional and national cancer organizations that serves as an informational clearinghouse, holds an annual conference on survivorship issues, publishes a newsletter, provides technical assistance to community cancer-support organizations, and advocates for the legal rights of cancer survivors.

National Consumers League
815 15th Street, N.W., Suite 516
Washington, DC 20005
(202) 639-8140

The National Consumers League is a nonprofit membership organization that represents consumers and workers on the federal level. It offers several publications on health issues (insurance, home health care, hospice care, etc.).

National Council Against Health Fraud Resource Center
P.O. Box 413213
Kansas City, MO 64141
(800) 821-6671

The National Council is a nonprofit organization that collects and disseminates publications on questionable health practices and organizations, including cancer treatment and cancer organizations. It prefers written inquiries.

National Hospice Organization
1901 North Moore Street, Suite 901
Arlington, VA 22209
(703) 243-5900

The National Hospice Organization is a nonprofit membership association dedicated to promoting and maintaining quality care for terminally ill people and their families. It provides educational programs, technical assistance, publications, and advocacy and referral services. It operates a toll-free help line. See p. 177.

National Lymphedema Network
2211 Post Street, Suite 404
San Francisco, CA 94115
(800) 541-3259

The National Lymphedema Network is a nonprofit resource center that provides information about prevention and treatment of lymphedema, swelling that is a common complication of lymph-node surgery. It helps organize local support groups focusing on the treatment and impact of lymphedema. It publishes a newsletter containing personal stories about dealing with lymphedema, as well as network news.

Ostomy Rehabilitation Program

This program provides rehabilitation support for people who have had ostomy surgery. Contact your local American Cancer Society unit for information about the Ostomy Rehabilitation Program in your area.

Patient Advocates for Advanced Cancer Treatment (PAACT)
P.O. Box 1656
Grand Rapids, MI 49501
(616) 453-1477

PAACT is an international organization that disseminates information on the latest developments in detection, diagnosis, treatment, and monitoring of prostate cancer.

Reach to Recovery Program

Reach to Recovery provides rehabilitation support for women who have had breast cancer, and offers hospital visits and temporary prosthesis. Contact your local American Cancer Society unit for information about Reach to Recovery in your area.

United Cancer Council, Inc.
1803 North Meridian Street
Indianapolis, IN 46202
(317) 923-6490

This organization is a federation of voluntary cancer agencies, funded through the United Way of Giving in most communities where they are located. Services include nursing, homemaking, housekeeping, medications, prostheses, and rehabilitation.

United Ostomy Association, Inc.
36 Executive Park, Suite 120
Irvine, CA 92714
(714) 660-8624

The United Ostomy Association sponsors local Ostomy Association chapters, which provide mutual support, visitor programs, educational materials, advocacy services, and a quarterly publication to those who have had ostomy surgery.

Well Spouse Foundation
17456 Drayton Hall Way
San Diego, CA 92128

Network of support groups and families that give emotional support to and advocates for the husbands, wives, and children of the chronically ill. Produces a quarterly newsletter.

Y-ME National Organization for Breast Cancer Information & Support
18220 Harwood Avenue
Homewood, IL 60430
(708) 799-8228
(800) 221-2141 (for callers outside of 708 area code)

Y-ME provides peer-support groups, volunteer matching, educational materials, and referrals to community resources. It also provides training and technical assistance to hotline staffs of other cancer support groups. It produces a detailed self-help manual for starting support groups (appropriate for Y-ME and other cancer support groups). Maintains a prosthesis bank for women with financial need.

Newsletters Published by Major Mutual-Aid Cancer Organizations

Many self-help organizations publish newsletters. Most newsletters focus on organizational news and local issues. The following newsletters provide information about cancer survivorship addressed to a national audience.

Cancer Communication
Patient Advocates for Advanced Cancer Treatment (PAACT)
P.O. Box 1656
Grand Rapids, MI 49501
(616) 453-1477

This six-to-eight-page seasonal periodical is written to educate men with prostate cancer about medical choices and advancements in treating prostate cancer.

Candlelighters Childhood Cancer Foundation Youth Newsletter
Candlelighters Childhood Cancer Foundation Quarterly Newsletter
1312 18th Street, N.W., Second Floor
Washington, DC 20036
(800) 366-2223

These quarterly publications contain information of interest to persons concerned with childhood cancer. The youth newsletter features stories and drawings by children who have or have had cancer and by their siblings.

Let's Face It
Let's Face It
Box 711
Concord, MA 01742
(508) 371-3186

This is a seasonal newsletter that presents resources for recovery from facial surgery or other facial disfigurements.

Living Through Cancer
Living Through Cancer Survivorship Center
323 Eighth Street, S.W.
Albuquerque, NM 87102
(505) 242-3263

This 10- to 12-page newsletter written by and for survivors and their families includes personal stories, poetry, book reviews, articles on survivorship, and resource lists.

NABCO News
National Alliance of Breast Cancer Organizations (NABCO)
1180 Avenue of the Americas, 2nd Floor
New York, NY 10036
(212) 719-0154

This quarterly publication contains information on breast cancer, breast-cancer organizations, and public and private policy in the areas of health insurance, funding priorities, and legislation.

NCCS Networker
National Coalition for Cancer Survivorship
323 Eighth Street, S.W.
Albuquerque, NM 87102
(505) 764-9956

This quarterly publication provides national news on cancer survivorship issues (conferences, legislation, etc.), book reviews, resource lists, and organizational news.

SEARCH
National Brain Tumor Foundation
323 Geary Street, Suite 510
San Francisco, CA 94102
(415) 296-0404

This quarterly publication reports stories of people who have been diagnosed with brain tumors and their families, as well as organizational news.

Surviving! A Patient Newsletter
Stanford University Medical Center
Patient Resource Center, Room H0103
Division of Radiation Oncology
300 Pasteur Drive
Stanford, CA 94305
(415) 723-6171

Created by Stanford University Medical Center patients primarily for survivors of Hodgkin's disease, this newsletter contains original personal stories, essays, and artwork by cancer survivors, as well as medical news.

Y-ME Hotline
Y-ME National Organization for Breast Cancer Information & Support
18220 Harwood Avenue
Homewood, IL 60430
(708) 799-8338
(800) 221-2141 (for callers outside of 708 area code)

This newsletter contains short articles of general interest to women dealing with breast cancer, resource lists, question-and-answer column, and organizational news.

Nonmedical Telephone Hotlines

Cancer Hotlines

Some cancer organizations operate telephone hotlines that match callers with staff or volunteers who are cancer survivors or family members. They provide callers with an opportunity to talk with a cancer survivor and/or family member who can offer emotional support and practical suggestions from personal experience. Unless otherwise noted, these hotlines provide services on a regional, not a national, basis. Most are staffed by trained volunteers.

Saint Vincent Infirmary and Medical Center
Saint Vincent Cancer Center
2 St. Vincent Circle
Little Rock, AR 72205
(501) 660-3900
(800) 632-4614 (within Arkansas)

This facility provides Arkansas residents with advice and emotional support by cancer survivors and their families.

Cancer Hotline
7201 North University Drive
Tamarac, FL 33321-2913
(305) 721-7600, (305) 547-6920

Cancer Hotline provides emotional, personal, and psychological support to callers in Dade and Broward counties in South Florida. Collect calls are accepted.

Cancer Wellness Center
9701 North Kenton, #18
Skokie, IL 60076
(708) 982-9789

The Cancer Wellness Center provides a 24-hour emotional hotline for hope, comfort, support, and encouragement, and also provides other support services.

Y-ME National Organization for Breast Cancer Information & Support
18220 Harwood Avenue
Homewood, IL 60430
(708) 799-8228
(800) 221-2141 (for callers outside the 708 area code)

This national hotline answers questions about breast cancer and matches callers with volunteers (primarily regional matches).

Cancer Support Network
802 E. Jefferson
Bloomington, IL 61701
(309) 829-CARE (2273)

Volunteer cancer survivors offer emotional support and practical advice.

Cancer Hot Line
4410 Main Street
Kansas City, MO 64111
(816) 932-8453

A service of the R. A. Bloch Cancer Foundation, Cancer Hot Line provides support to cancer survivors, family, and friends in the Kansas City area.

SHARE
817 Broadway, 6th Floor
New York, NY 10003
(212) 260-0580

SHARE is a hotline for women with breast cancer, their families, and health professionals. Whenever a volunteer is not available for immediate response, calls will be returned within 24 hours.

Cancer Hotline
2260 South Belvoir Street
Cleveland, OH 44118
(216) 292-8222

This hotline matches callers in the local calling area with volunteer cancer survivors.

Cancer Connection
Cancer Center of the Southwest
Baptist Medical Center
3300 Northwest Expressway
Oklahoma City, OK 73112
(405) 943-HOPE (4673)

Cancer Connection matches callers in southeastern, southwestern, and central Oklahoma with volunteer cancer survivors.

Cancer Hotline of the Cancer Guidance Institute

1323 Forbes Avenue
Pittsburgh, PA 15219
(412) 261-2211

This service provides emotional support and nonmedical information through a group of trained volunteers of cancer survivors and family members. It matches by sex, age, and type of cancer.

Cancer Hotline of Tarrant County, Inc.
3208 Flintridge Drive
Arlington, TX 76017
(817) 654-7222

This hotline provides understanding and tips on coping with cancer treatment, but does not provide medical advice, answers to questions about cancer, or financial assistance. It is staffed by volunteers, all of whom are either cancer survivors or family members. Callers are provided, free of charge, with a 47-page publication, *A Guide for Cancer Patients*.

Cancer Lifeline
500 Lowman Building
107 Cherry Street
Seattle, WA 98104
(206) 461-4542
(800) 255-5505 (Washington State only)

This is a 24-hour direct service providing telephone support and referrals for survivors, family, and friends.

National Health and Consumer Hotlines

Brain Tumor Information Services
Box 405, Room J341
5841 South Maryland Avenue
Chicago, IL 60637
(312) 684-1400

This hotline provides information about brain-tumor treatments and helps brain-tumor patients locate additional medical care.

Care Coordination Center
Kimberly Quality Care
695 Atlantic Avenue
Boston, MA 02111
(800) 645-3633

This 24-hour hotline describes services provided by Kimberly Quality Care (350+ private home-health-care offices in 44 states) and other agencies. It includes information about home nursing, hospice, rehabilitation facilities, equipment companies, and self-help groups in each community.

Department of Veterans Affairs
(formerly Veterans Administration)
(800) 422-8079

A national toll-free hotline provides information about insurance coverage for veterans.

Internal Revenue Service
(800) 424-1040

This number provides advice on completing tax returns and offers a wide variety of free consumer publications.

National AIDS Hotline
(800) 342-2437 (24 hours)
(800) 344-7432 Spanish-speaking (8:00 A.M. to 2:00 A.M.)
(800) 243-7889 hearing-impaired (8:00 A.M. to 10:00 P.M.)

American Social Health Association, a nonprofit organization, relays information, referral services, and publications about acquired immunodeficiency syndrome, through a contract with Centers for Disease Control.

National Health Information Clearinghouse
Office of Disease Prevention and Health Promotion
United States Public Health Service
(800) 336-4797

This health-information-and-referral service refers callers to appropriate national organizations, provides basic information about specific medical conditions, and offers publications.

National Hospice Organization Help Line
1901 North Moore Street, Suite 901
Arlington, VA 22209
(800) 658-8898

This service provides help to individuals who want to start a hospice or who need to find a hospice in their community.

National Lymphedema Network Hotline
2211 Post Street, Suite 404
San Francisco, CA 94115
(800) 541-3259

This hotline provides information about the prevention and treatment of lymphedema, swelling that is a common complication of lymph-node surgery.

United States Department of Health and Human Services
Health Care Financing Administration (HCFA)
Baltimore, MD 21207
(800) 888-1998

This service provides information about Medicare coverage.

Self-Help Clearinghouses

Self-help clearinghouses are nonprofit organizations that help callers locate self-help organizations that address cancer, general health, and other issues. Except where noted, clearinghouses disseminate information and provide services only in their geographic areas. Self-help clearinghouses provide some or all of the following services: training workshops, conferences, newsletters, speakers bureaus, consultation in developing and maintaining groups, development of group resource materials, assistance with coalition building, and outreach efforts with professionals and the media.

National Clearinghouses
National Self Help Clearinghouse
City University of New York
Graduate Center, Room 1206A
33 West 42nd Street
New York, NY 10036
(212) 840-1259

New Jersey Self Help Clearinghouse
St. Clares-Riverside Medical Center
Denville, NJ 07834
(201) 625-9565
(800) FOR-MASH (356-6274) (New Jersey only)

The Self Help Center
1600 Dodge Avenue #S-122
Evanston, IL 60201
(312) 328-0470
(800) 322-MASH (Illinois only)
(provides limited national information)

Regional Clearinghouses

California
California Self Help Center
UCLA Psychology Department
405 Hilgard Avenue
Los Angeles, CA 90024
(213) 825-1799
(800) 222-LINK (California only)

Northern Region Self-Help Center
Mental Health Association
5370 Elvas Avenue, Suite B
Sacramento, CA 95819
(916) 456-2070

Central Valley Self-Help Center
Mental Health Association
P.O. Box 343
Merced, CA 95341
(209) 723-8861

Southern Region Self-Help Center
Mental Health Association of San Diego

3958 Third Avenue
San Diego, CA 92103

Bay Area Self-Help Center
Mental Health Association
2398 Pine Street
San Francisco, CA 94115
(415) 921-4401

Self-Help Clearinghouse of Yolo County
Mental Health Association
P.O. Box 447
Davis, CA 95617

Connecticut
Connecticut Self Help/
Mutual Support Network
19 Howe Street
New Haven, CT 06511
(203) 789-7645

District of Columbia
Mental Health Association of Northern Virginia
100 North Washington Street, Suite 232
Falls Church, VA 22046
(703) 536-4100
(Washington, DC, northern Virginia, and southern Maryland)

Illinois
The Self Help Center
1600 Dodge Avenue #S-122
Evanston, IL 60201
(708) 328-0470
(800) 322-MASH (Illinois only)

Self-Help Center
Family Service of Champaign County
405 South State Street
Champaign, IL 61820
(217) 352-0092

Iowa
Iowa Self-Help Clearinghouse
Iowa Pilot Parents, Inc.
33 North 12th Street
Fort Dodge, IA 50501
(515) 576-5870
(800) 383-4777 (Iowa only)

Kansas
Self Help Network
The Wichita State University
Campus Box 34
Wichita, KS 67208-1595
(316) 689-3170

Massachusetts
Massachusetts Clearinghouse of Mutual Help Groups
University of Massachusetts Cooperative Extension Service
13 Skinner Hall
Amherst, MA 01003
(413) 545-2313

Michigan
Michigan Self Help Clearinghouse
Michigan Protection and Advocacy Service
109 West Michigan, Suite 900
Lansing, MI 48933
(517) 484-7373
(800) 752-5858 (Michigan only)

Center for Self Help
Riverwood Center
515 Ship S1485 Highway M-139
Benton Harbor, MI 49022
(616) 925-0594

Minnesota
Minnesota Mutual Help Resource Center
Wilder Foundation Community Care
919 Lafond Avenue
Saint Paul, MN 55104
(612) 642-4060

Missouri
Support Group Clearinghouse
Kansas City Association for Mental Health
1020 East 63rd Street
Kansas City, MO 64110
(816) 561-HELP

Nebraska
Self-Help Information Service of Nebraska

CANCER SURVIVORSHIP RESOURCES

1601 Euclid Avenue
Lincoln, NB 68502
(402) 476-9668

New Jersey
New Jersey Self Help Clearinghouse
Saint Clares–Riverside Medical Center
Denville, NJ 07834
(201) 625-9565
(800) 356-6274 (calls from New Jersey)

New York
Brooklyn Self-Help Clearinghouse
Heights Mills Mental Health Service
30 Third Avenue
Brooklyn, NY 11217
(718) 834-7341

Long Island Self-Help Clearinghouse
New York Institute of Technology
Central Islip Campus
Central Islip, NY 11722
(516) 348-3030

New York City Self-Help Clearinghouse
P.O. Box 022812
Brooklyn, NY 11020
(718) 596-6000

New York State Self-Help
Clearinghouse
New York Council on Children and
Families
Empire State Plaza, Tower 2
Albany, NY 12224
(518) 474-6293

Westchester Self-Help Clearinghouse
Westchester Community College
Academics Arts Building
75 Grasslands Road
Valhalla, NY 10595
(914) 247-3620

Oregon
Northwest Regional Self-Help
Clearinghouse
718 West Burnside Avenue
Portland, OR 97209
(503) 222-5555

Pennsylvania
Self-Help Group Network
710½ South Avenue
Pittsburgh, PA 15221
(412) 247-5400

Self-Help Information Network
Exchange
% Voluntary Action Center
225 North Washington Avenue
Park Plaza, Lower Level
Scranton, PA 18503
(717) 961-1234

Rhode Island
Support Group Helpline
Rhode Island Department of Health
Cannon Building
Davis Street
Providence, RI 02908
(401) 277-2231

South Carolina
Midland Area Support Group Network
Lexington Medical Center
2720 Sunset Boulevard
West Columbia, SC 29169
(803) 791-9227

Tennessee
Support Group Clearinghouse
Mental Health Association of Knox
County
6712 Kingston Pike, #203
Knoxville, TN 37919
(614) 584-6736

Texas
Texas Self-Help Clearinghouse
Mental Health Association
1111 West 24th Street
Austin, TX 78705
(512) 454-3706

Dallas Self-Help Clearinghouse
Mental Health Association
2500 Maple Avenue
Dallas, TX 75201-1998
(214) 871-2420

Self-Help Clearinghouse
Mental Health Association
2211 Norfolk, Suite 810
Houston, TX 77098
(713) 523-8963

Greater San Antonio Self-Help
Clearinghouse
Mental Health Association
1407 North Main Street
San Antonio, TX 78212
(512) 222-1571

Tarrant County Self-Help
Clearinghouse
Mental Health Association
3136 West 4th Street
Fort Worth, TX 76107-2113
(817) 335-5405

Vermont
Vermont Self-Help Clearinghouse
% Parents Assistance Line
103 South Main Street
Waterbury, VT 05676
(802) 241-2249
(800) 442-5356 (Vermont only)

Legal, Financial, and Insurance Resources

Sources of Insurance Information

American Council on Life Insurance
1001 Pennsylvania Avenue, N.W.
Washington, DC 20004

This office provides information about brokers who specialize in high-risk life insurance.

American Association of Retired Persons (AARP)
1909 K Street, N.W.
Washington, DC 20049
(202) 872-4700

AARP provides Medicare supplementary insurance for members age 65 and over, and hospital plans for members age 50 and over; newsletter, practical information, $5-a-year membership fee available to anyone 50 or older.

Blue Cross and Blue Shield Association
676 North Saint Claire Street
Chicago, IL 60611
(312) 440-6000

This office provides information regarding coverage offered in each state, or refers you to your local association. Blue Cross and Blue Shield plans differ from most commercial insurers in that they offer more options to high-risk individuals, are nonprofit, are usually billed directly by the provider (instead of your paying the provider and then seeking reimbursement from your insurance company), and are often required to get approval from the state before they raise rates.

Communicating for Agriculture
2626 East 82nd Street, Suite 325
Minneapolis, MN 55425
(612) 854-9005

Answers questions about state high-risk health-insurance pools.

Disabled American Veterans
807 Main Avenue, S.W.
Washington, DC 20024
(202) 554-3501

This national organization with approximately 3,000 chapters offers counseling, educational materials, support groups, transportation, conferences, and a newsletter.

Group Health Association of America
Membership Department

624 9th Street, N.W.
Washington, DC 20001
(202) 778-3200

This trade association provides information about eligibility for group health-plan coverage with commercial insurers. It represents HMOs and sells a national directory of HMOs.

Health Insurance Association of America
P.O. Box 41455
Washington, DC 20018

This trade association representing major health-insurance companies authors consumer publications about health insurance. It offers a free copy of a booklet called *The Consumer's Guide to Health Insurance* and a list of other consumer publications.

Medical Information Bureau Inc.
P.O. Box 105
Essex Station
Boston, MA 02112
(617) 426-3660

This bureau keeps data about your health on file for insurance companies. You can verify that any information they have about you is correct by writing for a form requesting disclosure of whatever information the bureau has on you. The records must be sent to a "licensed medical professional" whom you designate.

National Insurance Consumer Organization
121 North Payne Street
Alexandria, VA 22314
(703) 549-8050

This consumer-advocacy organization for insurance consumers provides books, newsletters, and information for high-risk insurance buyers. The annual membership fee is $30.

Pension and Welfare Benefits Administration
U.S. Department of Labor, Room N-5658
200 Constitution Avenue, N.W.
Washington, DC 20210
(202) 523-8521

This office enforces your rights under COBRA to continued health-insurance coverage and provides information about how to enforce your rights to equal job benefits under ERISA.

United States Department of Health and Human Services
Health Care Financing Administration (HCFA)
Baltimore, MD 21207
(800) 888-1998

This office provides consumer information about Medicare.

Government Agencies: Civil Rights and Rehabilitation

Coordination and Review Section
Civil Rights Division
United States Department of Justice
Washington, DC 20530
(202) 724-2235
(202) 724-7678 (for the hearing impaired)

Provides information about which federal agency you should contact to enforce your rights under the Rehabilitation Act of 1973.

Equal Employment Opportunities Commission
Office of Communications and Legislative Affairs
1801 L Street, N.W.
Room 9024
Washington, DC 20507
(800) USA-EEOC (872-3362)

Provides information, in English and Spanish, on how to enforce your rights under the Americans with Disabilities Act of 1990.

Job Accommodation Network (JAN)
President's Committee on Employment of the Handicapped
P.O. Box 468
Morgantown, WV 26505
(800) JAN-PCEH (526-7234)

JAN provides information to employers on how to accommodate a handicapped worker.

National Rehabilitation Information Center
8455 Colesville Road, Suite 935
Silver Spring, MD 20910
(800) 346-2742

Government-funded information service that provides access to comprehensive information on disability-related products, research, and resources. Provides publications and referrals to support groups.

United States Department of Education
Rehabilitation Services Administration
Office of the Commissioner
Office of Special Education and Rehabilitation Services
330 C Street, S.W.
Washington, DC 20202
(202) 732-1282

Responsible for ensuring that your state rehabilitation services agency complies with federal law.

State Enforcement Agencies

The following agencies handle handicap-discrimination complaints. See page 103 for a description of how these agencies enforce state law.

Alaska
State Commission for Human Rights
800 A Street, Suite 202
Anchorage 99501
(907) 276-7474

Anchorage Equal Rights Commission
620 E. 10th Avenue, Suite 204
Anchorage 99519
(907) 243-4342

Human Rights Commission
Southcentral Region
314 Goldstein Building
P.O. Box AH
Juneau 99811
(907) 465-4670
[*Temporarily closed*]

Arizona
Civil Rights Division
Attorney General's Office
1275 West Washington Street
Phoenix 85007
(602) 542-5263

Southern Arizona Office
402 West Congress Street, Suite 315
100 N. Stone Street
Tucson 85701
(602) 628-6500

Governor's Office of Affirmative Action
1700 West Washington Street,
State Capitol, Room 804
Phoenix 85007
(602) 542-3211

California
Department of Fair Employment and Housing
2000 O Street
Sacramento 95814
(916) 445-9918

District and Field Offices
1529 "F" Street
Bakersfield 93301
(805) 395-2728

1900 Mariposa Mall, Suite 130
Fresno 93721
(209) 445-5373

322 West First Street
Room 2126
Los Angeles 90012
(212) 620-2610

1330 Broadway
Oakland 94612
(415) 464-4095

375 W. Hospitality Lane
Room 280
San Bernardino 92408
(714) 383-4711

110 W. C Street, #1702
San Diego 92101
(619) 237-7405

30 Van Ness Avenue
San Francisco 94102
(415) 557-2005

111 N. Market Street, Suite 810
San Jose 95113
(408) 277-1264

28 Civic Center Plaza
Room 330
Santa Ana 92701
(714) 558-4159

5720 Ralston Street
Ventura 93303
(805) 654-4512

Colorado
Civil Rights Commission
Room 600C, State Services Building
1525 Sherman Street
Denver 80203
(303) 866-2621

Branch Offices
2860 S. Circle Drive
North Building, Suite 2103
Colorado Springs 80906
(719) 576-6386

222 S. 6th Street
Room 417
Grand Junction 81501
(303) 248-7329

800 8th Avenue, Suite 223
Greeley 80631
(303) 356-9221

720 N. Main, Suite 222
Pueblo 81003
(719) 545-3520

Connecticut
Central Office
Commission on Human Rights and Opportunities
90 Washington Street
Hartford 06106
(203) 566-3350

Capitol Region:
1229 Albany Avenue
Hartford 06112
(203) 566-7710

West Central Region:
50 Linden
Waterbury 06702
(203) 754-2108

Eastern Region:
100 Broadway
Norwich 06360
(203) 886-5703

Southwest Region:
1115 Main Street
Bridgeport 06604
(203) 579-6246

Delaware
Department of Labor
Anti-Discrimination Section
Wilmington State Office Building
820 North French Street, 6th Floor
Wilmington 19801
(302) 571-2900

State Human Relations Commission
William Service Center
805 River Road
Dover 19901
(302) 736-4567

Georgetown State Service Center
546 South Bedford Street
Georgetown 19947
(302) 856-5331

District of Columbia
D.C. Office of Human Rights
2000 14th Street, N.W., 3rd Floor
Washington, DC 20009
(202) 939-8740

Florida
Commission of Human Relations
325 John Knox Road, Suite 240, Bldg. F
Tallahassee 32399
(904) 488-7082; (800) 342-8170

Lee County Dept. of Equal Opportunity
P.O. Box 398
Fort Meyers 33902-0398
(813) 334-2166

Hillsborough County Office of
Community Relations
712 W. Ross Avenue
Tampa 33602
(813) 223-8241 or 8438

Georgia
Georgia Office of Fair Employment
Practices
156 Trinity Avenue S.W., Suite 208
Atlanta 30303
(404) 656-1736

Governor's Council on Human
Relations
270 Washington St., S.W., Suite 603
Atlanta 30334
(404) 656-6757

Augusta/Richmond County Human
Relations Commission
525 Telfair Street
Augusta 30902
(404) 821-2506

Hawaii
Department of Labor & Industrial
Relations
Enforcement Division
830 Punchbowl Street, Room 340
Honolulu 96813
(808) 548-3976

Idaho
Commission on Human Rights
450 W. State Street
Boise 83720
(208) 334-2873

Illinois
Department of Human Rights
One Illinois Center
100 West Randolph Street, Suite 10-100
Chicago 60601
(312) 814-6200

Springfield Regional Office
Stratton Office Building, Room 623
Springfield 62706
(217) 785-5100

Indiana
Civil Rights Commission
32 E. Washington Street, Suite 900
Indianapolis 46204
(317) 232-2600

Iowa
Civil Rights Commission
211 E. Maple Street, 2nd Floor, State
Office Building
Des Moines 50319
(515) 281-4121; (800) 457-4416

Ft. Dodge-Webster County
819 First Avenue S.
Municipal Building
Ft. Dodge 50501
(515) 576-2201

Kansas
Commission on Civil Rights
Landon State Office Building
900 S.W. Jackson, 8th Floor, Suite 851S
Topeka 66612
(913) 296-3206

Branch Offices
1071 S. Glendale
Parkland Office Park
Wichita 67218
(316) 681-2911

Wichita Civil Rights and Equal
Employment Opportunity Commission
455 North Main Street, 10th Floor
Wichita 67202
(316) 268-4487

EEOC
911 Walnut Street, 10th Floor
Kansas City 64106
(816) 426-5773

Kentucky
Commission on Human Rights
701 West Muhammad Ali Boulevard
P.O. Box 69
Louisville 40201
(502) 588-4024

832 Capitol Plaza Tower
Frankfort 40601
(502) 564-3550

Maine
Human Rights Commission
State House
Station No. 51
Augusta 04333
(207) 289-2326

Maryland
Commission on Human Relations
20 E. Franklin Street
Baltimore 21202
(301) 333-1700

514 Race Street
Cambridge 21613
(301) 228-0112

Professional Arts Building, Room 305
5 Public Square
Hagerstown 21740
(301) 791-4011

Massachusetts
Commission Against Discrimination
McCormack State Office Building
1 Ashburton Place, Room 601
Boston 02108
(617) 727-3990

145 State Street
Springfield 01103
(413) 739-2145

53 N. 6th Street, Room 203
New Bedford 02740
(508) 997-3191

22 Front Street
P.O. Box 8008
Worcester 01614
(508) 752-2272

Michigan
Department of Civil Rights
303 W. Kalamazoo
Lansing 48913
(517) 334-6079

Department of Civil Rights
Michigan Plaza Building
1200 Sixth Avenue
Detroit 48226
(313) 256-2663

District Offices:
221 East Roosevelt
Battle Creek 49014
(616) 964-7193

Grand Rapids State Office Building
350 Ottawa Street, N.W.
Grand Rapids 49503
(616) 456-7543

Town Center Building, 2d Floor
333 S. Capital Avenue
Lansing 48913
(517) 771-1701

State Office Building
411 East Genesee
Saginaw 48605
(517) 235-4655

242 Pipestone
Benton Harbor 49022
(616) 925-7044

State Office Building
125 E. Union Street
Flint 48502
(313) 235-4655

State Office Building
301 E. Louis B. Glick Highway
Jackson 49201
(517) 788-9550

2542 Peck
Muskegon Heights 49444
(616) 739-7168

Pontiac State Bank Building
28 N. Saginaw, 10th Floor
Pontiac 48058
(313) 334-1517

L'Anse-Baraga
Upper Peninsula
HCO 1, Box 281
U.S. 41 Arnheim
Pelkie 49958
(906) 353-7153

Minnesota
Department of Human Rights
500 Bremer Building
7th & Robert Street
St. Paul 55101
(612) 296-5663

Missouri
Commission on Human Rights
315 Ellis Boulevard
P.O. Box 1129
Jefferson City 65102
(314) 751-3325

Regional Offices:
625 N. Euclid, Suite 605
St. Louis 63108
(314) 444-7590

1601 E. 18th Street
Suites 320 and 340
Kansas City 64108
(816) 472-2491

526 D South Main
Sikeston 63801
(314) 471-7185

P.O. Box 1124
Jefferson City 65102
(314) 751-3325

Montana
Human Rights Commission
1327 Lockey
Helena 59601
(406) 444-2884

Nebraska
Nebraska Equal Opportunity
Commission
P.O. Box 94934
301 Centennial Mall, South
State Office Building, 5th Floor
Lincoln 68509
(402) 471-2024

Branch Offices:
1313 Farnam Street
Omaha 68102
(402) 595-2028

4500 Avenue I
Box 1500
Scottsbluff 69363
(308) 632-1340

Lincoln Commission on Human Rights
129 N. 10th Street, Room 323
Lincoln 68508
(402) 471-7624

Omaha Human Relations Department
1819 Farnam Street, Suite 502
Omaha 68102
(402) 444-5085

Nevada
Equal Rights Commission
1515 E. Tropicana Avenue, Suite 590
Las Vegas 89158
(702) 486-7161

2450 Wrondel Way, Suite C
Sparks 89502
(702) 789-0288

New Hampshire
Commission for Human Rights
163 Louden Road
Concord 03301
(603) 271-2767

New Jersey
Division on Civil Rights
Department of Law & Public Safety
Headquarters Office
1100 Raymond Boulevard, Room 400
Newark 07102
(201) 648-2700

Branch Offices:
383 W. State Street
Trenton 08608
(609) 292-4605

130 Broadway
Camden 08102
(609) 757-2850

370 Broadway
Paterson 07501
(201) 345-1465

New Mexico
Human Rights Commission
1596 Pacheco
Santa Fe 87501
(505) 827-6838

New York
State Division of Human Rights
55 West 125th Street
New York City 10027
(212) 870-8400

Branch Offices:
Alfred E. Smith State Office Building
25th Floor
Albany 12225
(518) 474-2705

State Office Building Annex
164 Hawley Street
Binghamton 13901
(607) 773-7713

Borough President's Office
851 Grand Concourse, 161st Street
Bronx 10451
(212) 870-8650

1360 Fulton Street, 4th Floor
Brooklyn 11216
(718) 622-4600

65 Court Street
Buffalo 14202
(716) 847-7621

State Office Building
Veterans Memorial Highway
Hauppauge 11787
(516) 360-6434

100 Main Street, 2nd Floor
Hempstead 11550
(516) 538-1360

270 Broadway, 9th Floor
New York City 10007
(212) 587-5041

N.Y.S. Harlem Office Building
163 W. 125th Street, 2nd Floor
New York City
(212) 870-8650

Borough President's Office
120-55 Queens Boulevard
Kew Gardens 11424
(516) 538-1360

259 Monroe Avenue
Rochester 14607
(716) 238-8250

351 S. Warren Street
Syracuse 13202
(315) 428-4633

30 Glenn Street, 3d Floor
White Plains 10603
(914) 949-4394

Borough President's Office
120 Borough Hall
Staten Island 10301
(718) 622-4600

North Carolina
Human Relations Council
121 W. Jones Street
Raleigh 27603
(919) 733-7996

Public Employees:
Office of Administrative Hearings
424 N. Blount

Raleigh 27601
(919) 733-2691

North Dakota
Department of Labor
600 E. Boulevard
State Capitol—5th Floor
Bismark 58505
(701) 224-2660

Ohio
Civil Rights Commission
220 Parsons Avenue
Columbus 43266
(614) 466-2785

Branch Offices:
615 West Superior Avenue, N.W.,
Suite 885
Cleveland 44113
(215) 622-3150

Southeast Regional Office
220 Parsons Avenue
Columbus 43266
(614) 466-5928

North Southwest Regional Office
800 Miami Valley Tower
40 West Fourth Street
Dayton 45402
(513) 449-6500

Northwest Regional Office
One Government Center, Room 936
Jackson and Erie Streets
Toledo 43604
(419) 244-2900

Southwest Regional Office
200 Goodall Complex
324 West 9th Street
Cincinnati 45202
(513) 852-3344

South Northeast Regional Office
Akron Government Center, Suite 205
161 South High Street

Akron 44308
(216) 379-3100

Oklahoma
Human Rights Commission
Room 480
2101 N. Lincoln Boulevard
Oklahoma City 73105
(405) 521-2360

Oregon
Bureau of Labor and Industries
Civil Rights Division
State Office Building
1400 S.W. Fifth Avenue
Portland 97201
(503) 229-5900 or (800) 452-7813 toll-free in Oregon

Branch Offices:
165 E. 7th Street, Room 220
Eugene 97401
(503) 686-7623

3865 Wolverine Street, N.E., Building E-1
Salem 97310
(503) 378-3296

700 E. Main
Medford 97504
(503) 776-6201

700 S.E. Immigrant
Pendleton 97801
(503) 276-7884

Pennsylvania
Human Relations Commission
101 S. Second Street, Suite 300
P.O. Box 3145
Harrisburg 17105-3145
(717) 787-4410

Branch Offices:
State Office Building, 11th Floor
300 Liberty Avenue
Pittsburgh 15222
(412) 565-5395

711 State Office Building
1400 Spring Garden Street
Philadelphia 19130
(215) 560-2496

2971 East N. 7th Street
Harrisburg 17110
(717) 787-9784

Puerto Rico
Department of Labor and Human Resources
Anti-Discrimination Unit
505 Munoz Rivera Avenue
Hato Rey 00918
(809) 754-5353

Rhode Island
Commission for Human Rights
10 Abbott Park Place
Providence 02903
(401) 277-2661

South Carolina
Human Affairs Commission
2611 Forest Drive
P.O. Box 4490
Columbia 29240
(803) 737-6570

South Dakota
Division on Human Rights
State Capitol Building
222 E. Capitol,
Suite 11
Pierre 57501
(605) 773-4493

Tennessee
Human Development Commission
Capitol Boulevard Building, Suite 602
226 Capitol Boulevard

Nashville 37219
(615) 741-2424

Field Offices:
170 N. Main Street, Room 1113
Memphis 38103
(901) 543-7389

540 McCallie Avenue
6th Floor West, Room 605
Chattanooga 37402
(615) 755-6222

Texas
Commission on Human Rights
P.O. Box 13493
Capitol Station
Austin 78711
(512) 837-8534

Austin Human Relations Commission
P.O. Box 1088
Austin 78767
(512) 499-3251

Corpus Christi Human Relations Commission
1201 Leopard
Corpus Christi 78408
(512) 880-3190

Fort Worth Human Relations Commission
600 Texas Street
Fort Worth 76102
(817) 870-7525

Utah
Industrial Commission
Anti-Discrimination Division
160 E. 3rd Street South
P.O. Box 510910
Salt Lake City 84151
(801) 530-6801

Vermont
Human Rights Commission
P.O. Box 997

Montpelier 05601
(802) 828-2480

Virginia
Dept. of Labor and Industry
P.O. Box 12064
Richmond 23241
(804) 786-2376

Alexandria Human Rights Office
2525 Mt. Vernon Avenue
Unit 11
Alexandria 22313
(703) 838-0890

Fairfax County Human Rights Commission
4085 Chain Bridge Road
Equity Building, Suite 300
Fairfax 22030
(703) 246-2953

Virgin Islands
Department of Labor
P.O. Box 3159 53A, 54A & B
Kronprindfens Gode
Charlotte, Amalie
St. Thomas 00801
(809) 776-3700

Washington
Washington State Human Rights Commission
402 Evergreen Plaza Building
711 South Capitol Way
Mail Stop FJ-41
Olympia 98504
(206) 753-6770

Branch Offices:
Columbia Building, Suite 400
1516 Second Avenue
4th Floor
Seattle 98101
(206) 464-6500

W. 905 Riverside Avenue, Suite 416
Spokane 99201
(509) 455-4473

32 N. 3rd Street, Suite 441
Yakima 98901
(509) 575-2772

West Virginia
Human Rights Commission
1036 Quarrier Street
215 Professional Building
Charleston 25301
(304) 348-2616

Wisconsin
Department of Industry, Labor and Human Relations
Equal Rights & Labor Standards
201 E. Washington Avenue
P.O. Box 8928
Madison 53708
(608) 266-6860

Branch Offices:
819 N. Sixth Street, Room 255
Milwaukee 53203
(414) 224-4384

1478 Kenwood Center
Midway Road
Menasha 54952
(414) 497-4170

718 W. Clairemont Avenue
Eau Claire 54701
(715) 836-5135

1328 Schofield Avenue
Schofield 54476
(715) 359-8157

Wyoming
Fair Employment Commission
Herschler Building, 2d Floor, E. Wing
Cheyenne 82002
(307) 777-7261

Commission of Labor & Statistics
Herschler Building, 2d Floor, E. Wing
Cheyenne 82002
(307) 777-7261

135 N. Ash Street, Room 180
P.O. Box 1134
Casper 82602
(307) 234-8650

Medical-Records Assistance

American Medical Record Association
Communications Director
875 North Michigan Avenue, Suite 1850
Chicago, IL 60611
(312) 787-2672

The office of the Communications Director of this association of medical-records personnel can answer questions about access to medical records from medical professionals.

Freedom of Information Clearinghouse
Public Citizen
2000 P Street, N.W.
Washington, DC 20036
(202) 293-9142

This is a project of Public Citizen, a consumer-rights group founded by Ralph Nader. It helps former patients obtain medical records from federal and state agencies under the Freedom of Information Act and other laws.

Sources of Financial Assistance

American Cancer Society
(800) ACS-2345

Many units have loan closets and transportation services that supply sickroom equipment, such as wheelchairs, walkers, and surgical dressings, as well as transportation to and from treatment. Contact your local American Cancer Society unit. If you are unable to locate an American Cancer Society unit in your area, call their national toll-free phone number for information.

National Association of Meal Programs
204 E Street, N.W.
Washington, DC 20002
(202) 547-6157

This office provides information about meal programs (Meals on Wheels, etc.) in your community. Such programs, which provide at least one hot meal a day to individuals who are housebound, may be run by private agencies; local departments of health, public welfare, or aging; church groups; or community volunteer organizations. Other Meals-on-Wheels programs may be listed in your telephone directory under "Meals-on-Wheels."

National Foundation for Consumer Credit, Inc.
8701 Georgia Avenue
Silver Spring, MD 20901
(301) 589-5600

This foundation provides referrals to local credit counseling services. NFCC is a nonprofit umbrella membership organization of more than 400 nonprofit consumer-credit counseling services that provides confidential financial counseling for people having trouble managing their bills. No one is turned away because of inability to pay.

Ronald McDonald House

Ronald McDonald houses provide low-cost lodging near many cancer-treatment centers for young cancer survivors and their families in over 120 locations in the United States and Canada. Each house is locally owned by a nonprofit organization. Rooms are provided only by referrals from your hospital staff.

Social Security Administration
(800) 234-5772

This national toll-free hotline answers your questions about available benefits.

Pharmaceutical Companies' Patient Assistance Programs

In addition to the above organizations, some pharmaceutical companies have limited programs that provide indigent patients with free medications. The following major manufacturers of oncology drugs have patient-assistance programs. Ask your physician to notify the appropriate company if you are unable to pay for your medication yourself.

Adria Laboratories, Inc.
Patient-Assistance Program
P.O. Box 16529
Columbus, OH 43216-6529
(614) 764-8100

Bristol Myers Mead Johnson
Pharmaceuticals
2400 Lloyd Expressway
Evansville, IN 47721
(812) 429-5595

ICI Pharmaceuticals
(formerly Stuart Pharmaceuticals)
Professional Services
Wilmington, DE 19897
(800) 456-5678

Lederle Laboratories
Professional Medical Services
Building 100, Third Floor
North Middletown Road
Pearl River, NY 19065
(914) 732-2133

Eli Lilly and Company
Lilly Corporate Center
Department MC492
Building 74-6

Indianapolis, IN 46285
(317) 276-2950

Merck, Sharpe & Dohme
West Point, PA 19486
(215) 661-6369

Miles, Inc., Pharmaceutical Division
Sales Services
400 Morgan Lane
West Haven, CT 06516
(203) 937-2376

Roche Laboratories
Professional Services Department
Indigent Patient Program
Nutley, NJ 07110-9988
(201) 235-3071

(For any Roche drug given to a private indigent patient out of hospital and receiving no third-party payment.)

Roche Laboratories
Cost Assistance Program
1800 Robert Fulton Drive
Reston, VA 22091-4346
(800) 227-7448

For patients on interferon (Roferon-A).

Legal Resources for the Latter Stages of Life

National Academy of Elder Law Attorneys
655 Alvernon, Suite 108
Tucson, AZ 85711
(602) 881-4005

This organization provides information about how to identify and select an elder law attorney (lawyer experienced in dealing with elderly clients and their families as well as the special areas of law that affect the elderly). Prefers written inquiries with a stamped, self-addressed envelope for replies.

Society for the Right to Die
250 West 57th Street
New York, NY 10107
(212) 246-6973

The Society for the Right to Die provides information about living-will laws. It is a not-for-profit organization working for recognition of an individual's right to die with dignity.

Appendix B

Common Cancers

You may be surprised to learn that, although cancer affects all age groups, it is primarily a disease of the elderly. The majority of cancers occur in persons older than 65 years of age. The four major kinds of cancers that occur in adults orginate in the breast, lung, large bowel (colon and rectum), and prostate. Other, less frequent types of cancer arise from the blood-forming organs (hematologic malignancies), the genitourinary tract (kidneys, bladder, and testes), female organs (uterus, ovaries, and cervix), other sites within the gastrointestinal tract (stomach, esophagus, pancreas, and liver), as well as in the head and neck (mouth, tongue, throat), brain, skin, and soft tissues.

Breast Cancer

Breast cancer is the most frequently occurring cancer in women. One out of ten American women will develop breast cancer during her lifetime. Breast cancer may occur (though rarely) in men as well. The specific causes of breast cancer in each individual are usually unknown, although hereditary factors, diet, and menstrual and pregnancy history all play some role in the development of this cancer. Usually, breast cancer is discovered by the woman herself, who finds a lump or a thickening in the breast tissue.

The majority of lumps women find are benign growths (are not cancers), but the only way to tell for certain is to remove a small amount of tissue from the lump and send it to the laboratory for examination. This can be done by needle aspiration or by surgical biopsy. Aspiration involves insertion of a very small needle into the lump, followed by suction of cells from the lump into a syringe. The cells are spread on a microscope slide and are examined by a pathologist. If a surgical biopsy is performed, a small amount of local anesthetic is injected into the tissues around the lump. The surgeon makes an incision in the skin, removes the lump, and sends it to the laboratory for microscopic examination. Both procedures can be performed in the doctor's office or a hospital outpatient unit.

Small cancers in the breast are often detected on a screening mammogram before they can be felt by the woman or her physician. These small cancers are usually described as an abnormal shadow or a calcium deposition. If a suspicious abnormality is found on the screening mammogram, a biopsy is recommended. If the shadow is not palpable, the biopsy must be performed using X-ray guidance.

Scientific studies during the past two decades have demonstrated that routine-screening mammography to detect breast cancer *before* it can be felt can improve survival rates. The American Cancer Society, the American College of Radiology, and the National Cancer Institute currently recommend that all women have a baseline mammogram performed between the ages of 35 and 40, and subsequent mammograms every one or two years between the ages of 40 and 50. After age 50, mammograms should be done annually. Many insurance companies pay for the cost of a screening mammography; some are required to do so by state law (see table on p. 202).

Once breast cancer is diagnosed as a result of clinical symptoms or through screening mammography, a treatment plan must be designed. Fortunately, most breast cancers found in women today are small and do not involve the entire breast or adjacent tissues. For this reason, women are usually given the choice of two different options for local treatment of the cancer.

One type of treatment is called a "modified radical mastectomy," which means that the surgeon removes all of the breast tissue from the involved breast and some lymph glands from under the armpit. This procedure removes all of the cancer that might be in the breast or in the lymph glands, and because all of the breast tissue is removed, there is only a small chance that the cancer might come back in the same area.

In another type of treatment, often referred to as "segmental mastectomy," "lumpectomy," "quadrantectomy," or "breast conservation surgery," only the portion of the breast grossly containing the cancer with a small margin of cancer-free tissue is removed, along with some lymph glands from under the armpit. Breast conservation surgery is almost always followed by radiation treatment to the remaining breast tissue in order to eliminate any microscopic cancer cells that may persist. The radiation treatments usually take five to six weeks to complete. After such surgery, the remaining breast tissue must be carefully checked through physical examination and mammography for the possibility of recurrent or new cancers. Scientific studies have shown that, for most women with breast cancer, both approaches (mastectomy or lumpectomy) to local treatment have the same survival rates. For women trying to decide between these two treatment approaches, it is often helpful to see both a surgeon and a radiation oncologist before making a decision. A woman's choice of treatment is often a difficult and personal decision that should be respected.

Following local surgical treatment, most women will receive some form of adjuvant therapy, additional treatment given to prevent the cancer from returning. The type of recommended treatment depends on whether the woman has gone through menopause, whether there was any cancer found in the lymph glands at the time of surgery, and the biologic characteristics of the cancer. Some women will receive chemotherapy, some will receive hormone treatment, and some may receive a combination of these treatments (see p. 15). Adjuvant therapy of breast cancer is actively being studied by international researchers, and their treatment recommendations are often in flux. Therefore, it is best to discuss your own unique medical situation with your doctor.

Lung Cancer

Lung cancer is the most common cancer in men and is becoming increasingly common in women. The vast majority of lung cancers are caused by smoking, and the risk of lung cancer increases directly in relation to the number of years someone smokes and the number of cigarettes smoked each day. Unlike breast cancer, lung cancer is usually discovered when the cancer has grown to a very large size in the lung or has spread outside the lung to a distant part of the body. Under these circumstances, the first symptom from lung cancer might occur in the bones, the liver, or the brain. Local symptoms from lung cancer include an unremitting cough, chest pain, shortness of breath, and coughing up blood.

The treatment plan for lung cancer depends on the specific cell type and whether the lung cancer has metastasized. If the cancer appears to be limited to the lung, then the surgeon must determine whether or not the cancer can be successfully removed by surgery. The two main types of lung cancer are small-cell cancer and non-small-cell cancer. Surgery is rarely used to treat small-cell lung cancer, even if the cancer seems to be localized to the lung. Chemotherapy and radiation treatments are successfully used to treat the majority of small-cell lung cancer patients. In contrast, surgery is the most effective form of treatment used for non-small-cell lung cancer, but surgery can only be considered if the cancer is confined to the lung. If the surgeon can successfully remove all or part of the cancerous lung, the cure rate is relatively high. Unfortunately, only a minority of persons with non-small-cell lung cancer can be helped by surgical treatment. The remainder, who have more extensive disease, are treated with radiation or chemotherapy, both of which may alleviate symptoms but rarely offer a cure.

Colon and Rectal Cancer

Cancers of the colon and rectum occur with equal frequency in men and women. These cancers are usually discovered because of a change in bowel habits (constipation, narrower stools, diarrhea), blood in the stool, abdominal pain, pain on having a bowel movement, or generalized weakness resulting from anemia (a low blood count resulting from loss of blood in the stool). Sometimes these cancers are found on a routine checkup during a rectal examination (the doctor examines the rectum with a gloved finger) or a sigmoidoscopic examination (visual inspection of the rectum and lower colon by a tubular instrument). In addition, a stool examination to test for microscopic evidence of bleeding is useful in the early detection of colorectal cancer. If blood is present, additional examinations will be necessary to find the source of bleeding and make sure it is not from a cancer. Cancers of the colon and rectum that are found when the individual has no symptoms are usually smaller, have not spread outside the bowel, and have an excellent chance of cure with surgery. In contrast, persons who have had prolonged or severe symptoms may have cancers that cannot be removed with surgery or that have spread outside the bowel wall to distant parts of the body. Thus, everyone should report any new bowel symptoms to the doctor for further investigation and should have regular checkups to look for colorectal cancer even when no symptoms are present.

Prostate Cancer

Each year, approximately 100,000 men are diagnosed with prostate cancer in the United States—nearly as many as those men found to have lung cancer. Prostate cancer is very common in elderly men. The prostate is a gland that is located at the base of the bladder in males. The size and consistency of the gland are easily evaluated by the physician by performing a rectal examination. If the examination reveals unusual firmness or focal swelling in the gland, a biopsy will be recommended. More often, prostate cancer is discovered because its local growth has caused urinary-tract symptoms (increasing difficulty passing urine or the complete inability to urinate, blood in the urine, need to urinate often) or symptoms from more distant spread of the disease, especially to the bones.

Only a few men with newly diagnosed prostate cancer have disease that is localized to the prostate gland. For those men, radiation therapy or surgical treatment is usually offered, and there is a good chance of cure with either treatment. As with breast cancer, radiation and surgery for prostate cancer have equivalent survival rates, but have different short- and long-term side effects. Therefore, it is important for the patient to consult with a urologist (a surgeon who specializes in treatment of the genitourinary tract) and a radiation therapist before making a treatment decision.

Most prostate cancers cannot continue to grow without the assistance of the male hormone testosterone. Prostate cancers that have spread outside the gland are usually treated with hormonal therapies aimed at reducing the amount of male hormones. There are several commonly used treatment approaches, which include removal of the primary source of male hormones (the testicles), the administration of female hormones, and giving other hormones that either suppress the production of male hormones in the testes or restrain the growth-promoting activities of male hormones within the cancer. All of these approaches have roughly the same likelihood of helping, but have different side effects, which should be discussed with the doctor when a treatment plan is being developed. Hormonal treatments, as well as radiation treatment, are usually very effective in slowing the growth of prostate cancer and alleviating pain, which is very common. Control of pain is a major problem for most patients with advanced prostate cancer and should be factored into the treatment plan.

Hematologic Cancers

Hematologic malignancies are cancers of the blood, blood-forming tissue (bone marrow), and the lymph-gland system. They affect a wide age range of adults and may vary from relatively slow-growing to rapidly fatal. Cancers of the blood include acute and chronic leukemia, lymphomas, and multiple myeloma.

Acute leukemia may occur at any age and is rapidly fatal if left untreated. Acute lymphocytic leukemia (ALL) is primarily a childhood cancer, but also occurs in young adults and older individuals. Acute nonlymphocytic leukemia (of which there are five or six subtypes) is primarily an adult cancer with an even distribution in all age groups. Acute-leukemia survivors may experience fatigue, easy bruising or bleeding, bone pain, and/or infections. These symptoms are the result of billions of cancerous white cells rapidly accumulating in the bone-marrow spaces and crowding out the normal cells that form red blood cells (which deliver oxygen to all tissues), white blood cells (which circulate in the bloodstream and fight infectious invaders), and platelets (tiny particles in the blood which plug up holes from cuts and bruises and initiate clotting). The cancerous white cells spill out of the bone marrow and enter the bloodstream, usually in large numbers, so that a simple blood test will often show an elevated white cell count, which is suspicious for a diagnosis of acute leukemia. A definitive diagnosis is usually made by removing and studying a bone-marrow sample.

A diagnosis of acute leukemia usually requires prompt hospitalization to start treatment with chemotherapy. Fever and acute infections must be treated immediately with antibiotics, because the patient has an inadequate number of healthy white cells to fight off the infection. Transfusions of red cells and platelets are often given as well. The specific choice of chemotherapy treatment depends on the type of acute leukemia, but in general the treatment is very intensive, with several weeks of hospitalization and a risk of death from infection or bleeding. The chemotherapy treatment affects both the cancerous white cells and the normal bone-marrow cells; however, the cancerous cells are more susceptible. This type of treatment means that the person will have low blood counts for several weeks after the treatment, and will not be discharged from the hospital until there are signs that the blood counts are returning to normal. Additional bone-marrow examinations will be necessary to make sure that the leukemic cells have been eliminated from the bone marrow.

Chronic leukemias grow more slowly than do acute leukemias. They are primarily diseases of older adults, though they may also be diagnosed in younger individuals. The three major types of chronic leukemias are chronic lymphocytic leukemia (CLL), chronic myelogenous leukemia (CML), and hairy-cell leukemia (HCL). As with the acute leukemias, the malignant white cells accumulate in the bone marrow and spill out into the bloodstream. In chronic leukemias, however, the pace at which this occurs is much slower, often developing over many years. Many individuals have no symptoms at the time of diagnosis. Often, the chronic leukemia is discovered during routine blood testing or because an enlarged spleen or lymph glands are found at the time of a regular physical examination. Just as with the acute leukemias, however, these individuals may have symptoms (infections, bleeding, fatigue) that will lead to a doctor visit.

Survivors can live with chronic leukemias for many years, but are rarely cured. Chemotherapy (for CLL, CML), interferon (for HCL, CML), and removal of the spleen (for HCL) are highly effective in controlling chronic leukemias. Bone-marrow transplantation is being explored as a potentially curative treatment in younger individuals with CML (see p. 16 for a discussion on bone-marrow transplantation).

Cancers of the lymph glands are called "lymphomas," and are generally divided into the Hodgkin's and non-Hodgkin's types. Hodgkin's lymphoma spreads from one lymph-node group to a neighboring one, rarely involving the bone marrow or sites outside the lymph-gland system. For this reason, elaborate staging procedures to determine exactly where the cancer is in the body are performed to determine the most effective treatment. Hodgkin's disease is highly curable using either radiation, chemotherapy, or a combination of treatments. The choice of specific treatment depends on the unique characteristics of the disease in the individual patient.

Non-Hodgkin's lymphomas have a high rate of bone-marrow involvement and can affect other organs in the body such as the tissues of the gastrointestinal tract, the bones, the breasts, and the head and neck. Some non-Hodgkin's lymphomas are extremely slow-growing, and are highly responsive to chemotherapy and radiation, but are very difficult to cure. Others grow rapidly and respond well to chemotherapy and radiation treatments, which often lead to a cure. Staging is a very important diagnostic procedure, because treatment choice depends on the exact cell type of non-Hodgkin's lymphoma.

Multiple myeloma is a form of bone-marrow cancer in which abnormal cells (plasma cells) accumulate in the bone marrow and gradually replace the other, normal bone-marrow cells, leading to a lowering of all the blood counts. These bone-marrow invaders gradually soften the bones, so that patients often develop bone pain and fractures. Other effects include increased risk of infection, excess levels of calcium in the blood, kidney problems, and abnormal proteins in the blood, which can lead to still other problems. Multiple myeloma responds very well to chemotherapy, and radiation is used to heal fractures or treat painful bony areas. This is largely a disease of older persons, for which treatment provides good symptomatic relief and longer life.

Genitourinary Cancers

Cancers of the genitourinary tract may arise anywhere in the kidneys, ureters (drainage system from the kidney to bladder), bladder, or testes. A number of environmental substances have been found to cause cancer in the lining system of the urinary tract, and smokers have a higher rate of developing bladder cancer. With the exception of testicular cancer, most cancers of the genitourinary system occur in older individuals.

The primary treatment for cancers of the kidney, ureter, and bladder is surgery, although both chemotherapy and radiation treatments are used as well. The type of treatment depends on how large the cancer is at diagnosis and whether it has spread. In contrast, testicular cancers, which are highly curable, are primarily treated with chemotherapy or radiation, after removal of the testicle to determine what type of cancer is present. Surgery is often performed to evaluate the extent of the cancer in the back of the abdomen. Because these cancers often travel to distant parts of the body, chemotherapy plays a major role in their treatment.

Gynecologic Cancers

Gynecologic cancers involve the cervix, uterus, and ovaries. Cervical cancer is primarily a disease of younger women, which can be easily diagnosed through Pap-smear examinations (cells from the cervix are spread on a glass slide and examined under the microscope) or by direct examination and biopsy of the cervix done in the gynecologist's office. The risk of cervical cancer is related to a number of behaviors, including early sexual intercourse with multiple partners and certain virus-caused genital infections associated with sexual intercourse. Fortunately, this cancer is detectable at an early stage by regular pelvic and Pap-smear examinations. With early detection and prompt treatment, few women should die from cervical cancer. Unfortunately, many high-risk women do not regularly obtain the screening examinations necessary to detect cervical cancer at an early stage.

Cancer of the uterine lining (endometrial cancer) usually occurs in older women, after menopause. The Pap-smear examination is not particularly useful in diagnosis, because the uterine-lining cells are infrequently found in the cervical smear. Usually, endometrial cancer is diagnosed because the woman has some abnormal uterine bleeding after regular menstruation has stopped. The doctor will usually perform a uterine examination under anesthesia, at which time samples of the endometrium are removed and sent to the laboratory for microscopic examination. If cancer is found in the sample, then surgical removal of the uterus is performed (hysterectomy), and the full extent of the cancer can be determined. The survival rate for most women with uterine cancer is excellent, because most such cancers are limited to the uterus and are cured with surgery alone.

Cancer of the ovaries usually occurs in women after menopause, although some rarer forms occur in young women. Ovarian cancers are difficult to detect when they are small and localized to the ovary. For this reason, ovarian cancer is usually diagnosed at an advanced stage, when the cancer cells have spread from the ovary to the lining surface of the abdomen. It is the most common cause of death from gynecologic cancers.

Most women with ovarian cancer will complain of vague abdominal symptoms (pain, bloating, gas, constipation, abdominal swelling) that increase over several months. At the time of detection, the surgeon often has difficulty removing all of the ovarian cancer from the abdomen, although an attempt is made to remove as much as possible. After surgery, most women receive chemotherapy, and some receive radiation treatments. The treatment plan is determined by the type of cancer and the extent of the disease. A newer approach to treatment (intraperitoneal therapy) involves placing drugs directly into the abdominal cavity through a soft catheter (tube). After several months of treatment for ovarian cancer, many women will be asked to consider some form of repeat examination of the abdominal cavity (second-look laparotomy) to see if all the cancer has disappeared.

Gastrointestinal Cancer

Cancers also occur in the digestive system or along the lining of the gastrointestinal tract (for example, pancreas, liver, stomach, esophagus, small intestine). The best chance of cure rests with surgery, because most of these cancers are not very effectively treated with chemotherapy or radiation. Unfortunately, a number of gastrointestinal cancers are diagnosed at an advanced stage, when surgery cannot completely remove the cancer. Under these circumstances, chemotherapy and radiation are often used to alleviate symptoms.

Head and Neck Cancer

Cancers of the head and neck involve the lining surfaces of the mouth, nose, sinuses, and throat, and the many glands that contribute to the production of saliva. With the exception of salivary-gland cancer, head and neck cancers are caused by tobacco use, and may be made worse by heavy alcohol consumption. Tobacco and alcohol are toxic to the lining membranes of the head and neck, and after many years precancerous and cancerous sores can arise in these areas.

Small and localized cancers of the head and neck have a good chance of cure with surgery or radiation. Cancers that have spread beyond the original site within the head and neck into draining lymph nodes have a poorer rate of cure. Chemotherapy to treat head and neck cancers is currently being evaluated.

Brain and Nervous-System Cancer

Cancers of the brain and nervous system are quite rare. They may occur at any age, but most are found in older adults. The mainstay of treatment is surgery, if the cancer is in an area of the brain or nervous system that is accessible and can be removed without serious side effects. Because many of these cancers cannot be surgically removed, radiation and drugs that decrease swelling (steroids) around the cancer are very commonly used. Chemotherapy has been tried in these cancers, but has demonstrated only modest benefit.

Skin Cancer

Skin cancers (squamous-cell and basal-cell) are the most common cancers. They are not generally included in discussions of other cancers, because they are almost always diagnosed early and rarely invade distant body parts. Skin cancers are caused by long-term sun exposure, especially in light-skinned, blue-eyed, and fair-haired individuals. Any nonhealing skin sore should be called to your doctor's attention, because it may represent an early skin cancer.

Melanoma, a rare but increasingly common form of skin cancer, is also related to sun exposure. Unlike the other forms of skin cancer, melanoma often spreads to other parts of the body and can be fatal. Melanomas are usually black or dark skin lesions that can occur on any part of the body. The risk of spread depends on how large it is and how deeply it has invaded the underlying tissues. Surgical removal of the melanoma is the major form of treatment. For melanomas that have spread to other parts of the body, chemotherapy and various immunologic therapies have been used.

Bone Cancer

A rare group of cancers (sarcomas) arise in the bones and connective tissues. Many sarcomas occur in children and young adults, but some are also found in adults. They can occur in any part of the body. Successful treatment depends on whether they are accessible and can be surgically removed. Some sarcomas are extremely slow-growing and tend to come back in the place where they originated, even after complete surgical removal. Additional operations may be needed. Other, faster-growing sarcomas spread through the bloodstream to distant parts of the body. These sarcomas are often treated with chemotherapy in addition to surgery. Because sarcomas are quite rare, treatment is best provided in a specialized cancer-treatment center.

Childhood Cancers

Cancer is the second most common cause of death (after accidents) in children. Much of the progress that has been made in cancer treatment during the past two decades has been accomplished in the treatment of childhood cancers. In part, this is because childhood cancers usually grow rapidly, and therefore respond well to chemotherapy and radiation. Additionally, physicians and researchers caring for children with cancer have worked cooperatively, so that most newly diagnosed children with cancer have been treated on research protocols. Consequently, the clinical treatment of some relatively rare cancers has progressed very rapidly. Overall childhood-cancer cure rates are much higher than cure rates for adults. Of the 6,600 children diagnosed with cancer in 1989, more than 60 percent can expect to be cured.

Hematologic malignancies, especially acute lymphocytic leukemia, are the most common cancers affecting children. Other common childhood cancers are neuroblastoma (cancer of the central nervous system that usually appears as a swelling in the abdomen), Wilms' tumor (found in the kidneys), brain tumors, osteogenic sarcoma (also called Ewing's sarcoma, a bone cancer), retinoblastoma (eye cancer), and rhabdomyosarcoma (soft-tissue cancer).

AIDS—Acquired Immunodeficiency Syndrome

Individuals infected with human immunodeficiency virus (HIV) are at high risk of developing cancer, as well as the many unusual infections that more often cause their death. The two most frequent types of cancer that occur in persons with HIV infection are non-Hodgkin's lymphomas and a rare skin and soft-tissue cancer called Kaposi's sarcoma. Both of these cancers respond to chemotherapy and radiation, but the outcome of treatment and survival is usually dominated by the other effects of AIDS, especially infections. Other unusual cancers have occurred in persons with AIDS, probably due to their weakened immune systems.

STATES WITH LAWS REQUIRING PHYSICIANS TO INFORM BREAST-CANCER PATIENTS ABOUT TREATMENT OPTIONS

Compiled with the assistance of the National Alliance of Breast Cancer Organizations

As of November 1989, the following states had laws that require physicians to inform breast-cancer patients about treatment options. These laws vary widely. Some require that the physician provide specific written information, while others instruct a physician how to obtain consent to breast surgery.

California	Michigan
Florida	Minnesota
Georgia	New Jersey
Hawaii	New York
Illinois	Pennsylvania
Kansas	Texas
Kentucky	Virginia
Louisiana	Wisconsin
Maine	
Maryland	
Massachusetts	

Bibliography

The listings in this bibliography do not signify our endorsement of the books, their authors, or the philosophies they espouse. The following books have been chosen from the thousands of books on cancer because they provide practical information and inspiration on coping with cancer. They represent a broad spectrum of approaches to cancer survivorship. Some may be appropriate to your personal needs. Although each book is listed under only one chapter, many books may be helpful on a variety of survivorship topics. Because cancer diagnosis, treatment, and survivorship are fields that are constantly changing, you should keep in mind the publication dates of the books you choose.

Introduction

Bayh, Marvella, with Kotz, Mary Lynn. *Marvella*. New York: Harcourt Brace Jovanovich, 1979. Cancer experience of former Senator Birch Bayh's wife.

Benjamin, Harold. *From Victim to Victor: The Wellness Community Guide to Fighting for Recovery for Cancer Patients and Their Families*. Los Angeles: Jeremy Tarcher, Inc., 1987. Approach of the California-based Wellness Community to facing cancer.

Bloch, Richard, and Bloch, Annette. *Cancer, There's Hope*. Kansas City, MO: Cancer Connection, Inc., 1981. Richard Bloch's (of H & R Block) personal story of his battle against lung cancer.

Blumberg, Rena. *Headstrong: A Story of Conquests and Celebrations . . . Living Through Chemotherapy*. New York: Crown Publishing, 1982.

Ford, Betty, and Chase, Chris. *The Times of My Life*. New York: Harper and Row, 1978. Former First Lady's account of breast-cancer experience.

Gaes, Jason. *My Book for Kids with Cansur*. Aberdeen, MD: Melius & Peterson Publishing Company, 1987. A young survivor's book for other children with cancer.

Glassman, Judith. *The Cancer Survivors: And How They Did It*. New York: Doubleday, 1983.

Hargrove, Anne. *Getting Better: Conversations with Myself and Other Friends While Healing from Breast Cancer*. Minneapolis: CompCare Publishers, 1988. Twenty-five witty vignettes of author's experience with breast cancer.

Harper, Randy, and Harper, Tom. *I Choose to Fight: Tom Harper's Courageous Victory over Cancer*. Englewood Cliffs, NJ: Prentice-Hall, 1984. Naval midshipman's fight to recover from testicular cancer, to play football, and to graduate.

Ireland, Jill. *Life Wish*. Boston: Little, Brown, 1987. Actress's experience with breast cancer.

Jaffe, Hirschel, et al. *Why Me? Why Anyone*. New York: St. Martin's Press, 1986. Experience of marathon-running rabbi with leukemia.

Kelley, Orville E. *Until Tomorrow Comes*. New York: Everest House, 1979. Story of Make Today Count founder.

Lifshitz, Leatrice H, ed. *Her Soul Beneath the Bone: Women's Poetry on Breast Cancer*. Urbana: University of Illinois Press, 1988. A collection of poems by breast-cancer survivors.

Lohmann, J. *Gathering a Life: A Journey of Recovery*. Santa Barbara, CA: John Daniel & Co., 1989. Personal experiences shared by the wife of a brain-tumor patient.

Lorde, A. *The Cancer Journals*. San Francisco: Spinsters, 1980. Notes from the diary of a black lesbian poet coping with breast cancer.

Moss, Ralph. *A Real Choice*. New York: St. Martin's Press, 1984. Novel-like stories of seven women with breast cancer who were treated by a New York breast surgeon.

Mullan, Fitzhugh. *Vital Signs: A Young Doctor's Struggle with Cancer*. New York: Farrar, Straus & Giroux, 1975. National Coalition for Cancer Survivorship president's story of facing cancer at the age of 32.

Patterson, James T. *The Dread Disease: Cancer and Modern American Culture*. Cambridge, MA: Harvard University Press, 1987. A historical, sociological, psychological, and political analysis of cancer in American culture since the 1880s.

Pepper, Curtis. *We the Victors: The Inspiring Stories of People Who Conquered Cancer and How They Did It*. New York: Doubleday, 1984. Personal stories of cancer survivors.

Photopolus, Georgia, and Photopolus, Bud. *Of Tears and Trimphs*. Chicago: Congdon and Weed, 1988. Couple reflects on wife's 20-year struggle with several cancers, including breast and brain.

Radner, Gilda. *It's Always Something*. New York: Simon and Schuster, 1989. Comedienne's story of her battle with ovarian cancer.

Rollin, Betty. *First, You Cry*. New York: Harper and Row, 1976. Personal story by news reporter who had a mastectomy.

Rosenthal, Ted. *How Could I Not Be Among You?* New York: Persea Books, 1973. A poetic and photographic account of one man's experience of dying from leukemia.

Sarton, M. *Recovering: A Journal*. New York: Norton, 1986. Personal journal recording the experience of mastectomy within the context of everyday life.

Schwerin, Doris. *Diary of Pigeon Watcher*. New York: Paragon House, 1986. Diary of postmastectomy experience.

Shook, Robert L. *Survivors: Living with Cancer*. New York: Harper and Row, 1983. Portraits of 12 people who overcame cancer.

Sontag, Susan. *Illness as Metaphor*. New York: Random House, 1977. Analysis of social attitudes toward cancer and tuberculosis.

Spingarn, Natalie Davis. *Hanging In There: Living Well on Borrowed Time*. New York: Stein and Day, 1982. Award-winning journalist's personal breast-cancer experience and suggestions for being a well-educated consumer of cancer services.

Trull, Patti. *On with My Life*. New York: Putnam, 1983. Long-term survivor of osteogenic sarcoma describes her experience with amputation, family life, school, and her work as an occupational therapist with children with cancer.

Tsongas, Paul. *Heading Home*. New York: Alfred A. Knopf, 1984. Former Senator Paul Tsongas's personal struggle with lymphoma.

1. Abolishing the Myths: The Facts About Cancer

American Cancer Society. *Questions and Answers About Pain Control*. Atlanta: American Cancer Society, 1988. Booklet for survivors and their families on causes of and solutions to pain.

Berger, Karen, and Bostwick, John. *A Woman's Decision: Breast Care, Treatment, and Reconstruction*. New York: Ballantine Books, 1984. Explanation of breast care, treatment, and reconstruction, with several personal stories.

Bloch, Richard, and Bloch, Annette. *Fighting Cancer*. Cancer Connection, Inc., 1985. Technical information about cancer and treatment resources.

Boston Women's Health Collective. *The New Our Bodies, Ourselves: A Book by and for Women*. New York: Simon and Schuster, 1984. Comprehensive information on women's health, including sexual physiology and sexuality.

Bradley, Jane, and Nass, Susan. *Nutrition of the Cancer Patient*. Dallas: NRC Publishing, 1988. Practical advice on nutritional needs of cancer patients.

Bruning, Nancy. *Coping with Chemotherapy*. New York: Ballantine Books, 1985. Describes effects of and ways to cope with chemotherapy.

Consumer Reports. *Drug Information for the Consumer*. Mount Vernon, NY: Consumers Union, 1988. Complete guide to prescription and over-the-counter drugs available to consumers in the United States and Canada.

Cox, Barbara, et al. *Living with Lung Cancer*. Gainesville: Triad Publishing, 1987. Answers practical questions about treatment and prognosis for lung cancer.

Dennerstein, Lorraine, et al. *Hysterectomy: A Book to Help You Deal with the Physical and Emotional Aspects*. Melbourne, Australia: Oxford University Press, 1982. Facts on adjusting to hysterectomy.

Fishman, Joan, and Anrod, Barbara. *Something's Got to Taste Good: The Cancer Patient's Cookbook*. New York: Signet Paperback, 1982. Includes 170 recipes selected for ease of preparation and nutrition.

Garee, Betty, ed. *Single-handed: Devices and Aids for One Handers and Sources of These Devices*. Bloomington, IL: Accent Special Publications, 1984. Reference booklet and bibliography on how to handle daily activities with one hand. Available from: Accent Special Publications, Cheever Publishing, P.O. Box 700, Bloomington, IL 61701.

Greenberger, Monroe, and Siegel, Mary-Ellen. *What Every Man Should Know About His Prostate*. New York: Walker, 1983. Answers questions about prostate cancer, surgery, and recovery.

Held, Doris, and Klosterman, Arlene. *Chris Has*

an Ostomy. Los Angeles: United Ostomy Association, 1983. Coloring book that explains ostomy care, and physical and emotional response to ostomy.

Holleb, Arthur, ed. *The American Cancer Society Cancer Book: Prevention, Detection, Diagnosis, Treatment, Rehabilitation, Cure.* New York: Doubleday, 1986. Detailed reference guide discussing prevention, detection, diagnosis, and treatment of common types of cancer.

Johnson, Jacquelyn. *Intimacy: Living as a Woman After Cancer.* Toronto: NC Press Ltd., 1987. Counselor and cancer survivor's suggestions for achieving and maintaining intimacy after cancer.

Kalter, Suzy. *Looking Up: The Complete Guide to Looking and Feeling Good for the Recovering Cancer Patient.* New York: McGraw-Hill, 1987. Advice with photos on hair care, wigs, makeup, and exercise.

Kreisler, Nancy, and Kreisler, Jack. *Catalog of Aids for the Disabled.* New York: McGraw-Hill, 1982. How to find hundreds of items to help with daily life.

Kushner, Rose. *Alternatives: New Developments in the War on Breast Cancer.* New York: Warner Books, 1986. Updated version of earlier book (*Why Me?*) describing breast-cancer treatment.

Laszlo, John. *Understanding Cancer.* New York: Harper and Row, 1987. Detailed reference guide discussing cancer prevention and treatment, and current social and political issues.

Levitt, Paul, and Guralnick, Elissa. *The Cancer Reference Book.* New York: Harper and Row, 1984. General medical information about cancer.

Macgregor, Francis Cooke. *After Plastic Surgery.* New York: Praeger, 1979. Case-history study of adaptation and adjustment to facial disfigurement and plastic surgery.

Margie, Joyce Daly, and Block, Abby. *Nutrition and the Cancer Patient.* Radnor, PA: Chilton, 1983. Practical guide to nutrition, including recipes.

Margolies, Cynthia, and McCredie, Kenneth. *Understanding Leukemia: What It Is, How It's Treated, How to Cope with It.* New York: Scribner's, 1983. Discusses causes of and treatments for leukemia, as well as suggestions for coping with the disease.

McGinn, Kerry. *Keeping Abreast: Breast Changes That Are Not Cancer.* Palo Alto: Bull Publishing Company, 1987. Description of breast changes through a woman's life and breast self-examination.

McLean, Marsha. *If You Find a Lump in Your Breast.* Palo Alto: Bull Publishing Company, 1986. Steps to take if you find a lump in your breast.

Morgan, Susanne. *Coping with a Hysterectomy.* New York: Dial Press, 1981. Suggestions for women who have undergone hysterectomy.

Morra, Marion, and Potts, Eve. *Choices: Realistic Alternatives in Cancer Treatment.* New York: Avon, 1987. Comprehensive questions and answers about cancer treatment with detailed resource lists.

Moss, R. *A Real Choice.* New York: St. Martin's Press, 1984. Choices in breast-cancer treatment.

Mullen, Barbara Dorr, and McGinn, Kerry Ann. *The Ostomy Book: Living Comfortably With Colostomies.* Palo Alto: Bull Publishing Company, 1980. Comprehensive resource for ostomates.

National Cancer Institute. *When Cancer Recurs: Meeting the Challenge Again.* Bethesda: National Institutes of Health, 1987. Booklet that addresses diagnosis, treatment, and how to cope with recurrence.

Oryx Press. *Directory of Pain Treatment Centers in the United States and Canada.* Phoenix: Oryx Press, 1989. Information about pain-treatment centers including address, telephone number, accreditation, personnel, financial coverage accepted, symptoms treated, and treatment procedures.

Rann, Patti. *Dinner Through a Straw: A Handbook for Oral Fixation.* Available from: Dinner Through a Straw, P.O. Box 5742, Cleveland, TN, 37320-5742. Practical guide to meals for people who cannot chew.

Renneker, Mark. *Understanding Cancer*, 3d ed. Palo Alto: Bull Publishing Company, 1988. Comprehensive guide to identification, treatment, prognosis, and prevention.

Rous, Stephen. *The Prostate Book.* Mount Vernon, NY: Consumers Union, 1989. A leading urologist explains all prostate disorders, their symptoms, and the latest treatments.

Schover, Leslie. *Sexuality and Cancer: For the Man Who Has Cancer, and His Partner.* Atlanta: American Cancer Society, 1988. Booklet that clearly describes impact of cancer treatment on sexuality and strategies for dealing with sexual problems.

Schover, Leslie. *Sexuality and Cancer: For the Woman Who Has Cancer, and Her Partner.* Atlanta: American Cancer Society, 1988. Booklet that clearly describes impact of cancer treatment on sexuality and strategies for dealing with sexual problems.

Seltzer, V. L. *Every Woman's Guide to Breast Cancer.* New York: Viking, 1987. Breast-cancer specialist's discussion of how the risks of developing cancer can be reduced by changing life-styles and diet.

Shipes, Ellen, and Lehr, Sally. *Sexual Counseling for Ostomates.* Springfield, IL: Charles C. Thomas, 1980. Although written for professionals, helpful guide to ostomates.

Siegel, Mary-Ellen. *The Cancer Patient's Handbook.* New York: Walker, 1986. Handbook of cancer diagnosis, treatment, and related resources.

Slayton-Mitchell, Joyce. *Winning the Chemo Battle.* New York: Norton, 1988. Personal account of chemotherapy treatment from a cancer survivor, including drug information and glossary.

Snyder, Marilyn. *Informed Decision: Understanding Breast Reconstruction.* New York: Evans, Little, Brown, 1989. Explanation of breast reconstruction.

Sobel, David, and Ferguson, Tom. *The People's Book of Medical Tests*. New York: Summit Books, 1985. Comprehensive guide to why tests are made, how to prepare for them, risks involved, and what the tests will show.

Stellman, Steven, ed. *Women and Cancer*. New York: Harrington Park Press, 1987. Essays on the medical and psychosocial consequences of cancer on women.

Tatelbaum, J. *You Don't Have to Suffer: A Handbook for Moving Beyond Life's Crisis*. New York: Harper & Row, 1990. An experienced psychotherapist discusses how to free oneself from suffering.

Walter, Carol, with Miller, Leonore. *Moving Free: A Total Program of Post Mastectomy Exercises*. New York: Bobbs-Merrill, 1981.

Weitzman, Sigmund, et al. *Confronting Breast Cancer: New Options in Detection and Treatment*. New York: Random House, 1986. Reviews partnership between patients and physicians in treating breast cancer.

Wilson, Randy. *Non-Chew Cookbook*. Glenwood Springs, CO: Wilson Publishing, 1985. Practical guidebook for people who have problems chewing or swallowing. Available from publisher: Wilson Publishing, Inc., P.O. Box 2190, Glenwood Springs, CO 81602.

2. Mind and Body: Harnessing Your Inner Resources

Anderson, Greg. *The Cancer Conqueror: An Incredible Journey to Wellness*. Dallas: Word Publishing, 1988. Lung-cancer survivor's thoughts on how to integrate body, mind, and spirit.

Benson, Herbert, and Klipper, Miriam. *The Relaxation Response*. New York: Avon, 1976. A guide to relaxation concepts and techniques.

Borysenko, Joan. *Minding the Body, Mending the Mind*. Menlo Park, CA: Addison Wesley, 1987. How to manage stress and anxiety and how to reframe life's problems into manageable situations.

Cantor, Robert. *And a Time to Live: Toward Emotional Well-Being During the Crisis of Cancer*. New York: Harper and Row, 1978. Psychotherapist's account of the emotional impact of cancer. Discusses patterns of relationships and common problems of survivors and families.

Carlson, Richard, and Shield, Benjamin, eds. *Healers on Healing*. Los Angeles: Jeremy Tarcher, 1989. Collection of essays on the art of healing.

Cousins, Norman. *Anatomy of an Illness as Perceived by the Patient*. New York: Bantam, 1981. Norman Cousins's story of forming a partnership with his doctor to combat serious illness with medicine and humor.

Cousins, Norman. *The Healing Heart: Antidotes to Panic and Helplessness*. New York: Norton, 1983. Norman Cousins's story of his participation in his recovery from a heart attack, the general principles of which are relevant to a cancer experience.

Fiore, Neil. *The Road Back to Health: Coping with the Emotional Side of Cancer*. New York: Bantam, 1984. Psychotherapist's personal experience with testicular cancer and suggestions for dealing with the psychosocial impact of cancer.

Garrison, Judith Garrett, and Shepherd, Scott. *Cancer and Hope: Charting a Survival Course*. Minneapolis: CompCare Publishers, 1989. Suggestions for surviving the emotional impact of cancer.

Graham, Jory. *In the Company of Others: Understanding the Human Needs of Cancer Patients*. New York: Harcourt Brace Jovanovich, 1987. Discussion of patients' rights, emotions, sex, and other cancer-related issues.

Green, Stephen. *Feel Good Again: Coping with the Emotions of Illness*. Mount Vernon, NY: Consumers Union, 1990. Accessible guide to the mind-body connection that shows how to adapt psychologically to illness by recognizing and acknowledging the emotional responses.

Greenberg, Mimi. *Invisible Scars: A Guide to Coping with the Emotional Impact of Breast Cancer*. New York: Walker, 1988. Practical suggestions as to how women can get involved in decisions about their treatment for breast cancer.

Jampolsky, Gerald G., and Taylor, P. *There Is a Rainbow Behind Every Dark Cloud*. Tiburon, CA: Center for Attitudinal Healing, 1978.

Johnson, Judi, and Klein, Linda. *I Can Cope: Staying Healthy with Cancer*. Minneapolis: DCI Publishing, 1988. Cofounder of I Can Cope describes how the program helps survivors learn to live well with cancer.

Jonsson Comprehensive Cancer Center. *Confronting Cancer Through Art*. Univ. of Calif., Los Angeles: Art That Heals (Jonsson Comprehensive Cancer Center), 1987. Sixty-page catalogue of art exhibit by artists who are cancer survivors. Available from: Art That Heals/UCLA, 1100 Glendon Avenue, Suite 711, Los Angeles, CA 90024.

Kellerman, Jonathan, ed. *Psychological Aspects of Childhood Cancer*. Springfield, IL: Charles C. Thomas, 1980. Nineteen articles on the psychological side effects of childhood cancer.

Koocher, Gerald, and O'Malley, John. *The Damocles Syndrome: Psychosocial Consequences of Surviving Childhood Cancer*. New York: McGraw-Hill, 1981. Assessment of intellectual functioning, social maturity, depression, anxiety, and other reactions to childhood cancer.

Kushner, Harold. *When Bad Things Happen to Good People*. New York: Avon, 1983. Discussion of guilt, blame, and other reactions by family members and cancer survivors.

LeShan, Lawrence. *You Can Fight for Your Life*. New York: M. Evans and Company, 1977. Emotional aspects of cancer treatment.

Noyes, Diane D. *Beauty and Cancer*. Los Angeles: AC Press, 1988. Practical information for improving physical appearance during chemotherapy and radiation treatments, designed to help women overcome treatment-related fear and isolation.

Ornstein, Robert, and Sobel, David. *The Healing Brain: Breakthrough Discoveries About How the Brain Keeps Us Healthy*. New York: Simon and Schuster, 1987. Discusses the central role of the brain in maintaining health.

Ritterman, Michele. *Using Hypnosis in Family Therapy*. San Francisco: Jossey Bass, 1983.

Rossman, Martin L. *Healing Yourself: A Step-by-Step Program for Better Health Through Imagery*. New York: Pocket Books, 1987. Guide to the use of imagery in improving health.

Siegel, Bernie. *Love, Medicine and Miracles*. New York: Harper and Row, 1986. Stories about self-healing from a former surgeon's experience with cancer patients and support groups.

Siegel, Bernie. *Peace, Love and Healing*. New York: Harper and Row, 1989. Sequel to *Love, Medicine and Miracles*.

Simonton, O. C.; Mathews-Simonton, S.; and Creighton, J. *Getting Well Again*. New York: Bantam Books, 1980. Encourages cancer patients to participate in recovery through medicine, visual imagery, exercise, relaxation, and psychotherapy.

Weisman, Avery. *Coping with Cancer*. New York: McGraw-Hill, 1979. Suggestions for professionals, family, and friends on how to cope with cancer.

3. The Cancer Survivor as Consumer

American Hospital Association. *American Hospital Guide to the Healthcare Field*. Chicago: American Hospital Association, annual. Lists all accredited hospitals in the United States, drug-abuse centers, ambulatory-care facilities, and long-term-care facilities. Available from the American Hospital Association (Catalogue #010089), 4444 West Ferdinand Street, Chicago, IL 60624, (800) 242-2626.

Coping Magazine, Pulse Publications (Franklin, TN: 1988). National consumer magazine that focuses on living with and beyond a cancer diagnosis. Available from: Coping Magazine, P.O. Box 41094, Nashville, TN 37204, (615) 377-3322.

Coping Magazine. *Cancer World: International Travel Guide and Glossary for Cancer Patients*. Franklin, TN: Pulse Publications, 1988. Lists international treatment centers and organizations.

Directory of Medical Specialists, Marquis Publications. Annual three-volume book that states background of medical specialists, including education, licenses, and certifications. For example, the American College of Surgeons accredits surgeons who have passed a series of written and oral tests. Board certification does not guarantee a surgeon's expertise, but it does signify his or her having met rigorous standards established by his or her peers. Available in major libraries.

Fink, John. *Third Opinion—An International Directory to Alternative Therapy Centers for the Treatment and Prevention of Cancer*. Garden City, NY: Avery Publishing Group, 1988. An uncritical listing of alternative practitioners.

Kauffman, Danette. *Surviving Cancer: A Practical Guide for Those Fighting to Win* (Revised Edition). Washington, DC: Acropolis Books, 1989. Updated practical resource guide for dealing with a cancer diagnosis.

Larschan, Edward. *The Diagnosis Is Cancer*. Palo Alto: Bull Publishing Company, 1986. Practical psychosocial and legal resource handbook.

Lerner, Michael. *Varieties of Integral Cancer Therapy—A Work in Progress on Alternative Cancer Therapies with a Primary Emphasis on Intelligent and Informed Personal Choice in the Integration of Conventional, Adjunctive and Alternative Treatment Systems*. Subjective review of selected unconventional international cancer treatments. Available from Commonweal, P.O. Box 316, Bolinas, CA 94924.

Morra, Marion, and Potts, Eve. *Triumph: Getting Back to Normal When You Have Cancer*. New York: Avon, 1990. Guide to living beyond a cancer diagnosis.

National Cancer Institute. *Facing Forward: A Guide for Cancer Survivors*. Bethesda, MD: National Institutes of Health (Publication #90-2424), 1990. Booklet of useful references and checklists for survivors' medical, emotional, and financial concerns. To obtain a copy, call 1-800-4-CANCER, or write to: Office of Cancer Communications, National Cancer Institute, Building 31, Room 10-A-24, Bethesda, MD 20892.

Nierenberg, Judith, and Janovic, Florence. *The Hospital Experience*. New York: Berkeley, 1985. Guide to understanding and participating in your hospital care.

Office of Technology Assessment of the United States Congress, *Unconventional Cancer Treatments*. Washington, DC: United States Government Printing Office, 1990. Objective descriptive review of the most popular unconventional cancer treatments used in the United States, with a discussion of related social and legal issues. Summary of report available for free or nominal charge. Available from: Office of Technology Assessment, Publications Office. U.S. Congress, Washington, DC 20510, (202) 224-8996.

Rosenbaum, Ernest, and Rosenbaum, Isadora. *A Comprehensive Guide for Cancer Patients and Their Families*. Palo Alto: Bull Publishing Company, 1980. Practical guide to common problems associated with cancer tratment.

4. Helping Therapies and Support Services

Aftel, Mandy, and Lakoff, Robin Tolmach. *When Talk Is Not Cheap, or How to Find the Right Therapist When You Don't Know How to Begin*. New York: Warner Books, 1985. Practical guidelines on choosing a psychotherapist.

Bruckner, Gordan, et al. *Making Therapy Work: Your Guide to Choosing, Using, and Ending Therapy*. New York: Harper and Row, 1988. Guide to choosing the right therapist and getting the most out of therapy.

Buckman, Robert. *I Don't Know What to Say: How to Help and Support Someone Who Is Dying*. Toronto: Key Porter Books, 1988. Suggestions on how to communicate with a friend or family member in the last stages of life.

Coleman, Barbara. *A Consumer Guide to Home Health Care*, 1985. A booklet that describes basic facts of home health care. Available from: National Consumers League, 815 15th Street, N.W., Suite 516, Washington, DC 20005, (202) 639-8140.

Coleman, Barbara. *A Consumer Guide to Hospice Care*, 1985. A booklet that describes basic facts of hospice care. Available from: National Consumers League, 815 15th Street, N.W., Suite 516, Washington, DC 20005, (202) 639-8140.

Colgrove, Melba; Bloomfield, Harold; and McWilliams, Peter. *How to Survive the Loss of a Love*. New York: Bantam, 1976. Practical suggestions for coping with loss.

Donnelly, Katherine. *Recovering from the Loss of a Child*. New York: Macmillan, 1982. Experiences of families, assuring readers that feelings of shock, anger, guilt, and helplessness are normal; includes resource guide.

Friedman, Jo-Ann. *Home Health Care: A Complete Guide for Patients and Their Families*. New York: Norton, 1986. Comprehensive resource guide for managing postsurgical recovery and daily complications of living with a chronic illness.

Golden, Susan. *Nursing a Loved One at Home: A Caregiver's Guide*. Philadelphia: Running Press, 1988. A practical guide to home care.

Jones, Monica Loose. *Home Care for the Chronically Ill or Disabled Child: A Manual and Sourcebook for Parents and Professionals*. New York: Harper and Row, 1985. Resource manual for addressing home-health-care needs of children.

Kennedy, Patricia. *Dying at Home with Cancer*. Springfield, IL: Charles C. Thomas, 1982.

Kübler-Ross, Elisabeth. *On Death and Dying*. New York: Macmillan, 1969. Psychiatrist tells her patients' stories of facing death and the emotional stages through which they pass.

Kübler-Ross, Elisabeth. *Questions and Answers on Death and Dying*. New York: Macmillan, 1974. Psychiatrist's answers to the most common questions posed in over 700 workshops she has conducted.

Moldow, D. Gay, and Martinson, Ida. *Home Care for the Seriously Ill Child: A Manual for Parents*. Alexandria: Children's Hospice International, 1984. Helps parents explore prospect of providing home care for dying child, providing practical resources. Available from: CHI, 1101 King Street, Suite 131, Alexandria, VA 22314.

Munley, Anne. *The Hospice Alternative: A New Context for Death and Dying*. New York: Basic Books, 1983. Description of daily world of patients, care givers, families, plus resources.

Nassif, Janet Zhun. *The Home Health Care Solution: A Complete Consumer Guide*. New York: Harper and Row, 1985. Step-by-step guidelines on using home-health-care services, plus resource guide.

Temes, Roberta. *Living with an Empty Chair: A Guide Through Grief*. New York: Irvington Publishers, 1984. Practical advice about the grieving process.

5. Survivors Helping Survivors: Peer-Support Networking

Clarke, Jean I. *Who, Me Lead a Group*. New York: Harper and Row, 1984.

Clyne, Rachael. *Coping with Cancer: Making Sense of It All*. Wellingsborough, England: Thorsons, 1986. Practical suggestions from a young adult who began a support group after her husband and sister were diagnosed with cancer. Lists support-group resources in Great Britain.

Cordoba, Catherine, et al. *Cancer Support Groups: Practice Handbook*. Oakland: American Cancer Society, California Division, 1984. Advice on creating a cancer-support group.

Dass, Ram, and Gorman, Paul. *How Can I Help: Stories and Reflections on Service.* New York: Alfred A. Knopf, 1985. Provides practical wisdom on how much one has to offer others by being oneself.

Directory of National Self-Help and Mutual Aid Resources. Lists of national self-help groups, clearinghouses, and toll-free phone numbers assembled by the American Hospital Association and the Illinois Self-Help Center. Available from: Hospital Research and Educational Trust, 840 North Lake Shore Drive, Chicago, IL 60611.

Green, Sharon. *Guidelines for Breast Cancer Support Programs.* Homewood, IL: Y-ME, 1989. Manual on how to establish a breast-cancer support group, appropriate for any health-oriented mutual-aid group. Available from: Y-ME, 18220 Harwood Avenue, Homewood, IL 60430, (708) 799-8228; (800) 221-2141 for callers outside the 708 area code.

Guzman, Carol. *Semillas de Prosperidad, or How to Cultivate Resources from the Private Sector.* Albuquerque, NM: Neighborhood Housing Services, 1982. Basic information on grassroots fund-raising.

Hill, Albert Fay. *I'm a Patient, Too.* New York: Nick Lyons Books, 1986. Story of the CanSurmont cancer-patient support program.

Kahn, Si. *Organizing: A Guide for Grassroots Leaders.* San Francisco: McGraw-Hill, 1982.

Nathanson, Minna Newman. *Organizing and Maintaining Support Groups for Parents of Children with Chronic Illness and Handicapping Conditions.* Washington, DC: Association for the Care of Children's Health, 1986. Organizational handbook for the Candlelighters Childhood Cancer Foundations, with practical advice on how to form support groups.

Self-Help Clearinghouse. *The Self-Help Sourcebook: Finding and Forming Mutual Aid Self-Help Groups.* Lists over 500 national self-help groups by name and with contact address. Available from: Sourcebook, Self-Help Clearinghouse, Saint Clares–Riverside Medical Center, Denville, NJ 07834.

6. Taking Care of Business: Employment, Insurance, and Money Matters

Bamford, Janet, et al. *Complete Guide to Managing Your Money.* Mount Vernon, NY: Consumer Reports Books, 1989. Comprehensive information and advice on investments, banking, tax planning, retirement planning, insurance, and financial planning.

Barofsky, Ivan, ed. *Work and Illness: The Cancer Patient.* New York: Praeger, 1989. Collection of articles on the psychosocial impact of cancer on employment.

Best Company, A. M. *Best's Insurance Reports.* A. M. Best Company (Oldwick, NJ: annual). Annual ratings of American insurance companies. Found in local libraries.

Communicating for Agriculture, Inc. *Comprehensive Health Insurance for High-Risk Individuals.* Minneapolis: Communicating for Agriculture, Inc., annual. Annual resource manual of health insurance mandated by state high-risk pools. Purchase from: Communicating for Agriculture, Inc., CA Support Services Office, 2626 East 82nd Street, Suite 325, Minneapolis, MN 55425, (612) 854-9005.

Esperti, Robert, and Peterson, Renno. *The Handbook of Estate Planning.* New York: McGraw-Hill, 1985. Practical guide to when you need an estate and how to plan accordingly.

Harrington, Geri. *The Health Insurance Fact and Answer Book.* New York: Harper and Row, 1985. Practical guide discussing group, individual, disability, and indemnity policies.

Hughes, Theodore, and Klein, David. *A Family Guide to Wills, Funerals, and Probate: How to Protect Yourself and Survivors.* New York: Charles Scribner's Sons, 1987. Handbook on how to prepare for protecting your family after your death.

Leiberman, Trudy. *Life Insurance: How to Buy the Right Policy from the Right Company at the Right Price.* Mount Vernon, NY: Consumers Union, 1988. Explains advantages and disadvantages of policies, when to purchase life insurance, and how to compare available policies.

Lipson, Benjamin. *How to Collect More on Your Insurance Claims.* New York: Simon and Schuster, 1985. Practical advice on how to collect insurance claims.

Mcloughlin, Caven, et al., eds. *Getting Employed, Staying Employed: Job Development and Training for Persons with Severe Handicaps.* Baltimore: Paul H. Brooks Publishing, 1987. A practical guide for securing employment for persons with severe handicaps.

Naeve, Pamela Priest, and Walker, Isabel. *Estates: Planning Ahead.* Belmont: Northern California Cancer Center, 1989. Practical guide to estate planning for cancer survivors in California; however, also contains useful informaton for all survivors. Available from: Northern California Cancer Center, P.O. Box 2030, Belmont, California 94002-5030.

National Underwriter Company. *Who Writes What in Life and Health Insurance.* Annual list of American insurance companies by type of life insurance issued. Includes a list of companies that issue policies for people with "unusual conditions," including cancer. Available in most libraries or from: The National Underwriter Company, 420 East 4th Street, Cincinnati, OH 45202, (513) 721-2140.

Polniaszek, Susan. *Managing Your Health Care Financing.* Washington, DC: United Seniors Health Cooperative, 1989. Advice on Medicare, Medicaid, and Medigap insurance. Available from United Seniors Health Cooperative, 1334 G Street, N.W., Room 500, Washington, DC 20005.

Public Citizen Health Research Group. *Medical Records: Getting Yours.* Washington, DC: Public Citizen Health Research Group, 1986. Step-by-step guide to obtaining your medical records and how to understand them. Available from: Health Research Group, 2000 P Street, N.W., Suite 708, Washington, DC 20036.

Russell, L. Mark. *Alternatives: A Family Guide to Legal and Financial Planning for the Disabled.* Evanston, IL: First Publications, 1983. Although written primarily for the mentally disabled, helpful to persons with physical disabilities in answering questions about wills, guardianship, trusts, government benefits, taxes, insurance, and financial planning.

Snyder, Harry, and Oshiro, Carl. *Medicare/Medigap: The Guide for Older Americans and Their Families.* Mount Vernon, NY: Consumers Union, 1990. Step-by-step handbook on how to receive maximum benefits under Medicare and Medicaid programs, and how to choose the right supplemental policy.

Society for the Right to Die. *Handbook of Living Will Laws.* New York: Society for the Right to Die, 1987. Comprehensive survey of living-will laws and resources to help you prepare a living will. Available from: Society for the Right to Die, 250 West 57th Street, New York, NY 10107, (212) 246-6973.

Soled, Alex J. *The Essential Guide to Wills, Estates, Trusts, and Death Taxes.* Washington, DC: American Association of Retired Persons, 1988. Practical guide that explains the fundamentals of a will, how to avoid unnecessary costs and taxes, and how to create the right will, trust, or estate for you.

Wisconsin Commissioner of Insurance. *Health Insurance: A Primer.* Short booklet summarizing types of health insurance in general, and details about Wisconsin insurance law. Available from: Office of the Commissioner of Insurance, P.O. Box 7873, Madison, WI 53707-7873.

7. Cancer and the Family

Adams, David, and Deveau, Eleanor. *Coping with Childhood Cancer: Where Do We Go From Here?* Reston, VA: Reston Publishing, 1984. Self-help guide on diagnosis, treatment, survival, and death issues in childhood cancer.

Baker, Lunn. *You and Leukemia: A Day at a Time.* Philadelphia: Saunders, 1978. Information for children in understanding the causes, treatment, and complications of leukemia.

Barbarin, Oscar, and Chesler, Mark. *Children with Cancer: School Experiences and Views of Parents, Educators, Adolescents and Physicians.* Oak Brook, IL: Eterna Press, 1983. Discussion of effect of cancer on school life, including references and bibliography. Available from: Eterna Press, Eterna International, P.O. Box 1344, Oak Brook, IL 60521.

Berstein, Joanne. *Books to Help Children Cope with Separation and Loss.* New York: Bowker, 1983, 2d ed. Review of more than 600 books, including bibliography.

Bracken, Jeanne Munn. *Children with Cancer: A Comprehensive Reference Guide for Parents.* New York: Oxford University Press, 1986. Guidebook of childhood cancers, treatments, coping strategies, and resources.

Chesler, Mark, and Barbarin, Oscar. *Childhood Cancer and the Family: Meeting the Challenge of Stress and Support.* New York: Brunner/Mazel, 1987. How families meet psychosocial challenges of childhood cancer, including relationships with care givers, friends, and teachers.

Dickens, Monica. *Miracles of Courage: How Families Meet the Challenge of a Child's Critical Illness.* New York: Dodd, Mead, 1985. Based on interviews with families, stories about addressing family concerns involved in critical illness.

Farkas, Susan. *Hospitalized Children: The Family's Role in Care and Treatment.* Washington, DC: Catholic University of America, 1983. Booklet on effect on family, how family can help, and principles of family-centered care. Available from: Family Impact Seminar, The National Center for Family Studies, The Catholic University of America, Washington, DC 20064.

Fassler, Joan. *Helping Children Cope: Mastering Stress Through Books and Stories.* New York: The Free Press (Macmillan), 1978. Reviews books and stories that help children deal with stress from events such as separation and loss.

Fine, Judylaine. *Afraid to Ask: A Book for Families to Share About Cancer.* New York: Lothrop, Lee & Shepard, 1984. Provides young people with answers about the physical and emotional impact of cancer.

Gallagher, James, and Vietze, Peter. *Families of Handicapped Persons: Research, Programs, and Policy Issues.* Baltimore: Paul H. Brooks Publishing, 1986. Investigates the adaptation and functioning of families with members who are disabled.

Goldfarb, Lori, et al. *Meeting the Challenge of Disability or Chronic Illness—A Family Guide.* Baltimore: Paul H. Brooks Publishing, 1986. Practical guide for making daily decisions for families living with family member who is disabled or chronically ill.

Gunther, John. *Death Be Not Proud: A Memoir.* New York: Harper and Row, 1949. A father's account of his teenage son's fight to overcome a brain tumor.

Ipswitch, Elaine. *Scott Was Here.* New York: Dell, 1979. Mother's story of her son's battle with Hodgkin's disease.

Kievman, B., and Blackmun, S. *For Better or Worse: A Couple's Guide to Dealing with Chronic Illness.* Chicago: Contemporary Books, 1989. Surviving partner offers practical advice for patients and caregivers coping with chronic illness.

Kruckeberg, Carol. *What Was Good About Today.* Seattle: Madrona, 1984. Mother's account of her eight-year-old daughter's battle with and death from leukemia.

LeShan, Eda. *When a Parent Is Very Sick.* Boston: Little, Brown, 1986.

LeShan, Lawrence. *Cancer as a Turning Point: A Handbook for People with Cancer, Their Families and Health Professionals.* New York: E. P. Dutton, 1989. A coordinated approach to mobilizing the survivor's self-healing abilities through involving families and helping professionals.

Lewis, C. S. *A Grief Observed.* New York: Seabury Press, 1963. Author's journal of his doubts, rage, and growing awareness of human frailty following the death of his wife from cancer.

Mathews-Simonton, Stephanie, and Shook, Robert. *The Healing Family: The Simonton Approach for Families Facing Illness.* New York: Bantam, 1984. Practical suggestions for a family's response to cancer.

McCollum, Audrey. *The Chronically Ill Child: A Guide for Parents and Professionals.* New Haven: Yale University Press, 1981. Strategies to meet needs of ill child and family, including resources for help.

Miles, Margaret. *The Grief of Parents: When a Child Dies.* Oak Brook, IL: Compassionate Friends, 1980. Suggestions for family members on how to respond to death of a child.

Miller, Angelyn. *The Enabler: When Helping Harms the One You Love.* Claremont, CA: Hunter House, 1988. Personal story of woman who discovers the difference between healthy and unhealthy "helping."

Murcia, Andy, and Stewart, Bob. *Man to Man: When the Woman You Love Has Breast Cancer.* New York: St. Martin's Press, 1989. Actress Ann Jillian's husband speaks frankly about the spouse's perspective on a woman's breast cancer.

National Cancer Institute. *When Someone in Your Family Has Cancer.* Bethesda: National Institutes of Health, 1987. Booklet addressed to family members, especially adolescents, of a survivor, answering basic facts about cancer.

Powell, Thomas, and Ogle, Peggy Ahrehold. *Brothers & Sisters—A Special Part of Exceptional Families.* Baltimore: Paul H. Brooks Publishing, 1985. Helps families, practitioners, and researchers recognize the special needs and powerful influence of the siblings of handicapped children and adults.

Pringle, Terry. *This Is the Child: A Father's Story of His Young Son's Battle with Leukemia.* New York, Alfred A. Knopf, 1983. Father's story of his family's experience with his four-year-old son's battle with leukemia.

Richter, Elizabeth. *The Teenage Hospital Experience: You Can Handle It!* New York: Coward, McCann and Geoghegan, 1982. Photographs and interviews with hospitalized teenagers about their experiences in the hospital.

Spinetta, John, and Deasy-Spinetta, Patricia, eds. *Living with Childhood Cancer.* Saint Louis: Mosby, 1981. Book resulting from three-day conference of professionals, parents, and children on issues of surviving childhood cancer.

Strong, Maggie. *Mainstay: For the Well Spouse of the Chronically Ill.* New York: Viking, 1989. Support and practical advice for the spouse of a person with a chronic illness.

Tucker, Jonathan. *Ellie: A Child's Fight Against Leukemia.* New York: Holt, Rinehart and Winston, 1982. Fictionalized composite of three cases takes a child and family through diagnosis, treatment, protocols, side effects, relapse, and bone-marrow transplantation.

Waller, Sharon. *Circle of Hope: A Child Rescued by Love from a Medical Death Sentence.* New York: M. Evans, 1981. A mother's story of coping with her daughter's diagnosis of osteosarcoma.

Whitfield, Charles L. *Healing the Child Within: Discovery and Recovery for Adult Children of Dysfunctional Families.* Deerfield Beach, FL: Health Communications, Inc., 1987. A guide to understanding the dynamics and steps of recovery for members of families that are not functioning well.

Zumwalt, Elmo, Jr.; Zumwalt, Elmo III. *My Father, My Son.* New York: Macmillan, 1986. Experiences of Admiral Zumwalt and his son's battle against hematic cancers.

About the National Coalition for Cancer Survivorship

In October 1986, three New Mexican cancer survivors (Catherine Logan, founder of Living Through Cancer, a statewide cancer support organization; Fitzhugh Mullan, a physician and the author of landmark articles on cancer survivorship; and Edith Lenneberg, an early leader in the United Ostomy Association), backed by two local institutions (Saint Joseph Healthcare Corporation in Albuquerque and Saint Vincent Hospital in Santa Fe), invited 21 representatives from a variety of survivorship groups and interests to meet in Albuquerque to discuss the growing national cancer survivorship movement. By the end of the three-day meeting, the group founded the National Coalition for Cancer Survivorship (NCCS). NCCS was established as a nonprofit organization designed to coordinate and support the growth of the cancer survivorship movement by creating a network of individuals and groups working to develop psychosocial resources for survivors and their families.

By 1990, the NCCS network had grown to a coalition of more than 2,500 individuals and organizations that represent tens of thousands of members and constituents in the cancer survivorship movement in the United States. NCCS members include community, regional, and national peer-support and professional cancer-related organizations, individual cancer survivors, family members and friends, health-care professionals, and major cancer-treatment institutions.

NCCS creates resources to meet the needs of cancer survivors and their families by:

- maintaining a survivorship network that links individuals, organizations, and resources
- serving as a national voice for cancer survivors before the media, government, and health communities
- sponsoring an Annual Assembly addressing issues of concern to survivors
- working to reduce cancer-based discrimination in employment and insurance
- disseminating information about life after a cancer diagnosis
- providing technical assistance to community cancer organizations
- publishing a national newsletter, *The NCCS Networker*
- sponsoring a national Speakers Bureau
- encouraging outreach to underserved survivor populations

Historically, the majority of formally organized cancer-support groups were founded by and served white middle-class women. A goal of NCCS is to expand peer-support resources to address the needs of men and women from all economic and social backgrounds.

NCCS welcomes new members and gratefully accepts contributions. If you are interested in joining or supporting NCCS, fill out and send the coupon on page 214.

JOIN/SUPPORT NCCS

ANNUAL MEMBERSHIP OPTIONS
- ☐ Individual Membership—$20 or more
- ☐ Individual Sustaining—$50 or more
- ☐ Individual Patron—$500 or more
- ☐ Other (individuals unable to pay the $20 fee are invited to join NCCS for any amount they can afford)
- ☐ Organizational and Institutional Members (recommended fees)
    - with budgets of less than $150,000—$50 or more
    - with budgets of $150,000 to $1,000,000—$150 or more
    - with budgets of $1,000,000 or more—$250 or more

DONATIONS ☐ $500 ☐ $250 ☐ $100 ☐ $50 ☐ Other

This donation is:
- ☐ In memory of
- ☐ In honor of the (specify milestones) of
- ☐ Send acknowledgment to

Please indicate whether you are contributing as an individual or an organization.

Name_____ Phone_____

Organization (if any)_____

Institution (if any)_____ Department_____

Address_____

City_____ State_____ Zip_____

NCCS is a 501(c)3, tax-exempt organization. Send checks payable to the NCCS to: NCCS, 323 Eighth St. SW, Albuquerque, NM 87102.

About the Editors

Fitzhugh Mullan, M.D., is a pediatrician, writer, and cancer survivor. In 1975, Dr. Mullan diagnosed a cancer in his own chest that proved to be a mediastinal seminoma and led to two years of intensive surgery, radiation, and chemotherapy, and the eventual publication of *Vital Signs: A Young Doctor's Struggle with Cancer* (1983). Dr. Mullan's writings and visits around the country with groups involved in cancer care led to the formation of the National Coalition for Cancer Survivorship, whose board of directors he chairs. He is a commissioned officer in the United States Public Health Service and has served as the director of the National Health Service Corps and as secretary for health and environment of the State of New Mexico. His other books include *Plagues and Politics: The Story of the United States Public Health Service* (1989) and *White Coat, Clenched Fist: The Political Education of an American Physician* (1976).

Barbara Hoffman, J.D., is a member of the adjunct faculty of Seton Hall University School of Law in Newark, New Jersey, and a private disability-rights consultant. She has published numerous articles and presented dozens of workshops on the legal rights of cancer survivors. She has testified as an advocate for survivors before congressional committees. Ms. Hoffman is the first vice-president of the National Coalition for Cancer Survivorship.

About the Authors

Katharine Gratwick Baker, D.S.W., L.C.S.W., is a family therapist in private practice in Washington, D.C. She conducted her postdoctoral work in family therapy at Georgetown University. She taught counseling at Catholic University School of Social Service and Trinity College, both in Washington, D.C. Dr. Baker has presented dozens of workshops and published numerous articles on family counseling.

Neil Fiore, Ph.D., is a management consultant and licensed psychologist in private practice in Berkeley, California. Dr. Fiore is the author of several books, including *The Road Back to Health: Coping with the Emotional Side of Cancer* (based on his experiences as a cancer survivor and psychologist) and *The Now Habit: Overcoming Procrastination and Enjoying Guilt-Free Play*. He has published and lectured throughout the country on health psychology, optimal performance, stress management, and hypnosis.

Patricia A. Ganz, M.D., is on the full-time faculty of the University of California at Los Angeles School of Medicine. Dr. Ganz completed postgraduate training in internal medicine and medical oncology at the UCLA Medical Center. She has published numerous articles and book chapters based on her research related to the rehabilitation needs and the quality of life of cancer patients.

Myra Glajchen, Ph.D., is an oncology social worker and assistant director of social service at Cancer Care, Inc., in New York City, where she supervises clinical social workers, leads a support group for young cancer patients, and has responsibility for program planning and research. Her doctoral dissertation addressed the psychosocial problems experienced by long-term survivors of Hodgkin's disease.

Annette Jolles, M.S.W., L.C.S.W., is a social worker at the Cancer Institute at Washington Hospital Center in Washington, D.C. She has served as an advocate in mutual-aid organizations as both a professional and a family member. Ms. Jolles has produced a video, "Practicing Survivorship," with patients at the Washington Hospital Center, which is used as an educational tool throughout the Washington area.

Catherine Logan, B.S., is the executive director of the National Coalition for Cancer Survivorship. In 1983, she founded Living Through Cancer, Inc., a mutual-aid community organization in Albuquerque, New Mexico, where she has developed innovative programs and print materials. She was a businesswoman and jeweler in Albuquerque when she was diagnosed with invasive cervical cancer in 1979.

Natalie Davis Spingarn is a prizewinning medical writer based in Washington, D.C. Her scores of publications include *Hanging In There: Living Well on Borrowed Time*, practical lessons from her personal experience with breast cancer. Her film *Patients and Doctors: Communication Is a Two-Way Street* won an Oscar in the 1988 John Muir Medical Film Festival. She is a member of the board of directors of the National Coalition for Cancer Survivorship and serves as editor of the organization's newsletter, *The Networker*.

Fitzhugh Mullan, Catherine Logan, Barbara Hoffman, Neil Fiore, and Patricia Ganz are five of the 24 co-founders of the National Coalition for Cancer Survivorship.

About the Artwork

The artwork at the beginning of each chapter of the book appeared in the first national art exhibition by artists with cancer. "Confronting Cancer Through Art 1987" assembled the work of 42 artists, both invited and juried, for a month-long showing at the Brand Library Art Galleries, a large community gallery in the Los Angeles area. The exhibition was conceived and organized by Art That Heals, a program created and directed by Devra Breslow, M.A., at the University of California at Los Angeles Jonsson Comprehensive Cancer Center. Exhibition books and posters, all in vibrant color, may be purchased from:

Art That Heals/UCLA
1100 Glendon Avenue, Suite 711
Los Angeles, CA 90024

Index

Adjuvant therapy, 15–16
   breast cancer, 195
AIDS, 201
   telephone hotline, 176
Alcohol consumption, 21
Allogeneic transplantation, 17
American Association of Retired Persons, 180
American Board of Medical Specialties, 167
American Cancer Society, 68, 81–82, 94, 169, 191–92
American College of Radiology, 167
American College of Surgeons, 167
American Council on Life Insurance, 180
American Medical Association (and medical records), 116, 117
American Red Cross, 169
American Society of Internal Medicine, 52
Americans with Disabilities Act, 102–3
Anxiety, 34–35
Appetite loss, 23, 24, 75
Association of Brain Tumor Research, 169
Attorneys
   and job-discrimination cases, 104
   and problems of elderly, 193
Autogenics, 39–41
Autologous bone-marrow transplantation, 17

Bell Telephone (cancer survivors as employees), 99
Benjamin, Harold, 66
Bereavement counseling, 158
Better Together Club, 169
Bill of Rights, cancer survivors' (American Cancer Society), 50, 51, 52
Bill of Rights, family members' (of cancer survivors), 148
Bladder cancer, 198
   incidence rates, 9
   mortality rates, 9
   survival rates, 9, 16, 18
   treatment, 198
Blood counts, low, 25
Blue Cross and Blue Shield, 122–23, 124, 180
Bone cancer, 200–201
Bone-marrow transplantation, 16–17
Brain, cancers of, 200
   newsletter, 174
   organizations for research and support services, 169, 171
   survival rates, 18
   treatment, 200
Brain Tumor Information Services, 176

Breast cancer, 194–95. *See also* Mammography; Mastectomy
  biopsy, 194
  causes, 194
  incidence rates, 9, 13
  mortality rates, 9, 13
  newsletter, 174
  organizations, alliance of, 171
  survival rates, 9, 16, 18
  telephone hotlines, 175
  treatment, 195
Breathing, improving, 26
Brennan, William, 102

Camps (children's) directory, 170
Cancer Care, Inc., 171
Cancer Communication, 173
Cancer Guidance Institute, Pittsburgh, 92–93
Candlelighters Childhood Cancer Foundation, 29, 80, 81, 104, 169
  newsletters, 173
CanSurmount (peer-support organization), 83, 169
Cassileth, Barrie R., 64, 67
Center for Medical Consumers, 169–70
Centering exercise, 41
Cervical cancer, 21, 199
  incidence rates, 9
  mortality rates, 9
  survival rates, 9, 16, 18
Chaplains, 76
Chemotherapy, 15, 16
  and depression, 74
  and fertility, 27–29
  hair loss, 23, 25
  nausea, 23
  for pain reduction, 22
  and sterility, 28–29
  for symptom relief, 12–13, 15
Childhood cancer, 29, 81, 169, 201
  and job discrimination, 98
  newsletter, 173
  support group, 29, 80, 81, 104, 169
  treatment, 201
Children (in families with cancer survivors), 152–54
Children's Oncology Camps of America, 170
Civil rights (state enforcement agencies), 182–91
Cleveland, Grover, 7
Clinical cancer centers, 58, 163–66
Clinical trials (treatment), 19, 49, 68
COBRA (Comprehensive Omnibus Budget Reconciliation Act), 119–20, 181
  and disabled, 120
College of American Pathologists, 167
Colon cancer, 196
  detecting, 196
  incidence rates, 9, 13
  mortality rates, 9, 13
  survival rates, 9, 16, 18
  symptoms, 196
Combined-modality therapy, 15
Communication problems (families), 147
Community Health Accreditation Program Inc., 167
Comprehensive cancer centers, 58, 163–66
Concentration (during treatment), 26
Consent form, 56
Consumer Health Information Research Institute, 170
Contagious (cancer as) myth, 8, 10, 99
Corporate Angel Network, 170
Counselors, 72–73
Cousins, Norman, 67
Credit counseling, 134–35, 192
Curative-intent treatment, 11

Death rates. *See* Mortality
Depression, 35–36, 74
  signs of, 74
DES Action U.S.A., 170
Diagnosis
  delay in, 113–14
  and family members, 146–50
  reactions to, 32–36
  recurrence, 156–57
Diagnostic phase (treatment), 13
Diet
  and cancer prevention, 19
  treatments, 63
Disability benefits (Social Security), 136–37
Disabled American Veterans, 180
Drugs
  free medications, 192–93
  information center for, 168

Employment
  blue-collar workers, 98
  co-workers, 38
  job discrimination, 38, 98–111
  work days lost due to cancer treatment (compared with disability), 101
Encore (YWCA), 170
Endometrial cancer, 199
Equal Employment Opportunities Commission, 102–3, 181
ERISA (Employee Retirement and Insurance Security Act), 119, 121–22, 181
Esophageal cancer, 199–200
  incidence rates, 9
  mortality rates, 9
  survival rates, 9, 18

Facial surgery, support-group, 171, 174
Families (of survivors)

Bill of Rights, 148
children, needs of, 152–54
communication barriers, 147
dealing with diagnosis, 146–50
involved in treatment, 150–52
support group, 173
Fatigue, 22–23
Federal Rehabilitation Act, 99–103, 109, 112, 181
Fertility (during treatment), 27–29
Financial assistance, 135, 191–93
Fobair, Pat, 95
Follow-up, long-term, 10, 29
Follow-up care phase (treatment), 13–14
Food and Drug Administration (FDA), 68
Fraud, health (resource center), 172
Freedom of Information Act, 117–18, 191

Government Life Insurance programs, 137
Gray, Lynn, 92
Group Health Association of America, 180–81

Hair loss, 23, 25
Halitosis (during treatment), 24
Hamilton, Paul K., 83
Head, cancers of, 200
Health Facts, 170
Health insurance. *See* Insurance, health
Health Insurance Association of America, 181
Health Maintenance Organizations (HMOs), 124, 181
Hematologic cancers, 197–98
Hematologist, 72
HMOs. *See* Health Maintenance Organizations
Hodgkin's disease, 198
newsletter, 95, 174
survival rates, 18
treatment, 198
Holland, Jimmie, 35, 65–66
Home-care services, 72, 74–75
accreditation, 167
Hormone medications, 15
Hospice services, 76
organization for, 172
telephone hotline, 177
Hospital equipment (for home use), 74–75
Hospitals
accreditation, 58–59, 168
admission process, 61
attitudes for dealing with stay, 61–62
choosing, 58–61
clinical cancer centers, 58, 163–66
community hospitals, 58
comprehensive cancer centers, 58, 163–66
discharge planning, 62
funding, 60
mortality rates, 59
physicians' affiliation, 50, 58

public, 60
services, 60–61
Hotlines. *See* Telephone hotlines
Housing (near treatment centers), 192
Hyperthermia treatment, 17–18

I Can Cope (peer-support organization), 82–83, 170
Imagery, 39–42, 63
Imagining exercise, 42
Immunologic system modification, 17
Incidence rates, 9
estimated, 17
sites, 13
United States, 12
Informed consent, 53–55
and children, 55
Insurance, consumer advocacy, 181
Insurance, disability, 125
Insurance, health
cancer insurance, 126
catastrophic insurance, 125
claims, 130–31
claims processing service, 131
COBRA (Comprehensive Omnibus Budget Reconciliation Act), 119–20, 181
contractual rights, 119
converting group policy to individual, 120, 121
and employment, 118
after employment termination, 119–20
and experimental drugs, 119
group plans, 126–27
high-risk pools, 122, 124, 180
hospital indemnity, 124
individual plans, 127
major medical, 124–25, 128
managed health-care plan, 124
Medicare supplementary, 180
records, maintaining, 130, 131
regulated by, 132
shopping for, 129–30
state laws, 122–23
types, 123–26
Insurance, life, 132–33
graded policy, 133
group plan, 133
high-risk, 180
Insurance agents, 129
Internal Revenue Service information, 176
International Association of Laryngectomees, 171
International Ostomy Association, 89
International Pain Foundation, 167–68

Job Accommodation Network, 112–13, 182
Job accommodations (for survivors), 111–13
Job discrimination, 38, 98–111

Job discrimination (cont'd)
  asserting rights, 110–11
  avoiding, 108–9
  blue-collar workers, 98
  childhood-cancer survivors, 98
  state enforcement agencies, 182–91
  state laws, 103–8
  union contracts, 108
Johnson, Judi, 82
Joint Commission on Accreditation of Healthcare Organizations, 58–59, 168

Kaplan, Mimi, 85
Kaplan, Henry S., 95
Kelly, Orville, 80
Kidney cancer, 198
  incidence rates, 9
  mortality rates, 9
  survival rates, 9, 18
  treatment, 198
Kimberly Quarterly Care (telephone hotline), 176

Laboratories (accreditation), 167
Laryngectomees, organization for, 171
Larynx cancer
  incidence rates, 9
  mortality rates, 9
  survival rates, 9, 18
Lasser, Terese, 82
Lawsuits
  and Federal Rehabilitation Act, 100–103
  malpractice, 113–15
Lerner, Michael, 65, 66
Let's Face It (peer-support organization), 171, 174
Leukemia
  acute, 197
  chronic, 197–98
  incidence rates, 9, 13
  mortality rates, 9, 13
  survival rates, 9, 16, 18
  symptoms, 197, 198
  treatment, 197, 198
Leukemia Society of America, Inc., 171
Life insurance. *See* Insurance, life
Liver cancer, 199–200
  survival rates, 18
Living Through Cancer Survivorship Center (LTC), Albuquerque, 93–94
Living Through Cancer (newsletter), 174
Living will, 138–39, 140
Long-term control, 12, 15
Lung cancer, 195–96
  cause, 195
  incidence rates, 9, 13
  mortality rates, 9, 13
  survival rates, 9, 16, 18
  symptoms, 195
  treatment, 196
  types, 196
Lymphedema
  resource center for, 172
  telephone hotline, 177
Lymphomas, 198
  incidence rates, 9, 13
  mortality rates, 9, 13
  survival rates, 9, 18
  treatment, 198

Macrobiotic diet, 63
Maintenance phase (treatment), 13
Make Today Count (peer-support organization), 80–81, 171
Malpractice cases, 113–15
  statute of limitations, 115
Mammography
  accredited facilities, 167
  insurance coverage mandated by states, 123
  recommendations, 194–95
Marcou, Ann, 85
Mastectomy, 195
  postmastectomy support organizations, 82–83, 85, 94–95, 170, 172–73
Meal programs, 192
Medicaid, 126
Medical Information Bureau, 129, 132, 181
Medical records, access to, 52, 115–18, 191
  state laws, 116–17
Medical societies, 166–68
Medicare, 125–26
  chemotherapy payments, 119
  information services, 177, 181
Melanoma, 200
  survival rates, 16, 18
Metabolic treatments, 62–64
Metastasis, 11, 14
Metropolitan Life Insurance (cancer survivors as employees), 99
Mortality rates, 9
  by cancer sites, 13
  estimated, 17
  worldwide, 20
Mount Sinai Hospital, New York City, 83
Mourning, premature, 147
Mouth, dry, 25
Mouth, inflammation of (during treatment), 24
Multiple myeloma, 198
  survival rates, 18
  treatment, 198
Mutual-aid organizations. *See* Peer-support organizations

Myths (about cancer), 8, 102
   and job discrimination, 98–99

National Alliance of Breast Cancer Organizations, 171
   newsletter, 174
National Brain Tumor Foundation, 171
National Cancer Institute, 58, 163
   Cancer Information Service, 48, 49, 58
National Coalition for Cancer Survivorship (NCCS), 2–4, 83–84, 171–72, 213
   newsletter, 174
   and peer-support organizations, 91
National Consumers League, 172
National Council Against Health Fraud Resource Center, 172
National Foundation for Consumer Credit, 134–35, 192
National Health Information Center, 168
National Hospice Organization, 172
National Information Center for Orphan Drugs and Rare Diseases, 168
National Insurance Consumer Organization, 181
National Lymphedema Network, 172
Nausea, 24
   and chemotherapy, 23
Neck, cancers of, 200
Neo-adjuvant therapy, 16
Nervous system, cancers of, 200
   survival rates, 18
   treatment, 200
Neurotoxicity (during treatment), 26
Newsletters, 173–74
Norby, Pat, 82
Nurses
   in doctors' offices, 50
   in hospitals, 61, 72
   visiting nurses association, 168
Nutrition (during treatment), 75

Oncologist, 71–72
Oncology, 49
Oral cancer, 200
   incidence rates, 13
   mortality rates, 13
   survival rates, 16, 18
Ostomy, organizations for support services, 80, 83, 169, 172, 173
Ostomy Rehabilitation Program, 172
Ovarian cancer, 199
   incidence rates, 9, 13
   mortality rates, 9, 13
   survival rates, 9, 16, 18
   symptoms and treatment, 199

Pain, 21–22
   research organization, 167–68
Pain relievers, 22
Pancreatic cancer, 199–200
   incidence rates, 9, 13
   mortality rates, 9, 13
   survival rates, 9, 16, 18
Pap-smear examination, 199
Patient Advocates for Advanced Cancer Treatment (PAACT), 172
   newsletter, 173
Peer-support organizations, 79–95, 169–73
   compared with professional counseling, 85
   evaluating, 87–88
   locating, 86–87
   organizing, 88–91
Pharmaceutical companies' drug assistance programs, 192–93
Physician Data Query (PDQ), 48, 49, 163
Physicians
   board certification, 49, 167
   choosing, 48–52
   communicating with, 52–53, 55–57
   credentials, 49
   hospital affiliation, 50
   in hospitals, 72
   surgeons, list of, 167
Pollard, Mary, 94–95
Power of attorney, 142
Prevention, 19, 21
Privacy Act, 117–18
Prostate cancer, 196–97
   incidence rates, 9, 13
   mortality rates, 9, 13
   newsletter, 173
   organization for information on, 172
   survival rates, 9, 16, 18
   symptoms, 196
   treatment, 197
Psychiatrists, 73
Psychologists, 73
Psychotherapy, 73
Public Citizen (consumer-rights group), 118, 191
Public-opinion poll (Is cancer contagious?), 10

QT alumni, 83

Radiation, excessive, avoiding, 19, 21
Radiation therapy, 15
   and depression, 74
   and fertility, 27–28
   hair loss, 23, 25
   for pain reduction, 22
   and sterility, 28–29
   for symptom relief, 12–13, 15
Radon, 21

INDEX

Rare diseases, information center for, 168
Reach to Recovery (peer-support organization), 82, 172–73
Rectal cancer, 196
    detecting, 196
    incidence rates, 9, 13
    mortality rates, 9, 13
    survival rates, 9, 16, 18
    symptoms, 196
Recurrence (of cancer), 156–57
Relaxation techniques, 39
Respiratory problems, 26
Ringer, Lynn, 83
Ronald McDonald House, 192

Sarcomas, 200–201
Schimmel, Selma, 84–85
SEARCH (National Brain Tumor Foundation), 174
Second opinions, 19, 52
Self-help clearinghouses, 177–80
Self-image, 36–38
Sexual activity (and cervical cancer), 21, 199
Sexual problems, 75
    and self-image, 38
    during treatment, 27–28
SHARE (telephone hotline), 175
Siegel, Bernie, 63, 66
Simonton, Carl, 63
Skin cancer, 200
    incidence rates, 9, 13
    mortality rates, 9, 13
    survival rates, 9
Skin problems (during treatment), 25–26
Skin stimulation (for pain reduction), 22
Smoking, 19
    and lung cancer, 195
Social Security Administration hotline, 138
Social Security benefits, 136–37
Social workers, 73
    in hospitals, 61
Society for the Control of Cancer, 81
Society for the Right to Die, 138–39, 193
Sperm banking, 29
Stages of survival, 2
Stanford University Hospital, peer-support group, 95
Sterility, 27–29
Stomach cancer, 199–200
    incidence rates, 9
    mortality rates, 9
    survival rates, 9, 18
Stomatitis (during treatment), 24
Straus, Charlotte Gerson, 63

Stress management, 38–39
Sun exposure, 19, 21, 200
Supplemental Security Income (SSI), 136
Support Centers of America, 91–92
Surgery, 15
    for pain reduction, 22
Survival rates, 8, 9, 50
    estimated, 17
    percentage of population, 1
    by race, 18
    by site, 16, 18
Survival stages, 2
Surviving, 95, 174
Symptom relief, 12–13, 15

Taste, changes in (during treatment), 24
Taxes
    IRS information, 176
    medical-expenses deductions, 137–38
Teenagers (and self-image), 36
Telephone hotlines, 85, 92–93, 174–77
Testicular cancer, 199
    survival rates, 16, 18
    treatment, 199
Thyroid gland, cancer of (survival rates), 18
Tobacco use, 19
Transportation (to treatment), 170, 191
Treatment. *See also* Unconventional therapy
    clinical trials, 19, 49, 68
    consent form, 56
    costs, 134
    family involvement, 150–52
    goals, 11–13
    informed consent, 53–55
    phases, 13–15
    right to choose, 53–55
    right to refuse, 55
    and sexual problems, 27–28
    work days lost, 101
Trusts, 141–42

Unconventional therapy, 62–68
    costs, 66–67
    and depression, 36
    estimate of participants, 64
    information sources, 68, 170
    and self-blame, 66
Unemployment-disability benefits, 135–36
United Cancer Council, Inc., 173
United Ostomy Association, 80, 173
University of California Medical Center, 33

Veterans
    benefits, 137
    organization for, 180

Veterans (*cont'd*)
   telephone hotline, 176
Visiting Nurses Association of America, 168
Vital Options (peer-support organization), 84–85
Vocational rehabilitation, 111–12

Warning signs (cancer), 21
Weight problems, 23, 24
Well Spouse Foundation, 173
Wigs, 25

Wildcat Ladies Breast Cancer Support Group, Washington, D.C., 94–95
Wills, 139–41
   validity, 141
   witnesses, 141
Worker's compensation, 135

YWCA (Encore program), 170
Y-ME (peer-support organization), 85, 173
   newsletter, 174
   telephone hotline, 175